Handbook of Gynecologic Oncology

Handbook of Gynecologic Oncology

Second Edition

Edited by
M. Steven Piver, M.D.
Clinical Professor of Gynecology, State University of New York at Buffalo School of Medicine and Biomedical Sciences; Chief, Department of Gynecologic Oncology, and Director, Gilda Radner Familial Ovarian Cancer Registry, Roswell Park Cancer Institute, Buffalo, New York

Little, Brown and Company
Boston New York Toronto London

Second Edition

Previous edition titled *Manual of Gynecologic Oncology and Gynecology* copyright © 1989 by M. Steven Piver

Library of Congress Cataloging-in-Publication Data

Handbook of gynecologic oncology / edited by M. Steven Piver. -- 2nd ed.
p. cm.
Rev. ed. of: Manual of gynecologic oncology and gynecology. 1st ed. c1989.
Includes bibliographical references and index.
ISBN 0-316-70939-5
1. Generative organs, Female--Cancer--Handbooks, manuals, etc. I. Piver, M. Steven. II. Manual of gynecologic oncology and gynecology.
[DNLM: 1. Genital Neoplasms, Female--handbooks. WP 39 H2357 1995]
RC280.G5M368 1995
616.99'265--dc20
DNLM/DLC
for Library of Congress 95-331
CIP

Printed in the United States of America
RRD-VA

Editorial: Nancy E. Chorpenning, Rebecca Marnhout
Production Services: Silverchair Science + Communications
Copyeditor: Elizabeth Willingham
Indexer: Elizabeth Willingham

With appreciation and love to my wife
and best friend, Susan

Contents

Preface

In 1989, we were pleased to write the *Manual of Gynecologic Oncology and Gynecology* for Little, Brown and Company's Spiral Manual Series. The completely new *Handbook of Gynecologic Oncology*, Second Edition, is intended not only to supply the most current and clinically relevant information but also to be easily accessible—be it in a coat pocket, on a desk, or close to a favorite reading chair. The chapters on ovarian, fallopian tube, uterine, cervix, vulvar, and vaginal cancers are designed to provide the reader with what we believe is the latest in diagnosis and treatment. The chapters on the principles of chemotherapy, radiation therapy, tumor immunology, pathology, diagnostic imaging, critical care, and tumor genetics we hope will provide the reader with information to shape improved diagnostic and therapeutic modalities for the future.

Lest we forget the enormous bravery of women during their battle with cancer, I have asked Gene Wilder to allow me to share some of his thoughts expressed nearly 3 years after the death of his wife, Gilda Radner, from stage IV ovarian cancer. "I used to think that Gilda was the biggest baby in the world. Even after she got cancer I thought she was a baby. I thought she wasn't making things easy for me as she so easily could have with a little more effort, a little more consideration for what her husband must be going through. The hair falling out I could sympathize with, but she was assured by so many doctors that it would grow back. Probably just as thick. The vomiting I could sympathize with, but it was, after all, a temporary discomfort. We all go through things like that and then realize later that it wasn't really so bad. The fear of the chemo—well, that I sympathized with the most. But, oh, so much crying before each treatment. When the bowels stopped working and the green bile came up all night and then she had the ileostomy—I was shaken in my belief that she wasn't taking it 'like a man.' But I still could not convince myself that she was fighting as bravely as she might . . . because it was all *temporary!* A horrible but temporary condition, from which she would emerge the tennis and eating champion of the neighborhood. Three weeks before she died, when she willed herself out of bed to record the audio cassettes of her book, *It's Always Something*, the thought occurred to me, for the first time, that she might die. And, shortly after, the thought occurred to me that she—not having my protective ignorance—must have lived with that fear from the beginning. And then, maybe halfway through her odyssey, she must have had the instinctive knowledge that she would, in fact, soon be dead. She died on May 20, 1989. Sometime in June—I forget the exact day, but it was warm and sunny and the flowers were in full bloom—I realized that she was the bravest woman I had ever known."

A special thanks to Nancy Chorpenning, Executive Editor of Little, Brown and Company's Medical Books and Journals Division, for her patience and support as we worked together to try to make this a truly outstanding handbook. My sincere appreciation to all the coauthors, whose time, effort, and expertise made this book possible. From an editor's perspective, one truly gets a global appreciation of the enormous effort made by the physicians and scientists who took time from their already frenetic schedules to work on this book. To them, I will always owe a great debt of gratitude. To the seven coauthors who, having made significant contributions while at Roswell Park, have moved on to record even bigger contributions elsewhere to the field of oncology, a special thanks. A very special thanks to Cheryl Blake, for without her extraordinary effort, this book would never have become a reality. Finally, thanks, Gene Wilder, for sharing some of your pain, lest we forget.

M. S. P.

Contributing Authors

Trudy R. Baker, M.D.
Clinical Associate Professor of Gynecology, State University of New York at Buffalo School of Medicine and Biomedical Sciences; Clinician II, Gynecologic Oncology, Roswell Park Cancer Institute, Buffalo, New York

Oscar A. de Leon-Casasola, M.D.
Assistant Professor of Anesthesiology, State University of New York at Buffalo School of Medicine and Biomedical Sciences; Director, Intensive Care Unit, Roswell Park Cancer Institute, Buffalo, New York

Richard A. DiCioccio, Ph.D.
Associate Professor of Biochemistry, State University of New York at Buffalo School of Medicine and Biomedical Science; Cancer Research Scientist IV, Gynecologic Oncology, Roswell Park Cancer Institute, Buffalo, New York

Kenneth A. Foon, M.D.
Professor and Chief, Division of Hematology and Oncology, and Director, Markey Cancer Center, University of Kentucky College of Medicine, Lexington, Kentucky

Ronald E. Hempling, M.D.
Clinical Associate Professor of Gynecology, State University of New York at Buffalo School of Medicine and Biomedical Sciences; Clinician II, Gynecologic Oncology, Roswell Park Cancer Institute, Buffalo, New York

Steven Herman, M.D.
Assistant Professor of Radiology, State University of New York at Buffalo School of Medicine and Biomedical Sciences; MRI Section Head, Diagnostic Radiology, Roswell Park Cancer Institute, Buffalo, New York

Michael L. Hicks, M.D.
Assistant Professor of Obstetrics and Gynecology, Case Western Reserve University School of Medicine, Cleveland, Ohio; Staff Gynecologic Oncologist, Henry Ford Hospital, Detroit, Michigan

Anthony Ho, Ph.D.
Assistant Professor of Radiation Oncology, State University of New York at Buffalo School of Medicine and Biomedical Sciences; Senior Medical Physicist, Radiation Medicine, Roswell Park Cancer Institute, Buffalo, New York

Donald L. Klippenstein, M.D.
Assistant Professor of Radiology, State University of New York at Buffalo School of Medicine and Biomedical Sciences; Ultrasound Section Head, Diagnostic Radiology, Roswell Park Cancer Institute, Buffalo, New York

John R. Lurain, M.D.
John and Ruth Brewer Professor of Gynecology and Cancer Research, Northwestern University Medical School; Chief, Gynecologic Oncology, Northwestern Memorial Hospital/Prentice Women's Hospital, Chicago, Illinois

John H. Malfetano, M.D.
Associate Professor of Obstetrics and Gynecology, Albany Medical College; Director, Gynecologic Oncology, Albany Medical Center, Albany, New York

Kathleen A. O'Leary, M.D.
Assistant Professor of Anesthesiology, State University of New York at Buffalo School of Medicine and Biomedical Sciences; Director, Post-Anesthesia Care Unit, Roswell Park Cancer Institute, Buffalo, New York

James Orner, M.D.
Assistant Professor of Radiation Medicine, State University of New York at Buffalo School of Medicine and Biomedical Sciences; Assistant Professor of Radiation Medicine, Roswell Park Cancer Institute, Buffalo, New York

Bruce Patsner, M.D.
Clinical Professor of Obstetrics and Gynecology, UMDNJ-New Jersey Medical School, Newark; Director, Gynecologic Oncology, Riverview Medical Center, Red Bank, New Jersey

M. Steven Piver, M.D.
Clinical Professor of Gynecology, State University of New York at Buffalo School of Medicine and Biomedical Sciences; Chief, Department of Gynecologic Oncology, and Director, Gilda Radner Familial Ovarian Cancer Registry, Roswell Park Cancer Institute, Buffalo, New York

Peter G. Rose, M.D.
Associate Professor of Reproductive Biology, Case Western Reserve University School of Medicine; Director, Gynecologic Oncology, MacDonald Women's Hospital, Cleveland, Ohio

Kyu Shin, M.D.
Director, Radiation Therapy, State University of New York at Buffalo School of Medicine and Biomedical Sciences; Chief, Radiation Medicine, Roswell Park Cancer Institute, Buffalo, New York

Thomas B. Shows, Ph.D.
Professor of Cellular and Molecular Biology, State University of New York at Buffalo School of Medicine and Biomedical Sciences, Roswell Park Graduate Division; Chair, Human Genetics, Roswell Park Cancer Institute, Buffalo, New York

Paul C. Stomper, M.D.
Associate Professor of Radiology, State University of New York at Buffalo School of Medicine and Biomedical Sciences; Acting Chief, Diagnostic Radiology, Roswell Park Cancer Institute, Buffalo, New York

Yoshiaki Tsukada, M.D.
Clinical Professor of Pathology and Obstetrics and Gynecology, State University of New York at Buffalo School of Medicine and Biomedical Sciences; Pathologist, Sisters of Charity Hospital, Buffalo, New York

I

Ovarian and Fallopian Tube Cancer

Notice

The indications and dosages of all drugs in this book have been recommended in the medical literature and conform to the practices of the general medical community. The medications described do not necessarily have specific approval by the Food and Drug Administration for use in the diseases and dosages for which they are recommended. The package insert for each drug should be consulted for use and dosage as approved by the FDA. Because standards for usage change, it is advisable to keep abreast of revised recommendations, particularly those concerning new drugs.

1

Ovarian Epithelial Cancer

M. Steven Piver

Incidence, Epidemiology, and Etiology

In spite of extraordinary efforts to improve the results of screening, diagnosis, and treatment of ovarian cancer, the annual incidence of ovarian cancer in the United States has increased from 18,200 in 1983 to 22,000 in 1993. Of even greater concern during the same period, the annual death rate increased 15.6% from 11,500 to 13,300. It is likely that the growth and increased age that have characterized the United States population in recent decades account for increased ovarian cancer burden, but incidence and mortality trends for this disease over the past two decades magnify its importance. In spite of seemingly significant progress in surgical staging for early-stage disease (I and II), radical debulking, and the effectiveness of platinum compounds for advanced-stage ovarian cancer (III and IV), the 5-year survival rate of all stages of ovarian cancer has remained constant at 39% over the past 30 years. Moreover, current 5-year disease-free (surviving without recurrence) survival rates of 12–14% for the 70% of women presenting with advanced-stage disease are consistent with those achieved when alkylating agents were used during the 1960s and 1970s. This apparent lack of significant progress notwithstanding, continued effort is of the utmost urgency because in the United States ovarian cancer (1) is the most common cause of death due to gynecologic malignancy (52%); (2) is the most common gynecologic cancer to occur at an advanced stage (67%); (3) occurs in one of every 55 (1.8%) women and causes death in one of every 100 women during their lifetime; (4) is the sixth most common female cancer (4%) following breast, colorectal, lung, uterine, and leukemia/lymphoma; and (5) is the fifth most common cause of female cancer deaths (5%), (after breast, lung, colorectal, and lymphomas).

It was revealed in the 1973–1987 National Cancer Institute Surveillance, Epidemiology, and End Results (SEER) data on 23,843 women that ovarian cancer incidence increases after age 40 and peaks between 75 and 79. This data demonstrated that incidence increased significantly as women aged: In women less than 30 years of age, the incidence was 3/100,000; in ages 30–50, 21/100,000; greater than 50 years, 37/100,000; greater than 60 years, 46/100,000; and for ages 75–79, 54/100,000. Median age at diagnosis is 61; it increases with advanced stage. Forty percent of women diagnosed with ovarian cancer are diagnosed after age 65. Those at highest incidence include (1) women with a family history of ovarian cancer, (2) middle- and upper-class women who live in highly industrialized nations, (3) nulliparous women, (4) women who have not used oral contraceptives, (5) women who have had difficulty conceiving, and (6) possibly those that have used fertility-stimulating drugs.

Etiology

HEREDITARY FACTORS

Site-Specific Familial Ovarian Cancer and Hereditary Breast-Ovarian Cancer Syndrome

Of all the etiologic factors in the development of ovarian cancer, none is more important than a family history (Table 1-1). Ovarian cancer can be inherited as (1) site-specific familial ovarian cancer in which two or more first-degree (mother, sister, daughter) or first- and second-degree (grandmother, aunt) relatives have epithelial ovarian cancer, or (2) breast-ovarian cancer syndrome, in which clusters of breast and ovarian cancer occur among first- and second-degree relatives. A third entity known as family cancer syndrome or Lynch syndrome II consists of nonpolyposis colorectal cancer and occurs primarily in association with endometrial cancer, but also with ovarian cancer and other adenocarcinomas. As of December 31, 1992, the Gilda Radner Familial Ovarian Cancer Registry had assessed 1,002 families in which two or more first- and second-degree relatives have ovarian cancer for a total of 2,409 cases of site-specific familial ovarian cancer (Fig. 1-1).

Inheritance Patterns

Results from pedigree analyses of families with familial ovarian cancer are consistent with autosomal dominant inheritance with variable penetrance that is derived from either the maternal or paternal genes. Since site-specific familial ovarian cancer (two or more first-degree or first- and second-degree relatives) is thought to be inherited this way, the probability for inheriting the gene is 50% in first-degree relatives, 25% in second-degree relatives, and 12.5% in third-degree relatives. Houlston et al. evaluated 462 pedigrees from women who attended an ovarian cancer screening clinic by a segregation analysis. Results from their study suggest an average lifetime penetrance of 0.74 and 0.79. That is, for women who inherit the gene,

Table 1-1. Etiology of ovarian cancer

Increased risk	*RR*	*Decreased risk*	*RR*
Talc	1.9	Pregnancy	0.6
High-fat diet	2.6	Oral contraceptives	0.6
Infertility	1.6	Tubal ligation	0.33
Fertility drugs	2.8		
Heredity			
Family history of breast cancer	1.7		
One first-degree relative with ovarian cancer	4.5		
<55	7.4		
≥ 55	3.7		
Site-specific familial ovarian cancer	39.1		

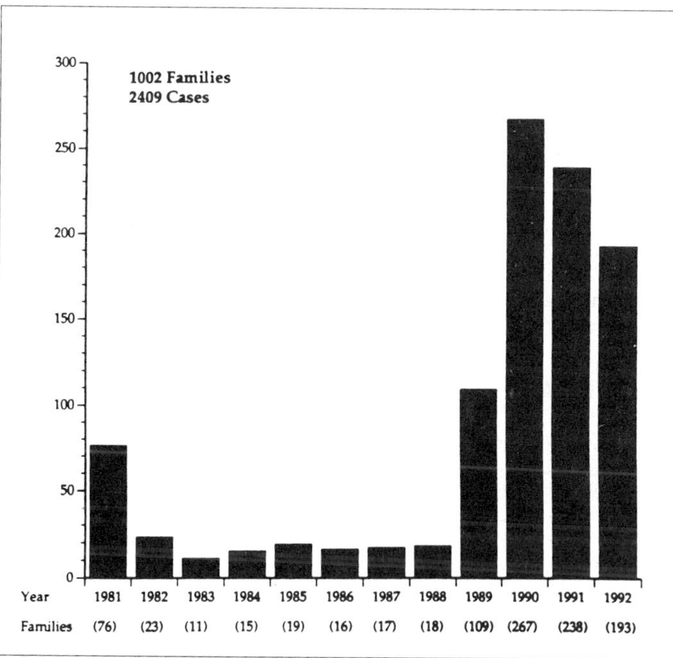

Fig. 1-1. Number of families and cases of familial ovarian cancer assessed into the Gilda Radner Familial Ovarian Cancer Registry from 1981 to 1992.

74–79% will develop ovarian cancer. Given the forenamed probabilities for inheriting the gene, lifetime risk is estimated at 37–40% among first-degree relatives, 18.5–20.0% among second-degree relatives, and 9.25–10.00% among third-degree relatives. Women who had one first-degree relative with ovarian cancer manifest a 4.5% relative risk and a 8% (4.5 × 1.8) lifetime risk of developing ovarian cancer. In addition, women who have two or more first-degree relatives with ovarian cancer were found to have a relative risk and lifetime risk of developing the disease at 39.1% and 55%, respectively. These figures are consistent with our understanding of site-specific familial ovarian cancer as an autosomal dominant inheritance with variable penetrance. This data may be criticized because these women have volunteered in an ovarian cancer screening clinic due to a large number of ovarian cancer cases in their families. Thus, inflated risk estimates may have resulted because the clinic was seeing mainly families with many sisters and daughters who had ovarian cancer, missing families with lower disease occurrence.

CLONAL ORIGIN OF OVARIAN CANCER

Jacobs and co authors studied the clonal origin of ovarian cancer by using p53 gene mutations, X-chromosome inactivation, and allelic deletion (loss of heterozygosity) on DNA specimens from cancers of the ovary and multiple sites of metastases from 17 patients with epithelial ovarian cancer. In 15 of the cases, allelic deletion, p53 gene mutation, and/or X-chromosome inactivation were consistent with a monoclonal origin. In two cases the pattern of allelic deletion and p53 mutation was compatible with monoclonal or dual primary origin from the right and left ovaries. These data suggest a unifocal or monoclonal origin of ovarian cancer with the same allelic deletion in the tumors from different sites and a similar X-chromosome inactivation. This monoclonal or unifocal origin of ovarian cancer is important because if the origin were from polyclonal peritoneal mesothelium, any effect would act simultaneously in the ovarian mesothelium (epithelium) and the peritoneal mesothelium and negate the value of prophylactic oophorectomy in high-risk women.

BRCA1 GENE AND OVARIAN CANCER

In collaboration with the University of Cambridge, the Gilda Radner Familial Ovarian Cancer Registry studied families with breast-ovarian cancer syndrome and documented that the candidate gene for breast-ovarian cancer susceptibility (BRCA1) has been localized to an interval of 1 cm or less on chromosome 17q12-21. The same investigators documented the first linkage for site-specific familial ovarian cancer to BRCA1 on 17q12-21 in 70% of the cases. Results from epidemiologic studies suggest that this may be a shared gene (breast and ovary). Women with breast cancer have twice the expected incidence of ovarian cancer, and women with ovarian cancer have three times the risk of developing breast carcinoma.

TALC

The use of talc (hydrous magnesium silicates) on the perineum is reported to increase the risk of developing ovarian cancer. Talc is implicated because of its relationship to asbestos, a known carcinogen. Cramer and co-authors reported a relative risk of 1.9% for perineal exposure to talcum powder compared to no exposure.

DIET

A major difference between women in industrialized countries and women in nonindustrialized countries is the high intake of dietary fat. Researchers from Roswell Park Cancer Institute (RPCI) reported results from a case-control study that suggest that women who drank only whole milk were at a significantly increased risk for developing ovarian cancer compared to those who drank only milk with a reduced fat content (OR = 2.6; 95% CI 1.7–4.0). This finding suggests that high fat content is responsible for the increased risk.

INFERTILITY

The Collaborative Ovarian Cancer Group reported that married infertile women who had 15 or more years of unprotected sexual intercourse had an increased risk for the development of ovarian cancer (OR = 1.6; 95% CI 1.2–2.2), suggesting some commonality between the inability to conceive and the development of ovarian cancer.

PREGNANCY

The Collaborative Ovarian Cancer Group reported that a decreased risk for the development of ovarian cancer is associated with pregnancy. Data from the population-based studies indicated a 40% decrease in risk for the first pregnancy (OR = 0.6; 95% CI 0.47–0.76) and an estimated 14% reduction in risk for each subsequent pregnancy. The odds ratio of 0.29 (95% CI 0.20–0.42) for women with six or more pregnancies supports the protective effect of pregnancy.

ORAL CONTRACEPTIVES

In 1987, results of a case-control study from the Centers for Disease Control revealed a 40% reduction (RR = 0.6) in the risk for developing ovarian cancer in women ages 20–54 who had used oral contraceptives. Results from the Collaborative Ovarian Cancer Group population study suggest that for any use of oral contraceptives, the odds ratio was a similar 0.6 (95% CI 0.55–0.70).

TUBAL LIGATION

In a prospective study of 121,700 female nurses, tubal ligation was found to significantly decrease the risk of developing ovarian cancer. A strong inverse association between tubal ligation and ovarian cancer persisted after adjustment for age, oral contraceptive use, parity, and other ovarian cancer risk factors (RR = 0.3; 95% CI 0.16–0.64). The mechanism remains unclear.

FERTILITY DRUGS

The most commonly used fertility drugs in the United States are clomiphene citrate (Clomid) and injected menotropins (Perganol). Of great concern from the Collaborative Ovarian Cancer Group is the reported increased risk of developing ovarian cancer in women who use fertility drugs. Although the number of cases is very small, among 31 women with physician-diagnosed infertility who took fertility drugs, there was a 2.8% (95% CI 1.3–6.1) increased risk of developing ovarian cancer compared with women with no clinical history of infertility.

Symptoms and Physical Findings

SYMPTOMS

Because ovarian cancer is often asymptomatic in its earliest stages, over 70% of women present with widespread (stage III and IV) disease at the time of diagnosis. Symptoms do not occur until the ovarian mass begins to encroach on other viscera or there is intraabdominal spread. At that time, patients most commonly report first vague abdominal discomfort, abdominal swelling or fullness, and early saity, most often secondary to ascites and spread to the omentum ("omental cake"). Pelvic discomfort, low back pain, and vaginal bleeding may also be noted and usually occur after these initial symptoms.

PHYSICAL FINDINGS

Since 95% of ovarian cancers measure more than 5 cm in diameter at initial diagnosis, when an ovarian mass of this size is found on pelvic examination, especially in women over 40 years of age, further evaluation is necessary. An exception to this dictum is a 5- to 7-cm mass in a young menstruating female, since most of these masses will be functional and 70% will regress spontaneously. An adnexal mass should not be considered a functional ovarian cyst (follicular or corpus luteum cyst) unless it has benign characteristics: smooth, cystic, mobile, unilateral, no larger than 5–7 cm in diameter, persists for less than 4–6 weeks, occurs during reproductive years, and is primarily cystic (anechogenic) on sonography. Since only 5% of benign tumors are bilateral at initial presentation, compared with 25% of malignant tumors, the presence of bilateral ovarian masses, even in the young age group, requires immediate evaluation to rule out ovarian cancer. Ascites and nodularity of the rectovaginal septum may be present with malignant tumors. Patients may rarely present initially with either (1) an umbilical mass (Sister Mary Joseph nodule); (2) an enlarged inguinal lymph node (spread from the ovary up the round ligament); or (3) a right-sided pleural effusion (secondary to involvement of the undersurface of the right diaphragm).

Diagnosis and Screening

ULTRASOUND AND COMPUTED TOMOGRAPHY

Pelvic ultrasonography and computed tomography (CT) are helpful for confirming the diagnosis of an ovarian mass. The ultrasonography may be preferential to CT due to its (1) lack of radiation exposure, (2) absence of possible reaction to contrast material, (3) superiority of differentiating cystic and solid tumors, and (4) lower financial cost. Even if there are no pathologic ultrasonographic findings, malignancy can be detected because increased percentages of echogenic (solid) material is associated with a stronger likelihood that the tumor is malignant. Conversely, with increased presence of anenchogenic (simple) cysts without internal echoes, there is a decreased likelihood of malignancy in the tumor. If an ovarian solid mass larger than 5 cm in diameter is found by ultrasonography, one may be suspicious of malignancy. Unfortunately, both techniques are hindered by inadequacy in the detection of masses less than 2 cm.

TRANSVAGINAL COLOR FLOW DOPPLER

Initially, it was thought that since transvaginal color flow imaging combines ultrasound with images of the blood flow velocity (pulsatile index) to the ovarian tumor, it would reduce the false-positive rate associated with the use of ultrasound. However, recent findings demonstrate that this is a false assumption because blood flow velocity and pulsatile index results overlap between benign and malignant tumors.

SERUM TUMOR MARKERS

CA125

CA125 is a high-molecular-weight glycoprotein antigenic determinant recognized by the murine monoclonal antibody OC125. CA125 is present in fetal tissue derived from coelomic epithelium and adult coelomic epithelium (fallopian tube, endometrium, endocervix). It was originally reported that serum levels of CA125 exceeded 35 μ/ml in 83% of patients with epithelial ovarian cancer compared with only 1% of healthy controls. CA125 levels were increased in patients with different stages of epithelial ovarian cancer (stage I, 50%; stage II, 90%; stage III, 92%; and stage IV, 94%). Unfortunately, the CA125 test is not the effective screen necessary to detect early ovarian cancer. Often levels are elevated in patients with carcinoma of the endometrium, fallopian tube, endocervix, and pancreas and less often in patients with lung, breast, or colorectal cancers. Also, elevated levels may result from laparotomy or many other nonmalignancy conditions such as menstruation, early pregnancy, endometriosis, pelvic inflammatory disease, adenomyosis, peritonitis, pancreatitis, hepatitis, and renal failure. Further results of CA125 assays may vary as much as 15% from day to day, and assay kits from different sources may contribute to more variable results. Among premenopausal women, the high false-positive rate, low specificity, and low predictive value negate the value of CA125 in screening. The questionable benefits do not justify the cost of the test and the resultant tens of thousands of unnecessary surgical procedures. Thus, CA125 is used primarily for monitoring disease status during therapy. Elevated CA125 is of value both in predicting persistent disease during therapy and after chemotherapy in patients with no clinical evidence of disease. However, a normal CA125 is not highly predictive of the presence or absence of disease.

OVXI and Macrophage Colony-Stimulating Factor

Researchers from Duke University evaluated CA125, OVXI, and macrophage colony-stimulating factor (M-CSF) in 46 patients with stage I ovarian cancer, 237 patients with benign pelvic masses, and 204 apparently healthy females. At least one of the three tumor markers was elevated in 98% of stage I cases, 11% of healthy individuals, and 51% of benign masses. The sensitivity of these three serum markers used in combination was significantly greater than CA125 ($p < .0005$).

Inhibin

Inhibin is a glycoprotein composed of an alpha and a beta subunit secreted by the granulosa cells of the ovary. Researchers have previously reported that women with granulosa cell tumor of the ovary had elevated serum inhibin concentrations. A more recent report demonstrated that 18 of 22 women (82%) with mucinous carcinomas and mucinous borderline carcinomas of the ovary had elevated serum inhibin concentrations. This finding is useful because CA125 is less frequently elevated in mucinous carcinomas of the ovary.

Staging

METASTATIC PATTERNS

There are three main spread patterns for ovarian cancer: (1) via direct continuity to pelvic and abdominal peritoneal structures by seeding from the primary tumor; (2) via lymphatic dissemination from the iliac lymphatics to the pelvic lymph nodes; and (3) via dissemination from the lymphatics along the ovarian vessels to the para-aortic lymph nodes in the region of the renal vessels. Hematogenous spread is rare and thus distant metastasis to the lung, kidney, bone, and liver is rare.

FIGO STAGING SYSTEM

In 1987, the International Federation of Gynecologists and Obstetricians (FIGO) adopted a revised staging system that classified tumors previously staged IAii, IBii, and IC as stage IC (Table 1-2).

Despite significant change adopted for the classification of stage III (A, B, and C), the most important prognostic factor in advanced stage ovarian cancer, the size of residual disease *after* debulking or cytoreductive surgery, is still not taken into account.

Pathology

TUMOR TYPES

Serous tumors are the most common benign and malignant ovarian tumors, and 90% of ovarian cancers are common epithelial (adenocarcinoma) tumors. Of the malignant neoplasms, serous carcinomas account for 40–45%, mucinous tumors 10%, endometrioid tumors 15%, undifferentiated carcinomas 17%, and clear-cell adenocarcinomas 6%. Five percent of endometrioid tumors arise in endometriosis, and one-fourth to one-third are associated with endometrial adenocarcinoma. For unknown reasons, clear-cell carcinomas have the worst prognosis. Rare common epithelial tumors include the Brenner tumor and small-cell carcinomas. Pseudomyxoma peritonei, the presence of mucinous ascites secondary to mucinous tumors of intraabdominal organs, are found primarily in tumors of the ovary or appendix. Primary peritoneal papillary serous carcinoma refers to a condition morphologically similar to papillary serous carcinoma of the ovaries but in the absence of other malignancy. The histologic features, spread patterns, elevated CA125, and response to cisplatin chemotherapy are essentially similar to those with serous papillary carcinoma of the ovary. Unlike the other four subtypes of common epithelial tumors that are endophytic tumors within the ovary, a small percentage of serous tumors are entirely exophytic and are designated surface

Table 1-2. FIGO stage grouping for primary carcinoma of the ovary, 1987

Stage I	Growth limited to the ovaries.
Stage IA	Growth limited to one ovary; no ascites. No tumor on the external surface; capsule intact.
Stage IB	Growth limited to both ovaries; no ascites. No tumor on the external surface; capsule intact.
Stage IC*	Tumor either stage IA or IB but with tumor on the surface of one or both ovaries or with capsule ruptured or with ascites present containing malignant cells or with positive peritoneal washings.
Stage II	Growth involving one or both ovaries with pelvic extension.
Stage IIA	Extension and/or metastases to the uterus and/or tubes.
Stage IIB	Extension to other pelvic tissues.
Stage IIC*	Tumor either stage IIA or IIB but with tumor on the surface of one or both ovaries with capsule(s) ruptured or with ascites present containing malignant cells or with positive peritoneal washings.
Stage III	Tumor involving one or both ovaries with peritoneal implants outside the pelvis and/or positive retroperitoneal or inguinal nodes. Superficial liver metastasis equals stage III. Tumor is limited to the true pelvis but with histologically verified malignant extension to small bowel or omentum.
Stage IIIA	Tumor grossly limited to the true pelvis with negative nodes but with histologically confirmed microscopic seeding of abdominal peritoneal surfaces.
Stage IIIB	Tumor of one or both ovaries with histologically confirmed implants of abdominal peritoneal surfaces, none exceeding 2 cm in diameter. Nodes negative.
Stage IIIC	Abdominal implants >2 cm in diameter and/or positive retroperitoneal or inguinal nodes.
Stage IV	Growth involving one or both ovaries with distant metastasis. If pleural effusion is present, there must be positive cytologic test results to allot a case to stage IV.

*To evaluate the impact on prognosis of the different criteria for allotting cases to stage IC or IIC. It would be of value to know whether rupture of the capsule was spontaneous or caused by the surgeon and whether the source of malignant cells detected was peritoneal washings or ascites.

Source: International Federation of Gynecologists and Obstetricians. Changes in definitions of clinical staging for carcinoma of the cervix and ovary. *Am J Obstet Gynecol* 156:263, 1987.

papillary serous tumors. Small-cell carcinomas, the most aggressive common epithelial tumors, occur in adolescence through the early 20s, are associated frequently with hypercalcemia, and are almost uniformly fatal.

BORDERLINE OVARIAN TUMORS

Approximately 10–15% of all common epithelial tumors are classified as borderline. This histology is characterized by an unusual degree of epithelial cell stratification, increased mitotic activity, nuclear abnormalities, and atypical cells in the absence of stromal invasion. Because these tumors are associated with a high cure rate and lack any histologic evidence of invasion, FIGO proposed that this intermediate group of ovarian tumors be classified as a separate entity designated "carcinomas of low malignant potential." Similarly, the World Health Organization (WHO) has labeled this category of tumors "borderline ovarian malignancies."

Histology

Borderline ovarian tumors can be serous, endometrioid, clear-cell, or Brenner with serous or, most commonly, mucinous. It is clinically important that approximately 25% of borderline tumors occur in patients under age 40, while less than 10% of invasive common epithelial tumors occur in this age group. Also important for younger patients who wish to preserve fertility is that 25–40% of serous borderline tumors are bilateral at initial presentation in contrast to only 8% of mucinous borderline tumors.

FIGO and WHO stressed that diagnosis of borderline tumors must be based only on the primary tumor, regardless of the histopathology of any extraovarian metastasis. This contradicts the general pathologic principle of grading a neoplasm from the worst area. Thus, if there are invasive peritoneal implants from a primary borderline ovarian tumor, this tumor is still classified as borderline, even though in reality, these implants behave like invasive cancer. This point was made in a recent study by Bell in which 56 borderline tumors associated with peritoneal implants were followed for 4 years or more or until death. Of the 50 patients with noninvasive implants, 94% had no progression of disease, but only 17% of the six patients with invasive implants showed no progression.

Stage

Although 70% of invasive epithelial ovarian tumors present as stage III and IV ovarian cancer, borderline tumors usually present at earlier stages. In a report of 370 borderline tumors treated at the Norwegian Radium Hospital, 84% (31) were stage I, 55% (20) were stage II, 11% (39) were stage III, and none were stage IV. Although 5-year actuarial survival rates for women diagnosed with stage I borderline tumors ranged from 90% to 100%, systematic surgical staging of stage I ovarian tumors demonstrates a significant incidence of subclinical metastasis. In 1988, Yazigi et al. reported that two of 25 patients (8%) had malignant peritoneal cytology, none of 20 had metastasis to the omentum, none of 11 had metastasis to the diaphragm, and none of 11 had peritoneal metastasis. However, three of 13 (23%) had pelvic lymph node metastasis, and one of 12 patients (8%) had aortic lymph node metastasis. Therefore, when one is considering conservative surgery (unilateral salpingo-oophorectomy or ovarian cystectomy) in young patients with borderline tumors, surgical staging should still be performed.

CA125

Rice et al. studied preoperative CA125 levels in 38 patients undergoing primary surgery for borderline tumors of the ovary. Elevated preoperative CA125 levels were found in 10 of 25 (40%) stage I cases, two of two (100%) stage II cases, nine of 10 (90%) stage III cases, and one of one (100%) stage IV cases.

Long-Term Survival

Although 5-year actuarial survival for stage I borderline tumors ranges from 90% to 100%, there are few reports of long-term survival. In a study conducted at Johns Hopkins University, it was found that among patients followed for 3–27 years with a median of 10 years, 6% of the 123 stage I ovarian cancer patients, 18% of the 17 stage II ovarian cancer patients, and 56% of the 16 stage III ovarian cancer patients had a recurrence.

Chemotherapy

The Gynecologic Oncology Group (GOG) reported on 32 patients with stage III borderline tumors of the ovary with less than 1 cm residual disease who were treated with either cisplatin and cyclophosphamide or cisplatin, cyclophosphamide, and Adriamycin. With a median follow-up of 31.7 months (1–75), only one patient had died, but cancer was present at that autopsy. The remaining patients were alive without clinical evidence of disease at a median of 30 months. Of special note was that of 15 patients who underwent second-look laparotomy, only six had no evidence of disease. Apparently, the lack of significant efficacy of chemotherapy was documented because only two of the eight (25%) patients with residual disease at the completion of the initial surgical procedure were disease-free at second-look laparotomy, and two of six patients with no gross disease at the completion of the initial surgery had a microscopically positive second-look laparotomy. This latter group had progressive disease on chemotherapy.

Stage I and II Invasive Ovarian Carcinoma

From 1960 to 1975, the 5-year survival rate for stage I and II ovarian cancer cases treated by total abdominal hysterectomy and bilateral salpingo-oophorectomy (TAH/BSO) was only 70% and 32%, respectively. The addition of postoperative irradiation directed primarily at the pelvis did not improve these survival statistics for the earliest stages of ovarian cancer. The reasons for these poor survival rates were elusive until the 1970s, when it was discovered that five areas within the peritoneal cavity harbored microscopic or unrecognized metastases from what appeared clinically to be localized ovarian cancer. These areas include the (1) diaphragm, (2) omentum, (3) para-aortic lymph nodes, (4) pelvic lymph nodes, and (5) malignant cytologic peritoneal washings. These new findings led to the use of surgical staging to more accurately define stage I and II ovarian cancer. This method facilitated upstaging to stage III those patients found to have subclinical metastasis above the pelvis.

SURGICAL STAGING

Roswell Park Cancer Institute: Collective Review

In 1978, researchers from the RPCI reported a collective review of the incidence of such microscopic metastases in patients with stage I or II ovarian cancer. Of the women with presumed stage I disease, it was determined that 11% had diaphragmatic metastasis, 13% had para-aortic lymph node metastasis, 8% had pelvic lymph node metastasis, 3% had omental metastasis, and 33% had malignant peritoneal cytologic washings (Table 1-3). Similar results were found in patients with FIGO stage II disease.

Ovarian Cancer Study Group

The first prospective studies of such surgical staging in clinically localized ovarian cancer were reported by the Ovarian Cancer Study Group (OCSG) that formed in 1976, composed of researchers from the Mayo Clinic, M.D. Anderson Cancer Center, RPCI, and the National Cancer Institute. Of the 100 women reported, 31% with presumed stage I or II ovarian cancer were upstaged after exploration and surgical staging, and 77% were reclassified as stage III. Moreover, of the 100 patients diagnosed with FIGO stage I or IIB ovarian cancer that were referred to member institutions within 4 weeks of their original surgery, 61 were considered to have no residual cancer after the initial operation. When restaging laparotomy was performed by the OCSG within 4 weeks of the initial surgery, metastasis was present in the diaphragm (3%), in the omentum (11%), in abdominal tissues (9%), in other pelvic tissues (9%), in the cul-de-sac peritoneum (3%), and in the para-aortic lymph nodes (9%) of those supposedly disease-free patients.

Gynecologic Oncology Group

In 1989, the results of a prospective study conducted by the GOG demonstrated findings similar to those found in studies performed by RPCI (1978) and the OCSG (1983). Therefore, complete surgical staging is required for apparent stage I and II ovarian cancer to identify those patients who truly have localized disease and to upstage the remaining patients to allow for appropriate treatment.

Surgical staging, in addition to TAH/BSO, should include peritoneal cytologic sampling from the pelvis, right and left paracolic gutters (obtained immediately after the peritoneal cavity is entered to avoid the red blood cell contamination that interferes with cytologic interpretation), and brushings for cytology from the undersurface of the diaphragm, bilateral pelvic lymphadenectomy, para-aortic lymphadenectomy, and omentectomy (Fig. 1-2).

TREATMENT OF STAGE I OVARIAN CARCINOMA

Intraperitoneal Chromic Phosphate

Physical Characteristics

Even before the data on surgical staging were reported, pelvic irradiation alone fell into disuse after it was recognized that most recur-

Table 1-3. Incidence of subclinical metastases in apparent stage I or II ovarian cancer

	Stage I		*Stage II*	
Sites	*RPCI*	*GOG*	*RPCI*	*GOG*
Diaphragm	11.0%	11.0%	23.0%	6.0%
Omentum	3.0%	0.0%	7.0%	19.0%
Para-aortic nodes	13.0%	4.0%	10.0%	19.5%
Pelvic nodes	8.0%	0.0%	—	19.5%
Malignant peritoneal cytology	33.0%	—	12.5%	—

RPCI = Roswell Park Cancer Institute; GOG = Gynecologic Oncology Group.
Source: MS Piver, JJ Barlow, SB Lele. Incidence of subclinical metastasis in stage I and II ovarian carcinoma. *Obstet Gynecol* 52:100, 1978; and HJ Buchsbaum, MF Brady, G Delgado et al. Surgical staging of carcinoma of the ovaries. *Surg Gynecol Obstet* 169:226, 1989. By permission of *Surgery Gynecology and Obstetrics.*

rences were in the abdominal cavity. Subsequently, researchers used first intraperitoneal gold-198 (^{198}Au) and then chromic phosphate (^{32}P) in patients not surgically staged. ^{32}P emits purely beta radiation and has a half-life of 14.5 days. ^{32}P's high beta energy (^{198}Au emits both beta and gamma rays) allows deep tissue penetration, and its pure beta emissions are not harmful to hospital personnel and obviate patient isolation. Currie et al. concluded that although intraperitoneal ^{32}P delivers a therapeutic dose to the superficial peritoneal surfaces (6,000–7,000 cGy), it does not deliver a therapeutic dose to the retroperitoneal lymph nodes.

In Stage I

In a 1988 report from RPCI, 25 evaluable patients with FIGO stage I ovarian cancer treated with intraperitoneal ^{32}P were studied. All patients had undergone TAH/BSO, with (28%) or without (72%) omentectomy; none had undergone other surgical staging procedures at the time of referral. Patients were restaged by laparoscopy, with inspection of the diaphragm, abdomen, and pelvis; biopsies of suspicious lesions; and cytologic peritoneal washings, all prior to ^{32}P therapy. The estimated 5- and 10-year recurrence-free survival rate was 84% and 75%, respectively. The long-term result (75%) perpetuates the question of whether adjuvant ^{32}P therapy has any true effect on disease-free survival in presumed stage I ovarian cancer.

Researchers at Duke University reported a lack of effectiveness of adjuvant intraperitoneal ^{32}P in stage I ovarian carcinoma even in patients who had undergone surgical staging by peritoneal washings for cytology, multiple biopsies of pelvic and abdominal peritoneum, and selective pelvic and para-aortic lymphadenectomy at their initial surgery. These authors reported a 5-year disease-free survival rate of only 65% in the 23 stage I ovarian cancer patients studied.

Whole Abdominal Radiation

The major drawback of whole abdominal radiation is that only limited doses to the upper abdomen of less than 2,250–2,800 cGy in 100- to 120-cGy daily fractions can be delivered safely due to the radiosensitivity of the intestine, liver, and kidney, requiring kidney shielding at 1,800 cGy.

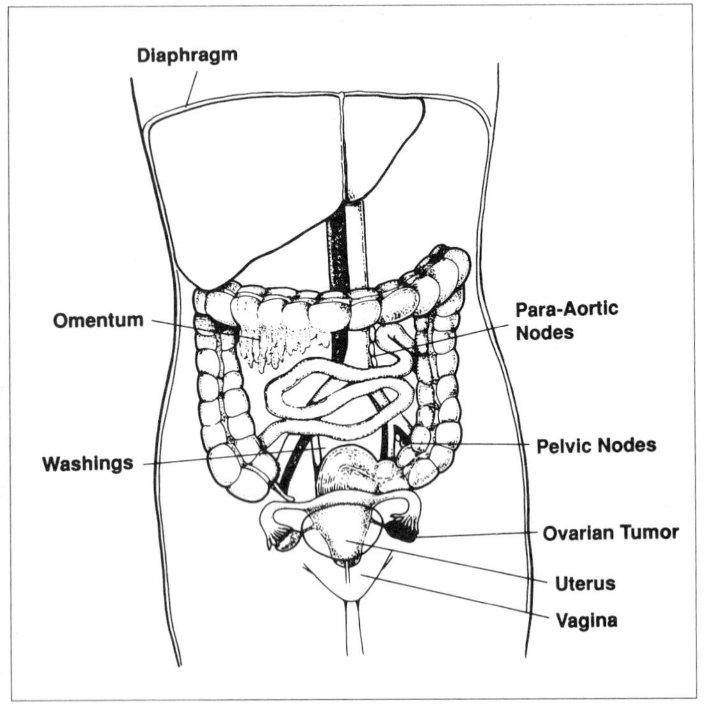

Fig. 1-2. Specific sites for surgical staging in presumed stage I or II ovarian cancer.

5-Year Survival in Stage I

Dembo from the Princess Margaret Hospital reported a disease-free survival rate of only 73% in 79 patients with stage I (not surgically staged) ovarian cancer treated by whole abdominal radiation. When MacBeth et al. used the whole abdominal radiation techniques described by Dembo et al. to deliver 2,500 cGy to surgically staged patients, they reported an estimated 5-year disease-free survival rate of 65% in 28 stage I ovarian cancer patients and 39% in 25 stage II patients. The authors concluded that these data do not seem to support a curative role for this dose of postoperative radiation in these early-stage patients.

Chemotherapy

Treatment of Stage IA or IB, Grade 1 or 2 Ovarian Cancer in Surgically Staged Patients

OVARIAN CANCER STUDY GROUP/GYNECOLOGIC ONCOLOGY GROUP. In a study conducted by the OCSG and GOG, surgically staged patients were entered into two prospective trials, protocols 7601 and 7602. Protocol 7601 included patients with stage IA, IB, grade 1 or 2 ovarian adenocarcinoma with no evidence of metastasis at complete surgical staging. Patients were randomly assigned to either observation or treatment with melphalan chemotherapy for 12 monthly cycles. With a median follow-up of over 6 years, the disease-free survival rate at 5 years was 95% for melphalan and 92% for observation, with no significant statistical difference. Based on the exceedingly high cure rates, it was concluded that patients with stage IA or IB, G1 or G2 ovarian adenocarcinoma and no evidence of metastasis at complete surgical staging do not require adjuvant therapy.

There are two important caveats to this study. First, although there were only five recurrences in 81 patients, four in the observation arm and one in the melphalan arm, 37 (46%) were reclassified as borderline carcinomas, leaving only 54 truly invasive cancers in this study. Also, since only five patients were grade 2, no conclusion on grade 2 can be made.

Treatment of Stage IC or Stage I, Grade 3 Ovarian Cancer in Surgically Staged Patients

ROSWELL PARK CANCER INSTITUTE/ALBANY MEDICAL CENTER. In a prospective trial from RPCI and Albany Medical Center (AMC), the authors reported on 32 stage IC or stage I, grade 3 ovarian cancer patients who were treated by induction cisplatin followed by cisplatin and cyclophosphamide with or without Adriamycin. With a median follow-up of 5 years, there were three recurrences (9%). The 5-year progression-free survival rate was 90.5%, and the 5-year survival rate was 93.3%. Of the 20 completely surgically staged patients, there was only one (5%) recurrence, suggesting that adjuvant cisplatin chemotherapy as administered in this trial following complete surgical staging is effective in lowering the recurrence rate in this high-risk group of patients.

ITALIAN ONCOLOGIC COOPERATIVE GROUP. The Italian Oncologic Cooperative Group (GONO) reported results from a prospective trial of adjuvant cisplatin and cyclophosphamide in patients with stage I and II epithelial ovarian cancer. Although patients in this trial underwent omentectomy and multiple biopsies and washings, the pelvic and para-aortic lymph nodes "were biopsied only if clinically suspicious." Since most lymph node metastasis in early-stage ovarian cancer is subclinical or microscopic and thus not clinically suspicious, the patients in this study were not completely surgically staged. Of the 48 stage IC patients, there were eight relapses (16.6%) and a 7-year actuarial relapse-free survival rate of only approximately 65%. This is not a significant improvement over surgery alone among this early-stage, poor-prognosis group of patients.

Prognosis

Results from a retrospective analysis from the Princess Margaret Hospital and the Norwegian Radium Hospital of 519 presumed stage I ovarian cancer patients suggest that histologic differentiation (grade 1 versus grades 2 and 3) is the most powerful predictor of relapse, with dense adherence of the tumor and large-volume ascites being second and third, respectively. The results also suggest that when these three factors were accounted for, bilaterality (stage IB), cyst rupture (stage IC), capsular penetration (stage IC), tumor size, histologic subtype, patient age, and postoperative therapy are not adverse prognostic factors. A 98% 5-year relapse-free survival rate was found for patients with stage I grade 1 tumors in the absence of dense adhesions or large-volume ascites. However, these patients were not surgically staged, nor did they have peritoneal cytology for evaluation.

Summary of Stage I

Because of the sensitivity of the small intestine, liver, and kidneys to radiation, it is theoretically doubtful that using 2,250 cGy in the whole abdomen would improve survival rate over surgery alone. This may account for the Princess Margaret Hospital's 5-year relapse-free rate of only 78%. Similarly, the RPCI 10-year disease-free survival rate of only 75% with the use of adjuvant intraperitoneal ^{32}P and the 5-year disease-free survival rate of 65% reported from Duke University with the use of adjuvant intraperitoneal ^{32}P are not significantly better than that of surgery alone. Based on the more than 90% 5-year survival rate reported by the OCSG and GOG in surgically staged IA or IB, G1 or G2, this subset of patients needs no adjuvant therapy. Because of the encouraging preliminary results of 5-year progression-free survival of over 90% in a small group of stage IC or stage I grade 3 patients from RPCI treated with induction cisplatin and cisplatin plus cyclophosphamide with or without Adriamycin, we recommend that all stage IC, stage I grade 3 patients receive 6 months of cisplatin-based combination chemotherapy. However, a larger series is required to verify these results.

TREATMENT OF STAGE II OVARIAN CARCINOMA

Whole Abdominal Radiation

The use of whole abdominal radiation for stage II patients by investigators from the Princess Margaret Hospital resulted in a relapse-free rate of 72% at 5 years and 65% at 10 years in patients who had no residual cancer after surgery.

Chemotherapy

Italian Oncologic Cooperative Group

The GONO reported the results from a prospective trial of cisplatin and cyclophosphamide on 35 stage II patients who were surgically staged with lymph node biopsy only if clinically suspicious. With 34% (12) developing a relapse and the actuarial 7-year relapse-free survival of only 55%, this study did not demonstrate significant improvement by adjuvant cisplatin-based chemotherapy.

Roswell Park Cancer Institute and Albany Medical Center

In the results of a prospective trial from RPCI and AMC, researchers reported on 20 consecutive patients treated with induction cisplatin followed by 6 months of cisplatin, Adriamycin, and cyclophosphamide. Of the 20 patients, 10 were completely surgically staged prior to therapy. The estimated 5-year progression-free survival of only 45% was not a significant improvement over no adjuvant treatment.

Ovarian Cancer Study Group and Gynecologic Oncology Group

OCSG and GOG recognized that a subset of completely staged patients with stage I and II ovarian cancer could not be entered into protocol 7601 due to their high risk for recurrence if they were randomized to the observation arm. Thus, this subset, which included patients with stage IC and stage II disease, were placed on protocol 7602, in which they were randomized to melphalan or intraperitoneal ^{32}P at a dose of 15 mCi. In a report of the 93 stage II surgically staged patients with no macroscopic residual disease and a mean follow-up of 6 years, OCSG and GOG reported a 5-year survival rate of 78% with no statistical significance between ^{32}P and melphalan. However, of the 93 patients studied, none of the 17 with borderline tumors were reported to have suffered recurrences. That leaves 76 patients with stage II invasive epithelial ovarian cancer, 24 (32%) of whom developed recurrent disease. The authors reported a 5-year survival rate of 74% when the patients with borderline tumors are excluded. Thus, it is probably for that reason that protocol 7602 was changed by the GOG to randomize these patients to either the new control arm of ^{32}P or cisplatin (100 mg/m^2) plus cyclophosphamide (1,000 mg/m^2) every 21–35 days for three cycles. Results from this study have not yet been reported.

Summary of Stage II

The OCSG-GOG report that only 74% 5-year survival was achieved with ^{32}P or melphalan in the surgically staged patients does not support the use of either of these treatments as adjuvant therapy in carefully staged patients. Even the use of cisplatin, Adriamycin, and cyclophosphamide (PAC) chemotherapy has not been reported to be as effective as hoped. We await results from the recent GOG study that will report on the use of cisplatin and cyclophosphamide in carefully staged stage IIB patients.

Treatment of Stage III and IV Ovarian Cancer

SURGERY

Studies consistently show that when compared to patients with large residual disease after initial surgery, those with small residual disease after radical surgery (referred to as *debulking* or *cytoreductive surgery*) for advanced ovarian cancer respond more frequently to chemotherapy and have significantly better survival.

Theoretical Models for the Benefit of Cytoreductive Surgery

Models to explain the benefit of maximum cytoreductive surgery include resection of preexisting resistant sub-clones and single random mutation. It is presumed that sensitive and resistant tumor cell populations are present at the initiation of chemotherapy, and thus resection may remove a significant number of de novo resistant populations. In the Goldie Coldman model it is assumed that an initial sensitive population of tumor cells undergoes subsequent mutation to cause treatment resistance to chemotherapy. In addition, when large tumors are reduced, the remaining tumor cells come closer to the blood supply, where they are more accessible to chemotherapy.

Improved Survival with Residual Disease of Less Than 1.5 Cm

Griffiths and Fuller reported one of the first and most compelling studies on the benefit of cytoreductive surgery. They demonstrated a 40-month survival rate of about 30% in patients with stage III or IV ovarian cancer with postoperative tumor nodules measuring less than 1.5 cm at initial presentation. This rate compared to a similar survival rate of 30% at 40 months for those patients who had undergone cytoreductive surgery that resulted in residual tumor of less than 1.5 cm. In sharp contrast, no patient survived 40 months with residual tumor measuring greater than 1.5 cm after cytoreductive surgery. Of special importance is the fact that this report was completed before the discovery of the effectiveness of cisplatin chemotherapy in epithelial ovarian cancer.

Improved Survival with Residual Disease Less Than or Equal to 2 Cm

Researchers from M.D. Anderson Cancer Center reported on 395 patients with stage III ovarian cancer who were treated with chemotherapy. They found that 40% of patients with 2 cm or less of residual disease survived 4 years, but only 14% of those with greater than 2 cm residual disease survived 4 years ($p = .01$).

Improved Survival with Residual Disease Less Than or Equal to 1 Cm

The Netherlands Joint Study Group (NJSG) reported on 191 stage III and IV patients with epithelial ovarian cancer who were treated with either cisplatin, Adriamycin, cyclophosphamide, and hexamethylmelamine (PAC-H or CHAP-5), or cisplatin and cyclophosphamide (PC). The 5- and 8-year survival rates for PAC-H were 32% and 21%, respectively, and for PC were 28% and 23%, respectively. These results suggest that no survival advantage can be attributed to the addition of hexamethylmelamine or Adriamycin. Most important, twice as many patients survived for 5 years after surgery who had tumors less than 1 cm compared to patients who had more than 1 cm residual disease.

Similarly, in a report on 136 patients with stage III and IV ovarian cancer who were treated with induction cisplatin followed by PAC chemotherapy, researchers at RPCI reported 5- and 8-year survival rates for patients with less than 1 cm of residual disease as 50% and 42%, respectively. However, these rates were only 19% and 10% for patients with 1–2 cm of residual disease, and 13% and 8.7% for patients with greater than 2 cm ($p = .001$). The 5- and 8-year progression-free survival rates were 40% and 36% for patients with less than 1 cm, 17% and 13% for patients with 1–2 cm, and 4% for patients with greater than 2 cm ($p = 0.001$) (Fig. 1-3).

Secondary Debulking Surgery

The principles that outline the value of primary debulking surgery theoretically also apply to patients whose tumors progress during or recur after initial cisplatin-based chemotherapy. Before reports of the value of paclitaxel (Taxol) as second-line therapy, most patients whose malignancy progressed during primary cisplatin-based chemotherapy for advanced ovarian cancer did not benefit from reoperation because there was then no second-line effective chemotherapy. Among patients who had an initial excellent response to cisplatin-based chemotherapy and especially among patients who had a long disease-free interval (>6–12 months), evidence suggests that they could re-respond to cisplatin-based chemotherapy. In the latter group of patients, the same principles used in initial debulking surgery should apply. The dictum that reoperation on patients who progressed during first-line chemotherapy with cisplatin is not beneficial may no longer be true due to the discovery of the activity of Taxol.

Second-Look Laparotomy

Evaluation of the cancer status of patients by second-look laparotomy was originally for patients with colon carcinoma. In the 1970s, when acute nonlymphocytic leukemia was reported to be associated with the prolonged treatment of ovarian cancer with alkylating agent chemotherapy, documentation of disease-free status with second-look laparotomy became a preventive measure and discontinuation of treatment became a priority. By the 1980s, cisplatin-based chemotherapy had replaced alkylating agent chemotherapy, and the use of second-look laparotomy became more controversial. The controversy was heightened by the fact that there were no prospective randomized trials to evaluate second-look laparotomy. More important, before the discovery of Taxol, there was no effective second-line chemotherapy if disease was present at second-look laparotomy. With the discovery of Taxol, patients can now be offered effective second-line treatment if they have not received it as initial therapy. Since the discovery of Taxol, the value of second-look laparotomy is to (1) discontinue all chemotherapy if no evidence of disease is found; (2) determine the actual surgical and pathologic response to previous cisplatin-based chemotherapy if cisplatin is again to be used as part of second-line therapy; and (3) debulk residual disease, if present, to minimal or microscopic disease if possible with the same theoretical benefit as at primary surgery. Approximately one-third of patients with stage III and IV ovarian cancer who undergo second-look laparotomy have no evidence of disease after careful restaging. However, approximately 50% of this group will subsequently develop recurrent disease.

Definition

By definition, second-look laparotomy is designed to determine whether cancer is still present in patients who were treated with surgery followed by adjuvant chemotherapy, who have no clinical or radiologic evidence of disease, and who have normal CA125 levels. It is not applicable to patients undergoing reoperation for persistent or recurrent disease.

Technique

The technique used for second-look laparotomy is similar to that used for initial staging laparotomy in early-stage ovarian cancer, but with the addition of the biopsy of all known sites of previous tumor from the initial surgery and all suspicious areas (usually white and granular), including adhesions that frequently contain small clusters of tumor cells.

CA125 and Second-Look Laparotomy

An elevated CA125 before second-look laparotomy is associated with persistent macroscopic disease nearly 100% of the time. However, in

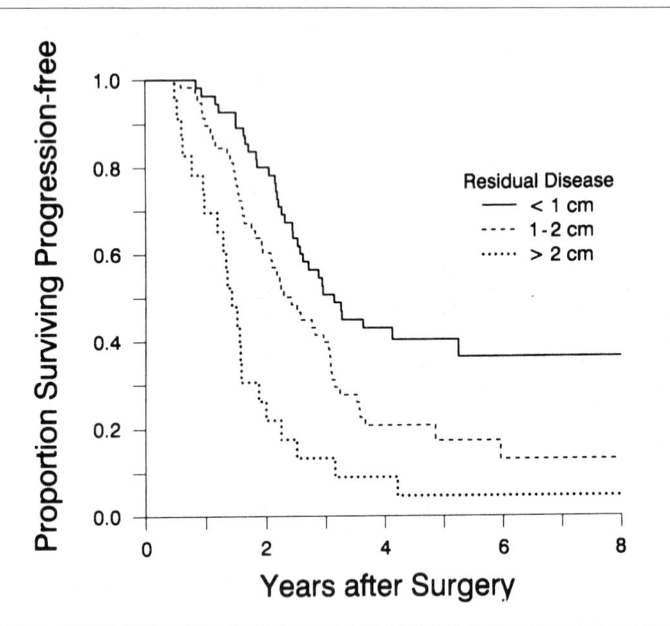

Fig. 1-3. Progression-free survival of 136 patients with stage III and IV ovarian carcinoma according to residual disease status after primary surgery. (From TR Baker, MS Piver, RE Hempling. Long-term survival by cytoreductive surgery to <1 cm, induction weekly cisplatin and monthly cisplatin, adriamycin, and cyclophosphamide in advanced ovarian adenocarcinoma. *Cancer* 74:656–663, 1994.)

patients with a normal CA125, approximately 50% will have persistent disease at second-look laparotomy. Jacobs and Bast found residual disease at second-look laparotomy in 96% of 243 patients with an elevated CA125 preoperatively, but only 46% of 336 patients with normal preoperative CA125. These results show an overall accuracy rate of 67% in 579 patients. Moreover, elevated CA125 levels correlate with the size of residual disease: microscopic = 21%; less than 1 cm = 38%; less than 2 cm = 46%; greater than 1 cm = 79%; greater than 2 cm = 70%; and greater than 10 cm = 100%.

OVX1 and Second-Look Laparotomy

Using a radioimmunoassay to detect an epitope on a high-molecular-weight mucin-like glycoprotein that is defined by the murine antibody OVX1, researchers from Duke University reported that 32% of patients at the time of a positive second-look laparotomy had normal CA125 but elevated OVX1.

Computed Tomography Scan and Second-Look Laparotomy

CT scans are not sensitive or specific enough to detect tumors of less than 2 cm. Researchers from Duke University reported that CT scans detect only 7% of tumor nodules 1 cm or smaller and only 37%

of tumors greater than 1 cm. Also, it was reported that some tumors as large as 4 cm were not detected by CT scan.

^{111}In-CYT-103 and Second-Look Laparotomy

^{111}In-CYT-103 (Oncoscint CR-OV) is an indium-labeled immunoconjugate of the murine monoclonal antibody B72.3. Surwit and coauthors reported that despite low specificity (57% versus 100%) and positive predictive value (83% versus 100%), immunoscintigraphy was more sensitive than CT scan (59% versus 29%). Therefore, the sensitivity of approximately 60% is not equal to the sensitivity of second-look laparotomy.

CHEMOTHERAPY

Results Before the Discovery of Cisplatin

Almost four decades ago, the successful use of chemotherapy using the alkylating agent 2-chloro-2-hydroxydiethyl sulfide (hemisulfur) for palliation of advanced ovarian cancer was first reported. Over the next 30 years, chemotherapy with alkylating agents, primarily phenylalanine mustard (melphalan), superseded irradiation as the most common adjuvant to surgery in advanced ovarian cancer. The realization that alkylating agent therapy may be curative came in a 1966 report from the M.D. Anderson Cancer Center in which Rutledge et al. reported that among 13 patients with advanced ovarian cancer who were treated with melphalan in which melphalan was subsequently discontinued, only two developed recurrent cancer. Single-agent melphalan therapy was replaced by combination chemotherapy in most institutions following a National Cancer Institute report of a randomized clinical trial comparing melphalan to hexa-CAF (hexamethylmelamine, cyclophosphamide, methotrexate, and 5-fluorouracil) in which 75% and 54% response rates to hexa-CAF and melphalan were found, respectively.

Five- and Ten-Year Survival Using Cisplatin-Based Chemotherapy

Although there are hundreds of cisplatin-based trials in advanced ovarian cancer (Table 1-4), most have small numbers, a small percentage of patients optimally debulked, and short follow-up. Compared to the 20–40% clinical response rate for alkylating agents alone, results from most of these cisplatin-based chemotherapy trials demonstrate a 60–80% clinical response rate and a 30–40% surgical complete response rate, with 50–70% of the latter group eventually developing progressive ovarian cancer. Since cisplatin-based trials are now maturing, 5-, 8-, and 10-year disease-free survivals can be evaluated to determine the true long-term curability of surgery and cisplatin-based chemotherapy in advanced ovarian cancer.

After the initial report using cisplatin, Adriamycin, and cyclophosphamide chemotherapy, some authors began to add hexamethylmelamine to the PAC regimen, while others deleted Adriamycin from the PAC regimen. In a randomized prospective trial of 191 patients with advanced ovarian cancer, researchers from NJSG compared PAC-H (or CHAP-5) to PC. It was found that there was no difference in response rate or survival after a median follow-up of 8 years, and significant added toxicity in the PAC-H patients suggested no additional survival value by hexamethylmelamine or Adriamycin. An analysis by the Ovarian Cancer Meta-Analysis Project, which pooled data from almost 1,200 patients from four chemotherapy trials in ovarian cancer, demonstrated a 7% survival advantage at 6 years that was statistically significant for PAC as compared to PC. This increase is especially important since most women with advanced ovarian cancer will eventually die of their disease. The true efficacy of cisplatin-based chemotherapy is the long-term 5-, 7-, 8-, and 10-year progression-free survival. However, regardless of whether patients receive cisplatin, adriamycin, and cyclophosphamide; cisplatin, adriamycin, cyclophosphamide, and hexamethylmelamine; or just cisplatin and cyclophosphamide, the 5-year progression-free survival ranged from a low of 10% to a high of only 27%. Moreover, even using cisplatin-based chemotherapy, it is primarily patients who have residual disease of 1 cm or less who have a significantly prolonged survival and progression-free survival.

Carboplatin-Based Chemotherapy in Advanced Ovarian Cancer

Two trials have compared cisplatin plus cyclophosphamide versus carboplatin and cyclophosphamide in stage III and IV ovarian cancer. In the Southwestern Oncology Group (SWOG) trial, with a median follow-up of 2.7 years, 80% of the patients were dead of disease. Neither the estimated median survival of 17.4 months for cisplatin and 20.0 months for carboplatin, nor the 3-year respective survival rates of 21% for cisplatin and 20% for carboplatin were statistically significant.

In the National Cancer Institute of Canada trial, there was no statistical difference in the median survival, with an estimated median survival for cisplatin of 25 months and for carboplatin of 27.5 months and an estimated median progression-free survival for cisplatin of 14 months and for carboplatin of 14.5 months. The approximate 3-year progression-free survival rates for cisplatin and carboplatin were 18% and 21%, respectively. It is clear in both of these trials, consisting primarily of patients with large residual disease, that 5- and 10-year survival rates will most likely be in the single digit range. This demonstrates little if any progress from the single-agent alkylating era of the 1960s and 1970s.

Taxol as First-Line Chemotherapy

Using Taxol as first-line chemotherapy, the GOG evaluated 394 patients with stage III and IV, suboptimally debulked disease (>1 cm). Researchers compared six 3-week cycles of Taxol, 135 mg/m^2, and cisplatin, 75 mg/m^2, to cyclophosphamide, 750 mg/m^2, and cisplatin, 75 mg/m^2. Of the 219 patients evaluable for clinical response, the Taxol arm was superior—79% versus 63% ($p = .02$). However, the rates of pathologically negative second-look laparotomies in the Taxol arm of 26% were not statistically different from the rates of 19% found in the cyclophosphamide arm ($p = .07$). This preliminary report of a 4-month increase in median progression-free survival of 17.9 months for Taxol versus 13.8 months for the cyclophosphamide arm has changed the primary therapy for advanced ovarian cancer in the United States.

Table 1-4. Five- to ten-year survival and progression-free survival in stage III and IV ovarian cancer treated with cisplatin-based chemotherapy

Author	*No. of Patients*	*Optimal surgery*	*Defini- tion*	*Chemo- therapy*	*5-year*		*7-year*		*8-year*		*10-year*	
					S	*PFS*	*S*	*PFS*	*S*	*PFS*	*S*	*PFS*
Netherlands, GOG	88	43%	<1.5 cm	PAC	33%	27%	—	—	—	—	—	—
Vanderbilt University, USA	55	36%	<2 cm	PAC-H	23%	18%	—	—	—	—	—	—
Vancouver Clinic, Canada	195	13%	<2 cm	PC	13%	10%	—	—	—	—	4%	8%
Indiana University, USA	56	30%	<3 cm	PAC	23%	18%	16%	11%	14%	9%	9%	7%
GICOG	175	33%	—	PAC	29%	—	22%	—	—	—	—	—
Italy	181	28%	<2 cm	PC	22%	—	17%	—	—	—	—	—
	173	30%	—	P	17%	—	12%	—	—	—	—	—
Netherlands	94	40%	<1 cm	PAC-H	32%	—	—	—	21%	—	21%	—
Joint Study		48%	<2 cm	PAC-H	—	—	—	—	—	—	—	—
Group	97	25%	<1 cm	PC	28%	—	—	—	23%	—	23%	—
		49%	<2 cm	PC	—	—	—	—	—	—	—	—
RPCI	136	40%	<1 cm	PAC	50%	40%	—	—	42%	36%	—	—
USA		43%	1–2 cm	PAC	19%	17%	—	—	10%	13%	—	—
		17%	>2 cm	PAC	13%	4%	—	—	9%	4%	—	—

GOG = Gynecologic Oncology Group; GICOG = Gruppo Interegionale Cooperativo Oncologico Ginecologica; RPCI = Roswell Park Cancer Institute; S = survival; PFS = progression-free survival; P = cisplatin; A = Adriamycin; C = cyclophosphamide; H = hexamethylamine.

However, this modest increase may not result in a significant increase in long-term survival in suboptimally debulked disease.

Second-Line Chemotherapy in Advanced Ovarian Cancer

In 1976, single-agent chemotherapy continued to evolve with the seminal observation by Wiltshaw and Kroner that 25% of patients responded to cisplatin as second-line chemotherapy after progression on alkylating agent chemotherapy. Regrettably, nearly 20 years later, it is clear that 90% and 97% of the patients with stage III and IV ovarian cancer, respectively, will develop recurrence and require second-line chemotherapy.

Retreatment with Cisplatin

Patients who have previously responded to cisplatin and have a long disease-free interval can be retreated with cisplatin. Of 18 patients retreated at MDAH with a treatment-free interval of more than 12 months, 100% responded (9 clinical complete responses and 9 clinical partial responses).

Taxol

In a study of the National Cancer Institute's first 1,000 patients with cisplatin-refractory ovarian cancer, it was found that among 652 evaluable patients treated with Taxol at a dose of 135 mg/m^2 for 24 hours every 3 weeks, a response rate of 22% (4% complete response, 18% partial response) was achieved. The median time of progression from treatment initiation was 7.1 months in responding patients and 4.5 months for all patients, while the median survival duration was 8.8 months. However, the eligibility criteria that patients had to have failed three former types of chemotherapy to be entered into this study probably contributed to the low overall response rate. There is some evidence that Taxol increased to 250 mg/m^2 with granulocyte colony-stimulating factor (G-CSF) may result in higher responses in cisplatin-refractory ovarian cancer. Of the 44 patients treated with 250 mg/m^2 of Taxol every 21 days with G-CSF, 21 (48%) had a greater than 50% reduction in tumor volume. However, because of the activity of Taxol, many clinicians now use it as first-line therapy with or without cisplatin and carboplatin, making it unavailable as salvage therapy.

Tamoxifen

Using tamoxifen at a high dose (80 mg/day for 30 days and then 40 mg/day), researchers from the Mid-Atlantic Oncology Program reported a 17% response rate in 29 patients treated with tamoxifen, 7% of which were complete responses and 10% of which were partial responses.

Oral Etoposide

Using oral etoposide, researchers from the British Columbia Cancer Agency reported on 31 evaluable patients who had progressed while on cisplatin or carboplatin or had achieved less than a complete response. The overall response rate was 26%, with one being a complete response.

In a report from the London Gynecologic Oncology Group of 41 patients who relapsed or had cisplatin-resistant ovarian cancer, it was found that using oral etoposide there were two complete and eight partial responses (24%).

Ifosfamide

A very small response (12%) in 41 patients with cisplatin-refractory ovarian cancer treated with ifosfamide was reported by researchers from the Memorial Sloan-Kettering Institute.

Hexamethylmelamine

A report from Sweden of 50 evaluable patients with cisplatin-resistant ovarian cancer showed a 14% response rate using oral hexamethylmelamine.

Second-Line Intraperitoneal Chemotherapy: Long-Term Survival

Because ovarian cancer primarily remains localized to the peritoneal cavity, the pharmacologic advantage of higher peritoneal fluid levels as compared with plasma levels after intraperitoneal chemotherapy administration was initially viewed as a rational method of salvage therapy in patients with persistent or recurrent ovarian cancer. Theoretically, the higher intraperitoneal dose might overcome tumor cell resistance to a lower-dose intravenous cisplatin-based chemotherapy. High-dose intraperitoneal chemotherapy became a theoretical method of dose intensification not dissimilar to bone marrow transplantation or high-dose intravenous chemotherapy with colony-stimulating factor protection. However, the depth of penetration of intraperitoneal chemotherapy in experimental tumor models is only 1.5 mm (1–2 mm), suggesting that the high local tumor drug interactions that occur with intraperitoneal therapy are not relevant and that any advantage from this approach primarily is related to higher drug levels within the systemic circulation.

Researchers from the University of California at San Diego, who were among the first to use intraperitoneal chemotherapy, reported on 90 patients treated on three sequential cisplatin-based chemotherapy protocols (with or without cytarabine, cytarabine and adriamycin, or cytarabine and bleomycin). The median survival was 8 months for patients with greater than 2 cm residual disease and increased to 49 months for patients with less than 2 cm.

In a study from RPCI of 63 patients with recurrent or persistent ovarian cancer after first-line cisplatin-based chemotherapy who were treated on a prospective protocol of cisplatin plus cytarabine, researchers reported a median survival from intraperitoneal chemotherapy of 29 months. For patients who responded to first-line chemotherapy and second-line intraperitoneal chemotherapy, the 5-year survival rate was 60%, but for patients who responded to first line chemotherapy and not to intraperitoneal chemotherapy, the 5-year survival rate was only 17%. No patient who did not have a response to first- or second-line therapy survived 5 years ($p < .0001$). There was significant improvement in 2-year survival (74%) from initiation of intraperitoneal therapy for patients with 5 mm or less of residual tumor compared with patients with residual disease of more than 5 mm but less than 2 cm (38%), and patients with residual tumors larger than 2 cm (0%) ($p < .001$) (Fig. 1-4).

High-Dose Chemotherapy with Autologous Bone Marrow Transplant

As is the case with first-line epithelial ovarian cancer, a fundamental principle for using autologous bone marrow transplant (ABMT) in ovarian cancer is that the best chance of success is in patients with minimal residual disease. Veins, Lotz, and Mulder, in three separate studies using high-dose chemotherapy with ABMT, reported a total of 39 evaluable patients with an overall response rate of 60% and a complete response rate of 30%. However, there has been no consistent use of the same drug in any large series, and there have been no long-term survival data.

PROGNOSIS IN STAGE III AND IV

Prognosis or poor survival in ovarian cancer is associated with the following:

1. Advanced stage (III and IV versus I and II)
2. Older age (>70 years)
3. High histologic grade (3 versus 1 and 2)
4. Mucinous and clear-cell histology
5. Residual disease in advanced stage (>1 cm)
6. Amplification of the HER-2/neu proto-oncogene
7. Overexpression of epidermal growth factor receptor
8. Tumor ploidy (aneuploid versus diploid)
9. Poor performance status
10. De novo or acquired drug resistance

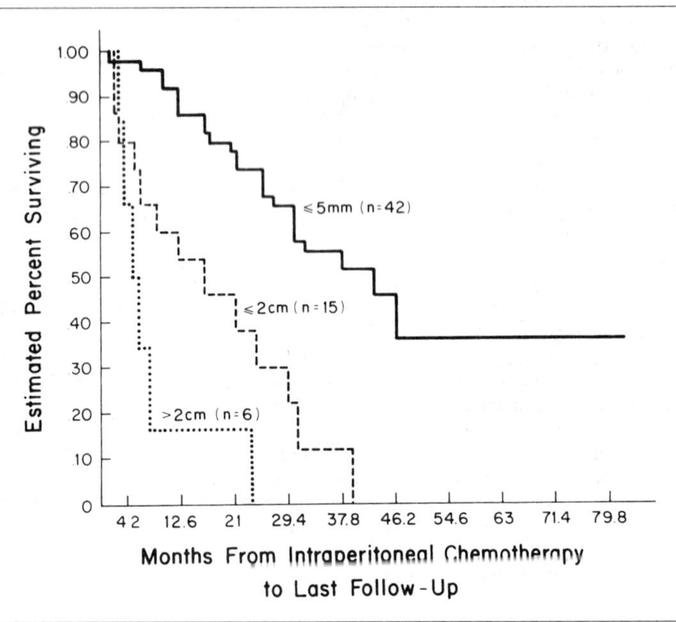

Fig. 1-4. Estimated percentage of survival according to size of residual tumor at second-look laparotomy in patients treated with intraperitoneal chemotherapy. (From MS Piver, FO Recio, TR Baker, D Driscoll. Evaluation of survival after second-line intraperitoneal cisplatin-based chemotherapy for advanced ovarian cancer. *Cancer* 73:1693, 1994.)

De novo or acquired drug resistance to cisplatin is made evident by the fact that although median survival is doubled or tripled as compared to that of the single alkylating agent era, most patients treated with cisplatin-based chemotherapy for advanced-stage disease eventually develop recurrence and die of their disease. However, of these poor prognostic factors, the only one clinically controllable in advanced-staged epithelial ovarian cancer is the size of residual disease (≤ 1 cm). Research is being done to overcome acquired drug resistance to cisplatin compounds.

Summary

It is clear that if long-term (5–10 years) disease-free survival is to be significantly improved, even in the short term, patients with suspected stage III or IV ovarian cancer (by age, physical findings, elevated CA125, and CT findings) must be provided with primary surgery that results in residual disease < 1 cm in most cases. In the long term, we must await the initial trials using Taxol and cisplatin with or without colony-stimulating factors as first-line therapy. The latter may require many years before these results can be compared to those of cisplatin and cyclophosphamide, cisplatin, Adriamycin, and cyclophosphamide, or carboplatin and cyclophosphamide. However, the true impact on lessening the ever increasing death rate from what is euphemistically known as the "silent killer" must await molecular analyses to determine genetic lesions (new germ line mutations) that occur early in the development of tumors that would make it feasible to screen women in the general population for such predisposing mutations. With the recent cloning of the BRCA1 gene, this may be more of a reality than just a wish.

Selected Readings

Ahlgren JD, Ellison NM, Gottlieb RJ et al. Hormonal palliation of chemoresistant ovarian cancer: Three consecutive phase II trials of the Mid-Atlantic Oncology Program. *J Clin Oncol* 11:1957, 1993.

Alberts DS, Green S, Hannigan EV et al. Improved therapeutic index of carboplatin plus cyclophosphamide versus cisplatin plus cyclophosphamide: Final report by the Southwest Oncology Group of a phase III randomized trial in stages III and IV ovarian cancer. *J Clin Oncol* 10:706, 1992.

Baker TR, Piver MS, Hempling RE. Long-term survival by cytoreductive surgery to <1 cm, induction weekly cisplatin and monthly cisplatin, Adriamycin and cyclophosphamide in advanced ovarian adenocarcinoma. *Cancer* 74:656, 1994.

Bell DA, Weinstock MA, Scully RE. Peritoneal implants of ovarian serous borderline tumors. Histologic features and prognosis. *Cancer* 62:2212, 1988.

Buchsbaum HJ, Brady MF, Delgado G et al. Surgical staging of carcinoma of the ovaries. *Surg Gynecol Obstet* 169:226, 1989.

Chiara S, Mammoliti S, Oliva C et al. Adjuvant cisplatin-based chemotherapy for stage I and II ovarian cancer: A 7-year experience. *Eur J Cancer Clin Oncol* 27:1211, 1991.

Cramer DW, Welch WR, Scully RE et al. Ovarian cancer and talc: A case-control study. *Cancer* 50:372, 1982.

Currie JL, Bagne F, Harris C et al. Radioactive chromic phosphate suspension: Studies on distribution, drug absorption and effective therapeutic radiation in phantoms, dogs, and patients. *Gynecol Oncol* 12:193, 1981.

Dembo AJ. Abdominopelvic radiotherapy in ovarian cancer: Ten-year experience. *Cancer* 55:2285, 1985.

Dembo AJ, Davy M, Stenwig AE et al. Prognostic factors in patients with stage I epithelial ovarian cancer. *Obstet Gynecol* 75:263, 1990.

Gershenson DM, Kavanagh JJ, Copeland LJ et al. Retreatment of patients with recurrent epithelial ovarian cancer with cisplatin-based chemotherapy. *Obstet Gynecol* 73:798, 1989.

GICOG. Long-term results of a randomized trial comparing cisplatin with cisplatin and cyclophosphamide with cisplatin, cyclophosphamide, and Adriamycin in advanced ovarian cancer. *Gynecol Oncol* 45:115, 1992.

Griffiths CT, Fuller AF. Intensive surgical and chemotherapeutic management of advanced ovarian cancer. *Surg Clin North Am* 58:131, 1978.

Hainsworth JD, Grosh WW, Burnett LS et al. Advanced ovarian cancer: Long-term results of treatment with intensive cisplatin-based chemotherapy of brief duration. *Ann Intern Med* 108:165, 1988.

Hankinson SE, Hunter DJ, Colditz GA et al. Tubal ligation, hysterectomy, and risk of ovarian cancer: A prospective study. *JAMA* 270:2813, 1993.

Healy DL, Burger HG, Mamers P et al. Elevated serum inhibin concentrations in postmenopausal women with ovarian tumors. *N Engl J Med* 329:1539, 1993.

Hoskins PJ, O'Reilly SE, Swenerton KD et al. Ten-year outcome of patients with advanced epithelial ovarian carcinoma treated with cisplatin-based multimodality therapy. *J Clin Oncol* 10:1561, 1992.

Hoskins PJ, Swenerton KD. Oral etoposide is active against platinum-resistant epithelial ovarian cancer. *J Clin Oncol* 12:60, 1994.

Houlston RS, Collins A, Slack J et al. Genetic epidemiology of ovarian cancer: Segregation analysis. *Ann Hum Genet* 55:291, 1991.

Howell SB, Zimm S, Markman M et al. Long-term survival of advanced refractory ovarian carcinoma patients with small-volume disease treated with intraperitoneal chemotherapy. *J Clin Oncol* 5:1607, 1987.

Jacobs I, Bast RC. The CA125 tumor associated antigen: Review of the literature. *Human Reprod* 4:1, 1989.

Jacobs IJ, Kohler MF, Wiseman RW et al. Clonal origin of epithelial ovarian carcinoma. Analysis of loss by heterozygosity, p53 mutation and X-chromosome inactivation. *J Natl Cancer Inst* 84:1793, 1992.

Koern J, Trope CG, Abeler VM. A retrospective study of 370 borderline tumors of the ovary treated at the Norwegian Radium Hospital from 1970–1982: A review of clinicopathologic features and treatment modalities. *Cancer* 71:1810, 1993.

Kohn EC, Sarosy G, Bicher A et al. Dose-intense taxol: High response rate in patients with platinum-resistant recurrent ovarian cancer. *J Natl Cancer Inst* 86:18, 1994.

Leake JF, Currie JL, Rosenshein NB et al. Long-term follow-up of serous ovarian tumors of low malignant potential. *Gynecol Oncol* 47:150, 1992.

Lotz JP, Machover D, Bellaich EA et al. Tandem high dose chemotherapy with VM26, ifosfamide and carboplatin with autologous bone marrow transplantation for patients with stage IIIC–IV ovarian cancer. *Proceed ASCO* 12:257, 1993.

MacBeth FR, MacDonald H, Williams CJ. Total abdominal and pelvic radiotherapy in the management of early stage ovarian carcinoma. *Int J Radiat Oncol Biol Phys* 15:353, 1988.

Markman M, Hakes T, Reichman B et al. Ifosfamide and mesna in previously treated advanced epithelial ovarian cancer. Activity in platinum-resistant disease. *J Clin Oncol* 10:243, 1992.

McGuire WP, Hoskins WJ, Brady MF et al. A phase III trial comparing cisplatin and Cytoxan and cisplatin/taxol in advanced ovarian cancer. *Proceed ASCO* 12:285, 1993.

Mettlin C, Piver MS. A case-control study of milk drinking and ovarian cancer risk. *Am J Epidemiol* 132:871, 1990.

Mulder POM, Villemse PHB, Aalders JB et al. High dose chemotherapy with autologous bone marrow transplantation in patients with refractory ovarian cancer. *Eur J Cancer Clin Oncol* 25:654, 1989.

Neijt JP, ten Bokkel Huinink WW, van der Burg MEL et al. Long-term survival in ovarian cancer: Mature data from The Netherlands Joint Study Group for Ovarian Cancer. *Eur J Cancer Clin Oncol* 27:1367, 1991.

Ovarian Cancer Meta-Analysis Project. Cyclophosphamide plus cisplatin versus cyclophosphamide, doxorubicin and cisplatin chemotherapy of ovarian carcinoma: A meta-analysis. *J Clin Oncol* 9:1668, 1991.

Piver MS, Baker TR, Jishi MF et al. Familial ovarian cancer: A report of 658 families from the Gilda Radner Familial Ovarian Cancer Registry (1981–1991). *Cancer* 71:582, 1993.

Piver MS, Barlow JJ, Lele SB. Incidence of subclinical metastasis in stage I and II ovarian carcinoma. *Obstet Gynecol* 52:100, 1978.

Piver MS, Lele SB, Bakshi S et al. Five and ten year estimated survival and disease-free rates after intraperitoneal chromic phosphate: Stage I ovarian adenocarcinoma. *Am J Clin Oncol* 11:515, 1988.

Piver MS, Malfetano J, Baker TR et al. Five-year survival for stage IC or stage I grade 3 epithelial ovarian cancer treated with cisplatin-based chemotherapy. *Gynecol Oncol* 46:357, 1992.

Piver MS, Malfetano J, Hempling RE et al. Cisplatin-based chemotherapy for stage II ovarian adenocarcinoma: Preliminary report. *Gynecol Oncol* 39:249, 1990.

Piver MS, Recio FO, Baker TR, Driscoll D. Evaluation of survival after second-line intraperitoneal cisplatin-based chemotherapy for advanced ovarian cancer. *Cancer* 73:1693, 1994.

Rice LW, Lage JM, Berkowitz RS et al. Preoperative serum CA125 levels in borderline tumors of the ovary. *Gynecol Oncol* 46:226, 1992.

Rutledge F, Burns BC. Chemotherapy for advanced ovarian cancer. *Am J Obstet Gynecol* 96:761, 1966.

Seymour MT, Mansi JL, Gallagher CJ et al. Protracted oral etoposide in epithelial ovarian cancer: A phase II study in patients with relapsed or platinum-resistant disease. *Br J Cancer* 69:191, 1994.

Soper JT, Berchuck A, Dodge R et al. Adjuvant therapy with intraperitoneal chromic phosphate (^{32}P) in women with early ovarian carcinoma after comprehensive surgical staging. *Obstet Gynecol* 79:993, 1992.

Steichen-Gersdorf E, Gallion HH, Ford D et al. Familial site–specific ovarian cancer is linked to BRCA1 on 17q12-21. *Am J Hum Genet* 55:870, 1994.

Surwit EA, Childers JM, Craig DN et al. Clinical assessment of ^{111}CYT-103 immunoscintigraphy in ovarian cancer. *Gynecol Oncol* 48:287, 1993.

Sutton GP, Bundy BN, Omura GA et al. Stage III ovarian tumors of low malignant potential treated with cisplatin combination therapy: A gynecologic oncology group study. *Gynecol Oncol* 41:230, 1991.

Sutton GP, Stehman FB, Einhorn LH. Ten-year follow-up of patients receiving cisplatin, doxorubicin and cyclophosphamide chemotherapy for advanced epithelial ovarian carcinoma. *J Clin Oncol* 7:223, 1989.

Swenerton K, Jeffrey J, Stuart G et al. Cisplatin-cyclophosphamide versus carboplatin-cyclophosphamide in advanced ovarian cancer: A randomized phase III study of the National Cancer Institute of Canada Clinical Trials Group. *J Clin Oncol* 10:718, 1992.

The Cancer and Steroid Hormone Study of the Centers for Disease Control and the National Institute of Child Health and Human Development. The reduction in risk of ovarian cancer associated with oral contraceptive use. *N Engl J Med* 316:650, 1987.

Trimble EJ, Adams JD, Vena D et al. Paclitaxel for platinum-refractory ovarian cancer: Results from the first 1,000 patients registered to National Cancer Institute Treatment Referral Center 9103. *J Clin Oncol* 11:2405, 1993.

Veins P, Maraninch ID, Legros M et al. High dose melphalan and autologous marrow rescue in advanced epithelial ovarian carcinomas: A retrospective analysis of 35 patients treated in France. *Bone Marrow Transplant* 5:227, 1990.

Vergote I, Himmelmann A, Frankendal B et al. Hexamethylmelamine as second-line therapy in platin-resistant ovarian cancer. *Gynecol Oncol* 47:282, 1992.

Walton LA, Yadusky A, Rubinstein L et al. Stage II carcinoma of the ovary: an analysis of survival after comprehensive surgical staging and adjuvant therapy. *Gynecol Oncol* 44:55, 1992.

Wharton JT, Edwards CL, Rutledge FN. Long-term survival after chemotherapy for advanced epithelial ovarian carcinoma. *Am J Obstet Gynecol* 148:997, 1984.

Whittemore AS, Harris R, Itnyre J et al. Characteristics relating to ovarian cancer risk. Collaborative analysis of 12 U.S. case-control studies. II. Invasive epithelial ovarian cancer in white women. *Am J Epidemiol* 136:1184, 1992.

Wils JA. Long-term follow-up of patients with advanced ovarian carcinoma treated with debulking surgery and chemotherapy consisting of cisplatin, doxorubucin, and cyclophosphamide. *Oncology* 47:115, 1990.

Wiltshaw E, Kroner T. Phase II study of cis-dichlorodiammine-platinum (II) (NSC-119875) in advanced adenocarcinoma of the ovary. *Cancer Treat Rep* 60:55, 1976.

Woolas RP, Xu FJ, Jacobs IJ et al. Elevation of multiple serum markers in patients with stage I ovarian cancer. *J Natl Cancer Inst* 85:1748, 1993.

Xu FJ, Yu YH, Daly L et al. OVXI radioimmunoassay complements CA125 for predicting the presence or residual ovarian carcinoma at second look surgical surveillance procedures. *J Clin Oncol* 11:1506, 1993.

Yazigi R, Sandstad J, Munoz AK. Primary staging in ovarian tumors of low malignant potential. *Gynecol Oncol* 31:402, 1988.

Young RC, Chabner BA, Hubbard SP et al. Advanced ovarian adenocarcinoma. A prospective clinical trial of melphalan (L-PAM) versus combination chemotherapy. *N Engl J Med* 299:1261, 1978.

Young RC, Decker DG, Wharton JT et al. Staging laparotomy in early ovarian cancer. *JAMA* 250:3072, 1983.

Young RC, Walton LA, Ellenberg SS et al. Adjuvant therapy in stage I and stage II epithelial ovarian cancer: Results of two prospective randomized trials. *N Engl J Med* 322:1021, 1990.

2

Ovarian Germ Cell Tumors

Trudy R. Baker

Incidence

Germ cell tumors of the ovary account for approximately 20% of all ovarian neoplasms. These neoplasms, which include a number of histologic types, are ultimately derived from the primitive germ cell. The benign forms, almost all of which are benign cystic teratomas, comprise almost 95% of the germ cell tumors. The malignant germ cell tumors, which comprise less than 3% of all ovarian cancers in the Western world, account for the remaining germ cell tumors. Although germ cell tumors occur in all age groups—from infancy to old age—the peak incidence is seen in the early 20s. More than 60% of ovarian neoplasms in patients under 20 years of age are germ cell tumors; the younger the patient, the more likely it is that the germ cell tumor is malignant.

Classification and Staging

The World Health Organization classification of ovarian germ cell tumors appears in Chap. 18. Staging of the malignant germ cell tumors follows the International Federation of Gynecologists and Obstetricians (FIGO) staging for epithelial ovarian carcinomas.

Clinical Features and Pattern of Spread

Patients with germ cell tumors often present with abdominal pain, usually in association with a pelvic and/or abdominal mass. These neoplasms, which may enlarge rapidly (excluding benign cystic teratomas), are associated with acute abdominal pain in approximately 10% of cases because of rupture, hemorrhage, or torsion of the tumor. Less common symptoms include abdominal distention, vaginal bleeding, and fever. If the tumor produces human chorionic gonadotropin (hCG), isosexual precocious pseudopuberty may occur in prepubertal girls, or menstrual irregularity may occur in older women.

Tumor spread occurs via the lymphatics as well as by peritoneal surface dissemination. Although lymphatic spread appears to occur more readily in germ cell tumors than in epithelial adenocarcinomas, data are lacking on the exact incidence of lymph node involvement. Hematogenous spread to the liver and lung can occur but usually does so late in the disease process. Approximately two-thirds of patients with germ cell tumors are diagnosed while disease is still confined to the ovary, while approximately 25% of patients

Table 2-1. Serum tumor markers in malignant germ cell tumors of the ovary

Histology	*AFP*	*hCG*	*LDH*	*CA125*	*NSE*
Dysgerminoma	−	±	±	±	±
Endodermal sinus tumor	+	−		±	
Immature teratoma	±	−		±	±
Mixed germ cell tumor	±	±		±	
Choriocarcinoma	−	+			
Embryonal carcinoma	±	+			
Polyembryoma	±	+			

AFP = alpha-fetoprotein; hCG = human chorionic gonadotropin; LDH = lactic dehydrogenase; NSE = neuron-specific enolase.

present with stage III disease. The malignant germ cell tumors are typically unilateral except for dysgerminoma, which is bilateral in 10–15% of cases.

Tumor Markers

Malignant germ cell tumors often produce serum tumor markers that not only facilitate diagnosis but also can be used to follow a patient's response to therapy and to detect recurrence after treatment (Table 2-1).

HUMAN CHORIONIC GONADOTROPIN

hCG is typically produced by the syncytiotrophoblastic cells of choriocarcinomas. A small percentage of dysgerminomas contain syncytiotrophoblastic giant cells and thus may be associated with low levels of hCG. However, the presence of other germ cell elements such as choriocarcinoma or embryonal carcinoma should be carefully ruled out, as their presence may alter treatment. Other malignant germ cell tumors that may produce hCG include polyembryoma and mixed germ cell tumors.

ALPHA-FETOPROTEIN

Elevations of the glycoprotein alpha-fetoprotein (AFP) are noted in yolk sac tumors in which the AFP can be demonstrated, by immunohistochemical techniques, to be localized to hyaline bodies or the cytoplasm of the cell. Although immature teratomas are not usually associated with production of tumor markers, elevated AFP levels have been reported. Embryonal carcinomas, polyembryomas, and mixed germ cell tumors may be associated with elevated AFP levels as well.

LACTIC DEHYDROGENASE

Levels of the glycolytic enzyme lactic dehydrogenase (LDH) are elevated in some patients with dysgerminoma. Isoenzyme analysis demonstrates elevated LDH-1 and LDH-2 fractions.

CA125

Elevated levels of CA125 have been reported for mixed germ cell tumors, dysgerminomas, immature teratomas, and yolk sac tumors. Mature cystic teratomas and mature cystic teratomas with malignant transformation also have been associated with elevation of this marker.

NEURON-SPECIFIC ENOLASE

Neuron-specific enolase (NSE) was found to be elevated in 50% of patients with immature teratoma and 80% of patients with dysgerminoma.

Preoperative Evaluation

The preoperative evaluation of any girl or young woman suspected of having a malignant germ cell tumor should include routine laboratory studies, chest radiograph, and measurement of tumor markers. Karyotyping should be carried out in patients with ovarian masses, as dysgerminomas can be found in association with dysgenetic gonads. Phenotypic females with gonadal dysgenesis who have a Y chromosome present (pure XY or XY mosaicism) run an approximately 25% risk of developing a malignant germ cell tumor. Therefore, dysgenetic gonads should be removed at the time of laparotomy.

Surgical Therapy

PRIMARY SURGERY

Patients with malignant germ cell tumors should undergo a full staging laparotomy similar to that for epithelial ovarian cancer. Evaluation of the pelvis begins with the involved ovary. Bilateral ovarian involvement is rare if advanced disease is not present, except in the case of pure dysgerminoma, in which bilaterality occurs in 10–15% of patients. In most cases, therefore, unilateral salpingo-oophorectomy (USO) is all that is necessary. While biopsy of the opposite ovary should not be performed if that ovary appears normal, biopsy should be considered in the case of pure dysgerminoma, as microscopic spread is present in 5% of such cases. If the opposite ovary appears abnormal, biopsy with frozen section should be carried out. The diagnosis of malignant disease or a dysgenetic gonad necessitates removal of that ovary also. Benign cystic teratomas, which occur in the contralateral ovary in 5–10% of patients with malignant germ cell tumors, can be removed via ovarian cystectomy, preserving the remaining normal ovary. In this generally young population in which future fertility is a consideration, it may be possible to conserve a normal uterus and opposite ovary even in the presence of extraovarian disease given the chemosensitivity of this group of tumors. In older women in whom fertility is not a consideration, total abdominal hysterectomy and bilateral salpingo-oophorectomy (TAH/BSO) should be carried out with other tumor resection, if necessary.

CYTOREDUCTIVE SURGERY

The role for primary cytoreductive surgery in patients with malignant germ cell tumors has not been scrutinized as closely as that for epithelial ovarian cancers. However, Slayton et al. noted a failure rate of 28% for 54 patients with malignant germ cell tumors treated with vincristine, actinomycin-D, and cyclophosphamide (VAC) after removal of all gross disease, versus a failure rate of 68% for those patients with incompletely resected disease. Williams et al. found that patients with nondysgerminomatous tumors treated with vinblastine, bleomycin, and cisplatin (VBP) with clinically nonmeasurable disease had a greater likelihood of remaining progression-free than those patients with measurable disease. Also, patients who had undergone optimal (<2 cm residual) debulking surgery prior to chemotherapy had better disease-free survival than those patients with suboptimal disease (>2 cm residual). While these results do not prove the value of cytoreductive surgery in malignant germ cell tumors, they do suggest that cytoreduction may improve the chance for disease-free survival.

Chemotherapy

NONDYSGERMINOMATOUS TUMORS

Before the era of combination chemotherapy, the nondysgerminomatous tumors were associated with a dismal prognosis, with most patients dying of their disease after surgical therapy alone. However, with the identification of effective chemotherapeutic regimens, sustained remissions can be induced in not only patients with early-stage disease but also patients with advanced or recurrent tumors. Also, with the use of conservative surgery and effective chemotherapy, the possibility of fertility preservation exists for most patients.

Vincristine, Actinomycin-D, and Cyclophosphamide

Reports of VAC's effectiveness in nondysgerminomatous tumors of the ovary were first published in the 1970s. Treatment results from several groups have now been reported. Gershenson et al. noted that 86% of their stage I patients were cured with this regimen, but only 48% of those with metastatic disease achieved a sustained remission. In an early Gynecologic Oncology Group (GOG) trial, Slayton et al. found that 72% (39 of 54) of patients who had removal of all gross disease prior to VAC administration remained disease-free. Only 32% (7 of 22) of those patients with incompletely resected germ cell tumors achieved remission, however. A more recent GOG study, as well as others, have reported findings similar to those noted above.

Vinblastine, Bleomycin, and Cisplatin

After the reports documenting the effectiveness of VBP in testicular germ cell tumors, reports of this regimen's efficacy in ovarian malignant germ cell tumors were published. Cumulative results in stage I disease from several different centers indicate a remission rate of 94% (15 of 16) with the use of this combination. In a GOG study reported by Williams et al., 53% of patients (47 of 89) with

Table 2-2. BEP regimen for malignant germ cell tumors of the ovary

Cisplatin	100 mg/m^2 IV day 1
Bleomycin	10–15 mg days 1–3 (24-hour infusion)
Etoposide	100 mg/m^2 IV days 1–3

stages II–IV or recurrent nondysgerminomatous tumors with residual unresected disease were continuously disease-free with a median follow-up of 52 months. At 2 years, a 71% survival rate was noted in this high-risk group, all of whom had residual disease prior to VBP administration and 27% of whom had received previous chemotherapy. While no randomized prospective trials have been performed to compare VAC with VBP, VBP appears superior to VAC in patients with advanced disease.

Bleomycin, Etoposide, and Cisplatin

In 1987, Williams et al. reported that the substitution of etoposide for vinblastine in the VBP regimen for testicular germ cell tumors produced equally effective results and was associated with less toxicity. Two reports of bleomycin, etoposide, and cisplatin (BEP) use in ovarian germ cell tumors have noted excellent results. Gershenson et al. found that 92% (11 of 12) patients with nondysgerminomatous lesions (stages I–III and recurrent disease) remained in sustained remission after treatment with this combination. The GOG reported a trial of stage I–III patients with nondysgerminomatous tumors with completely resected disease prior to chemotherapy. Three courses of adjuvant BEP were administered. Of 93 patients, 89 (96%) remained free of germ cell cancer. Two patients were found to have immature teratoma (grade 1) at second-look laparotomy but remained without clinical evidence of disease. Two other patients developed second neoplasms 22 months and 69 months after diagnosis of germ cell tumor. BEP is considered the regimen of choice at this time for patients with malignant germ cell tumors requiring therapy (Table 2-2).

Dysgerminoma

Dysgerminoma is the most common malignant germ cell tumor, accounting for approximately 45% of these tumors. Unlike the other malignant germ cell tumors, the dysgerminoma is bilateral in 10–15% of cases. Most retrospective studies have noted that approximately three-fourths of patients will have stage I disease at diagnosis; however, as these patients were not surgically staged, it is likely that approximately two-thirds of patients would have had stage I disease. Fifteen to 20% of dysgerminomas are diagnosed during pregnancy or in the immediate postpartum period. Dysgerminomas in most cases arise sporadically in genetically normal individuals, although they may arise in phenotypic women with gonadal dysgenesis either alone or in combination with other tumors. Although the gonadoblastoma is the most commonly associated tumor in these patients, it is associated with dysgerminoma in approximately 50% of cases.

Few cytogenetic studies involving dysgerminoma have been performed. However, dysgerminoma and seminoma have been shown to share the same chromosomal marker, an isochromosome for the short arm of chromosome 12. A pattern of chromosome imbalance similar to that seen in seminoma has been demonstrated as well, suggesting a common developmental pathway. Overexpression of the tumor suppressor gene, p53, was noted in all seven dysgerminomas evaluated by Dietl et al.

TREATMENT

Before the 1980s, the treatment of choice for dysgerminoma was radiation therapy, based not only on the tumor's marked radiosensitivity but also on its nodal spread pattern. However, this mode of therapy rendered patients, most of whom were or were soon to be of childbearing age, infertile. Based on the demonstration of chemosensitivity of metastatic testicular seminoma as well as scattered reports of responses of dysgerminoma to chemotherapy, patients with dysgerminoma became eligible in 1984 for GOG trials involving therapy of malignant germ cell tumors. Williams et al. reported the results of 20 evaluable patients with advanced or recurrent incompletely resected dysgerminoma treated on two such GOG protocols. Patients received VBP or BEP, and some of the latter group also received consolidation therapy with VAC. Of 11 patients with clinically measurable disease, 10 completely responded and all second-look laparotomies performed were negative. With a median follow-up of 26 months, 95% (19 of 20) of patients remained disease-free. Gershenson et al. treated 17 patients with dysgerminoma (12 with advanced disease) with BEP and all remain in sustained remission.

With the demonstration of dysgerminoma's chemosensitivity and the capability of fertility preservation, chemotherapy is now considered the treatment of choice for this group of tumors. In selected individuals, radiation therapy, equally as effective as chemotherapy, may be selected as the primary treatment modality. Radiation therapy may also play a role in salvage therapy for these patients.

Early studies of patients with stage IA dysgerminoma treated with USO only revealed a postsurgical recurrence rate of 24%. With proper surgical staging, this recurrence rate should be reduced, although the exact relapse rate in staged stage IA patients is unknown. For properly staged patients with disease confined to one ovary who undergo USO, careful follow-up with physical examinations, computed tomography (CT) scans, and tumor marker assessment is a management option. Adjuvant therapy consisting of three courses of BEP has been suggested for those patients with unstaged stage IA disease to reduce or prevent recurrences. In a limited number of reported patients so treated, no relapses have been noted.

Yolk Sac Tumor (Endodermal Sinus Tumor)

The yolk sac tumor accounts for approximately 20% of all malignant germ cell tumors.

TREATMENT

Two-year survival rates of less than 15% have been associated with surgical therapy alone in patients with this neoplasm. Therefore, all patients will require combination chemotherapy. Patients with completely resected disease (all stages) should receive adjuvant treatment with three to four cycles of BEP. For patients with residual disease after surgery, four to six cycles of that combination is recommended. In patients who have positive serum AFP, however, chemotherapy should be continued for two cycles after a negative AFP level is obtained. In those patients with elevated AFP levels at the start of chemotherapy, tumor marker levels should be followed after remission is induced to evaluate disease status. Levels should be obtained monthly for the first 2 years, every other month for the next 3 years, and twice a year thereafter.

Embryonal Carcinoma

The embryonal carcinoma of the ovary accounts for approximately 5% of malignant ovarian germ cell tumors. It was not until 1976 that Kurman and Norris described it and distinguished it from the endodermal sinus tumor, recognizing it as a separate clinical pathologic entity. The embryonal carcinoma is rarely found in pure form and usually exists as part of a mixed germ cell tumor.

TREATMENT

Combination chemotherapy should follow surgical therapy as discussed in the section on treatment of yolk sac tumor.

Choriocarcinoma

Choriocarcinoma of the ovary can be divided into gestational and nongestational types. Gestational ovarian carcinomas are associated with an ovarian pregnancy or, more commonly, represent a metastasis from another primary lesion that has developed in association with some pregnancy event. They are usually included under the gestational trophoblastic disease category. The rare nongestational ovarian choriocarcinoma can be diagnosed with certainty only when it occurs in premenarchal girls or when it is seen as a component of a mixed germ cell tumor. Although it is generally held that nongestational choriocarcinoma carries a worse prognosis than the gestational type, this issue has not been resolved.

TREATMENT

Combination chemotherapy follows surgical management as discussed in the section on treatment of yolk sac tumor.

Polyembryoma

TREATMENT

The paucity of cases does not allow an accurate description of the tumor's true clinical course. Treatment at this time should be similar to that for the other germ cell tumors—surgical staging followed by combination chemotherapy.

Teratoma

IMMATURE TERATOMA

The immature teratoma comprises approximately 20% of the malignant germ cell tumors. Bilateral involvement is rare without extraovarian spread. In one large series, approximately 10% of immature teratomas were associated with a mature cystic teratoma in the contralateral ovary. Immature teratomas will demonstrate chromosomal abnormalities in approximately 50% of cases, although no specific marker has been identified.

Grading System

The current grading system proposed by Norris et al. not only takes into consideration the amount of immature tissue but it also quantifies the amount of neural tissue within the tumor. Prognosis is directly related to the grade of the tumor. Norris et al. demonstrated the relationship between grade and survival in stage I disease, as well as the relation between grade of metastatic disease in advanced stages and survival. Of the stage I patients, survival for grade 1 was 100%, grade 2 was 55%, and grade 3 was 33%. Of the stage II and III patients whose metastases were graded, all those with grade 0 metastases were alive without disease, but only half of those with grade 1 or 2 metastases were living. None of the patients with grade 3 metastatic disease were alive.

Treatment

Grade 0 ovarian teratomas are benign tumors associated with long-term survival and require only surgical removal. Most patients with a stage I, grade 1 immature teratoma also survive progression-free and do not require adjuvant therapy. However, patients with stage I, grade 2 or 3 disease do require adjuvant therapy based on the high risk of recurrence. As well, all patients with more advanced disease will require postoperative therapy with combination chemotherapy.

Treatment with three to four cycles of BEP has been recommended for those with completely resected disease. In a GOG trial, of 42 patients treated with BEP, 41 were alive without evidence of disease. Two of these 41 patients had grade 1 implants noted at second-look laparotomy but remained clinically free of disease. One patient was noted to be free of disease at second-look laparotomy but had a recurrence shortly after and died. For those patients with incompletely resected disease, four to six cycles of BEP have been recommended, though some suggest that 1 year of combination chemotherapy might be more effective in those patients with advanced-stage immature teratomas. Based on the excellent results obtained using adjuvant VAC chemotherapy in those with stage I disease, this regimen continues to be recommended in some centers as primary adjuvant therapy following surgical treatment for stage IA, grade 2 or 3 disease.

MATURE TERATOMA

Solid Teratoma

Solid mature teratoma, composed entirely of mature tissue derived from the three germ cell layers, is benign and associated with long survival rates. All reported cases have been unilateral.

Cystic Teratoma

The mature cystic teratoma or dermoid cyst is the most common ovarian teratoma as well as the most common ovarian germ cell neoplasm. It represents up to one-fourth to one-third of all ovarian neoplasms and is bilateral in up to 15% of cases. Although it is found in all age groups, more than 75% of these benign tumors occur in women age 20–30 years. It is composed of maturely differentiated derivatives of all three germ cell layers, although the ectodermal component is the most prominent. These cystic neoplasms typically contain sebaceous material or hair, although other mature tissues may be present, including teeth or bones. The inner surface of the cyst typically contains a solid nodule known as a Rokitansky protuberance, generally composed of adipose tissue. The most highly developed form of dermoid cysts resembles a human monster and is called a *fetiform teratoma* or *homunculus*. Treatment for dermoid cysts is ovarian cystectomy with careful inspection of the opposite ovary.

Dermoid Cyst with Secondary Tumor Formation

Malignant transformation of benign cystic teratomas occurs in 1–2% of cases and tends to occur in older age groups. Squamous cell carcinoma is the malignancy found in about 80% of cases, although other tumors can occur, including adenocarcinomas, sarcomas, carcinoids, and melanomas.

MONODERMAL TERATOMAS

The monodermal or monophyletic teratomas are those in which there is a predominance of a single tissue element.

Struma Ovarii

The most common of the monodermal teratomas is the struma ovarii, in which 50% or more of the tumor is composed of thyroid tissue. The tumor occurs primarily within benign cystic teratomas and most often in women between 50 and 60 years of age. Approximately 5% of patients show evidence of hyperthyroidism. A proliferative struma ovarii has been described that differs from the usual struma ovarii in that areas of densely packed follicles or papillary formations are present. These tumors lack histologic evidence of malignancy such as ground glass nuclei, vascular space invasion, or mitotic activity, however. In one report, all such patients were free of recurrence after treatment with either USO or TAH/BSO. The diagnosis of malignant struma ovarii has been confined to those tumors that exhibit classic features of thyroid carcinoma or show evidence of recurrence or metastasis. The majority of cases of malignant struma ovarii tend to follow a benign clinical course, although deaths can occur, particularly with metastatic disease. Recurrence may be a late event, however, and associated with a prolonged clinical course.

The treatment of struma ovarii, benign and malignant forms, consists of USO, if fertility is desired, or TAH/BSO. Metastatic lesions and recurrences have been successfully treated with radioactive iodine.

Carcinoid

The second most common monodermal teratoma is the ovarian carcinoid. These primary ovarian tumors should be distinguished from carcinoid tumors metastatic to the ovary, which carry a grave prognosis. The primary ovarian carcinoid may occur in pure form but more often presents in association with other teratomatous elements.

Insular Carcinoid

The most frequently seen carcinoid is the insular carcinoid, which is similar to tumors arising from the mid-gastrointestinal tract.

CLINICAL PRESENTATION. One-third of the insular carcinoids are associated with the carcinoid syndrome produced by the release of serotonin, histamine, and catecholamines from the argentaffin cells. Symptoms include diarrhea, wheezing, cutaneous flush, and edema of the head and neck. Cardiac valvular disease may also be present. The ovarian carcinoid, unlike other types, can produce this syndrome while confined to the ovary because ovarian venous drainage bypasses the portal circulation and inactivation by the liver. For this reason, patients tend to have symptoms early in their disease and can be cured by surgical removal alone. Urinary 5-hydroxyindoacetic acid (5-HIAA), which is used to measure serotonin secretion, returns to normal levels within 24 hours after removal of tumor.

TREATMENT. Insular carcinoids are unilateral and have no evidence of metastasis. Robboy et al. reported an actuarial survival rate of 95% at 5 years and 88% at 10 years. Although the median age of occurrence is 58 years, younger women who wish to retain fertility may be treated by USO alone. Recurrences are rare; however, treatment of recurrence is combined surgical removal with chemotherapy. The BEP regimen, which has been used with success for immature teratomas, is a logical choice.

DIFFERENTIAL DIAGNOSIS. It is important to differentiate a primary ovarian carcinoid from the carcinoid metastatic to the ovary. The latter almost always involves both ovaries and is associated with the presence of other metastatic disease. Approximately one-third of those metastatic to the ovary are associated with the carcinoid syndrome; however, unlike primary ovarian carcinoids, 5-HIAA remains elevated in most patients 6 months after surgery. Most patients with metastatic carcinoids are dead of their disease within 5 years.

Trabecular Carcinoid

The trabecular carcinoid, similar to tumors arising from the hindgut or foregut, is the second most common primary ovarian carcinoid. It is not associated with the carcinoid syndrome, in contrast to the insular type. However, it, too, is a unilateral tumor with no evidence of metastasis at surgery. Treatment is the same as for the insular carcinoid.

Strumal Carcinoid

Strumal carcinoid is an admixture of both struma and carcinoid, with a median age of occurrence of 53 years. Carcinoid syndrome as well as thyroid hyperfunction has been reported in association with strumal carcinoid. One large study noted that almost half of these strumal carcinoids were immunoreactive for peptide hormones, pancreatic polypeptide and glucagon being the ones most often identified. This unilateral tumor can be treated by USO alone in the young patient who wishes to retain fertility. Only two cases of malignant strumal carcinoid have been reported.

Mucinous Carcinoid

The least common type of ovarian carcinoid is composed of goblet and argyrophil cells and resembles the same tumor that arises in the appendix. Signet ring cells may be present. Mucinous carcinoid may occur in association with an epidermoid or a dermoid cyst. It has been stated that this tumor exhibits aggressive behavior and metastatic spread unlike the other ovarian carcinoids.

Neuroectodermal Tumors

Neuroectodermal tumors, which resemble primary tumors of the nervous system, include a differentiated form (usually ependymomas), a primitive form (resembling medullo-epithelioma, medulloblastoma, ependymoblastoma, or neuroblastoma) and an anaplastic form (resembling glioblastoma). Kleinman et al. noted that the average age at diagnosis varies with each type (differentiated, 30 years; primitive, 23 years; anaplastic, 16 years), and differentiated tumors carry a better prognosis than the other two types. Extraovarian spread is often seen with the primitive and anaplastic types, and they are usually associated with an aggressive clinical course.

Sebaceous Tumors

Eight cases of this teratoma, characterized by a sebaceous neoplasm usually arising within a dermoid cyst, have been reported. Average age at diagnosis was 58 years. All cases were unilateral and associated with a good prognosis, with only one patient suffering a recurrence more than 2 years after diagnosis.

Mixed Germ Cell Tumors

Mixed malignant germ cell tumors contain more than one malignant germ cell type. They have been reported to comprise 8–19% of all malignant germ cell tumors.

TREATMENT

Because dysgerminoma is a common component of these tumors, the contralateral ovary should be carefully evaluated at laparotomy. BEP chemotherapy should be administered after surgical therapy.

Gonadoblastoma

Although classified by the World Health Organization in a category separate from the germ cell tumors, the gonadoblastoma deserves special mention. It is a rare tumor composed of tumor cells mixed with immature sex cord elements of Sertoli or granulosa type and Leydig or lutein cells. Calcification is commonly present. The tumor occurs almost exclusively in dysgenetic gonads and, in fact, is the tumor most commonly associated with gonadal dysgenesis. Ninety percent of patients with this tumor have a Y chromosome. The tumor has never been shown to metastasize; its importance lies in its association with dysgerminoma (50% of cases) and with the presence of other malignant germ cell components (less than 10% of cases). As most of these tumors arise in dysgenetic gonads in the presence of a Y chromosome, removal of both gonads is indicated in most cases. In those cases in which there is an associated dysgerminoma or any other mixed germ cell element, treatment is based on the type of tumor present.

Role of Second-Look Laparotomy

A GOG review of second-look laparotomy in germ cell tumors was performed to help define the role of this procedure in this setting. Of 46 patients with germ cell tumors who had complete resection of their disease followed by three courses of adjuvant BEP therapy, either no tumor or mature teratoma was noted in 44 patients at second-look laparotomy while immature teratoma (grade 1) was found in two patients. Of those two patients, one refused further therapy and one received further chemotherapy with VAC. All 46 patients remained disease-free.

Of 72 patients with germ cell tumors treated with either VBP or BEP for advanced incompletely resected tumor, 48 patients had a nonteratomatous primary tumor. Second-look laparotomy was negative in 45 of 48 patients, and three patients who had persistent tumor at second-look ultimately died of their disease despite further therapy.

Twenty-four of the 72 patients had teratoma elements in their primary tumor. At second-look laparotomy, 16 had mature teratoma, which in seven was bulky or progressive. Of those 16, 14 remained disease-free after surgical resection. Four patients had negative second-look surgery and remained with no evidence of disease, and four patients had immature teratoma noted at second-look, two of whom were rendered disease-free with surgery and postoperative VAC. The authors concluded that second-look laparotomy is of little benefit in patients with completely resected tumor who receive adjuvant BEP therapy and for those who do not have teratoma elements in their primary tumor. For those patients with incompletely resected disease or teratomas, however, second-look surgery and resection of residual masses did appear beneficial. Others suggest that in patients who have positive tumor markers at the start of therapy that fall to normal levels during therapy, second-look laparotomy is unlikely to provide benefit.

Surgery may be of benefit, however, in those patients who are tumor marker–negative at diagnosis.

Salvage Therapy

Patients with ovarian germ cell tumors who fail to respond or who have recurrences after primary VAC therapy have salvage rates of approximately 50% to cisplatin-based regimens. Most patients are now treated primarily with cisplatin-based therapy, however, and salvage therapy becomes more problematic. In patients who have failed primary cisplatin-based therapy without etoposide, successful salvage has been reported with the use of etoposide-based regimens or VAC. In testicular germ cell tumor patients who relapse from a complete response to first-line cisplatin-based regimens (including BEP or VBP), salvage therapy with ifosfamide combination therapy (plus etoposide and cisplatin or vinblastine and cisplatin) will result in durable complete response rates in 25–30% of patients. Reports of ifosfamide salvage therapy in ovarian germ cell tumors are sparse, but success has been reported.

For those testicular germ cell tumor patients who are cisplatin-resistant or not cured by ifosfamide salvage chemotherapy, treatment with high-dose chemotherapy followed by autologous bone marrow transplant will result in long-term disease-free survival in 10–20% of patients. Chemotherapeutic agents used most often in combination with autologous bone marrow transplant have been carboplatin and etoposide with or without ifosfamide.

A subset of patients who have persistent disease or relapse after therapy will have tumor confined to one or two sites that is amenable to surgery. Surgical resection with or without further chemotherapy can result in cure for some of these patients.

Long-Term Effects

The development of acute nonlymphocytic leukemia in association with alkylating chemotherapy given for epithelial ovarian cancer has been documented. Reports of this leukemia have been noted as well in male and female germ cell tumor patients treated with either VBP or VAC. More recently, an association between etoposide use and leukemia has been reported. The development of leukemia, which is usually monocytic or myelomonocytic, may be dose-dependent, and onset seems to occur sooner after treatment than that associated with the use of alkylating agents. However, a study of over 1,000 patients with testicular germ cell tumors that investigated the occurrence of secondary malignancies following chemotherapy found that chemotherapy containing standard-dose etoposide was not associated with an increased risk of secondary neoplasms.

The menstrual and reproductive function of a group of ovarian germ cell tumor patients treated with combination chemotherapy has been reviewed. Of the 44 patients who had an intact uterus and contralateral tube and ovary, normal menstrual function resumed in 33. Of 16 patients who attempted pregnancy, 12 were successful and 22 infants have been delivered. In general, reports seem to indicate that most patients will have resumption of menstrual function and that fertility can be preserved in patients who have undergone treatment for malignant germ cell tumors of the ovary.

Selected Readings

Assadourian LA, Taylor HB. Dysgerminoma: An analysis of 105 cases. *Obstet Gynecol* 33:370, 1969.

Bokemeyer C, Schmoll HJ. Secondary neoplasms following treatment of malignant germ cell tumors. *J Clin Oncol* 11:1703, 1993.

Carlson RW, Sikic BI, Turbow MM, Ballon SC. Combination cisplatin, vinblastine, and bleomycin chemotherapy (PVB) for malignant germ cell tumors of the ovary. *J Clin Oncol* 10:645, 1983.

Chumas JC, Scully RE. Sebaceous tumors arising in ovarian dermoid cysts. *Int J Gynecol Pathol* 10:356, 1991.

Depalo G, Zambetti M, Pilotti S et al. Nondysgerminomatous tumors of the ovary treated with cisplatin, vinblastine, and bleomycin: Long-term results. *Gynecol Oncol* 47:239, 1992.

Devaney K, Snyder R, Norris HJ, Tavassoli FA. Proliferative and histologically malignant struma ovarii: a clinicopathologic study of 54 cases. *Int J Gynecol Pathol* 12:333, 1993.

Dietl J, Horny HP, Ruck P, Kaiserling E. Dysgerminoma of the ovary. An immunohistochemical study of tumor-infiltrating lymphoreticular cells and tumor cells. *Cancer* 71:2562, 1993.

Germa JR, Izquierdo MA, Segui MA et al. Malignant ovarian germ cell tumors: The experience at the Hospital de la Santa Creu i Sant Pau. *Gynecol Oncol* 45:153, 1992.

Gershenson DM, Copeland LJ, Deljunco G et al. Second look laparotomy in the management of malignant germ cell tumors of the ovary. *Obstet Gynecol* 67:789, 1986.

Gershenson DM, Copeland LJ, Kavanagh JJ et al. Treatment of malignant nondysgerminomatous germ cell tumors of the ovary with vincristine, dactinomycin and cyclophosphamide. *Cancer* 56:2756, 1985.

Gershenson DM, DelJunco G, Copeland LJ, Rutledge FN. Mixed germ cell tumors of the ovary. *Obstet Gynecol* 64:200, 1984.

Gershenson DM, Kavanagh JJ, Copeland LJ et al. Treatment of malignant nondysgerminomatous germ cell tumors of the ovary with vinblastine, bleomycin and cisplatin. *Cancer* 57:1731, 1986.

Gershenson DM, Morris M, Cangir A et al. Treatment of malignant germ cell tumors of the ovary with bleomycin, etoposide, and cisplatin. *J Clin Oncol* 8:715, 1990.

Gershenson DM. Menstrual and reproductive function after treatment with combination chemotherapy for malignant ovarian germ cell tumors. *J Clin Oncol* 6:270, 1988.

Gershenson DM. Update of malignant ovarian germ cell tumors. *Cancer* 71:1581, 1993.

Gibas Z, Talerman A. Analysis of chromosome aneuploidy in ovarian dysgerminoma by flow cytometry and fluorescence in situ hybridization. *Diagn Molecular Pathol* 2:50, 1993.

Kawai M, Kano T, Kikkawa F et al. Seven tumor markers in benign and malignant germ cell tumors of the ovary. *Gynecol Oncol* 45:248, 1992.

Kleinman GM, Young RH, Scully RE. Primary neuroectodermal tumors of the ovary. A report of 25 cases. *Am J Surg Pathol* 17:764, 1993.

Kurman RJ, Norris HJ. Embryonal carcinoma of the ovary: a clinicopathologic entity distinct from endodermal sinus tumor resembling embryonal carcinoma of the adult testis. *Cancer* 38:2420, 1976.

Kurman RJ, Norris HJ. Malignant germ cell tumors of the ovary. *Hum Pathol* 8:551, 1977.

Norris HJ, Zirkin HJ, Benson WL. Immature (malignant) teratoma of the ovary—A clinical and pathologic study of 58 cases. *Cancer* 37:2359, 1976.

Robboy SJ, Norris HJ, Scully RE. Insular carcinoid primary in the ovary: a clinicopathologic analysis of 48 cases. *Cancer* 36:404, 1975.

Robboy SJ, Scully RE, Norris HJ. Carcinoid metastatic to the ovary: A clinicopathologic analysis of 35 cases. *Cancer* 33:798, 1974.

Robboy SJ, Scully RE. Ovarian teratoma with glial implants on the peritoneum. An analysis of 12 cases. *Hum Pathol* 1:643, 1970.

Robboy SJ, Scully RE. Strumal carcinoid of the ovary: an analysis of 50 cases of a distinctive tumor composed of thyroid tissue and carcinoid. *Cancer* 46:2019, 1980.

Scully RE. Gonadoblastoma, a review of 74 cases. *Cancer* 25:1340, 1970.

Sessa C, Bonazzi C, Landoni F et al. Cisplatin, vinblastine, and bleomycin combination chemotherapy in endodermal sinus tumor of the ovary. *Obstet Gynecol* 70:220, 1987.

Slayton RE, Park RC, Silverberg SG et al. Vincristine, dactinomycin, and cyclophosphamide in the treatment of malignant germ cell tumors of the ovary. A Gynecologic Oncology Group study (a final report). *Cancer* 56:243, 1985.

Smith EB, Clark-Pearson DL, Creasman WT. A VP-16-213 and cisplatin-containing regimen for treatment of refractory ovarian germ cell malignancies. *Am J Obstet Gynecol* 150:927, 1984.

Sporrong B, Falkmer S, Robboy SJ et al. Neurohormonal peptides in ovarian carcinoids: an immunohistochemical study of 81 primary carcinoids and of intraovarian metastases from six mid-gut carcinoids. *Cancer* 49:68, 1982.

Taylor MH, Depetrillo AD, Turner AR. Vinblastine, bleomycin and cisplatin in malignant germ cell tumors of the ovary. *Cancer* 56:1341, 1985.

Willemse PHB, Oosterhuis JW, Aalders JG et al. Malignant struma ovarii treated by ovariectomy, thyroidectomy and ^{131}I administration. *Cancer* 60:178, 1987.

Williams S, Blessing J, DiSaia P et al. Second look laparotomy in ovarian germ cell tumors: The Gynecologic Oncology Group experience. *Proc Am Soc Clin Oncol* 12:254, 1993.

Williams S, Blessing JA, Liao SY et al. Adjuvant therapy of ovarian germ cell tumors with cisplatin, etoposide, and bleomycin: A trial of the Gynecologic Oncology Group. *J Clin Oncol* 12:701, 1994.

Williams SD. Current management of ovarian germ cell tumors. *Oncology* 8:53, 1994.

Williams SD, Birch R, Einhorn LH et al. Treatment of disseminated germ cell tumors with cisplatin, bleomycin, and either vinblastine or etoposide. *N Engl J Med* 316:1435, 1987.

Williams SD, Blessing J, Slayton R et al. Ovarian germ cell tumors: adjuvant trials of the Gynecologic Oncology Group. *Proc Am Soc Clin Oncol* 8:150, 1989.

Williams SD, Blessing JA, Hatch KD, Homesley HD. Chemotherapy for advanced dysgerminoma: trials of the Gynecologic Oncology Group. *J Clin Oncol* 9:1950, 1991.

Williams SD, Blessing JA, Moore DH et al. Cisplatin, vinblastine, and bleomycin in advanced and recurrent ovarian germ cell tumors. A trial of the Gynecologic Oncology Group. *Ann Intern Med* 111:22, 1989.

Yanai-Inbar I, Scully RE. Relation of ovarian dermoid cysts and immature teratomas: an analysis of 350 cases of immature teratoma and 10 cases of dermoid cyst with microscopic foci of immature tissue. *Int J Gynecol Pathol* 6:203, 1987.

3

Ovarian Sarcomas

Bruce Patsner

General

Ovarian sarcomas are rare neoplasms comprised of a myriad of different malignant tumors. As with all sarcomas, ovarian sarcomas may be low grade or high grade and may contain elements of purely müllerian origin or may have nonovarian elements ("heterologous"). Although no official classification system for ovarian sarcoma exists, any of the current schema used for uterine sarcomas are acceptable.

The diagnosis of ovarian sarcoma is virtually never made preoperatively, and the vast majority of ovarian sarcomas are highly aggressive, high-grade lesions that, in most cases, will present with metastatic intraabdominal disease at the time of diagnosis. The International Federation of Gynecologists and Obstetricians (FIGO) staging system for ovarian sarcomas is the same as for all other ovarian malignancies (both epithelial and germ cell), and stage is assigned on the basis of either intraoperative findings in the presence of metastatic disease or pathologic analysis of tissue obtained during staging laparotomy when patients have disease that appears to be confined to the ovary.

Due to the rarity of ovarian sarcomas—fewer than 1% of all ovarian malignant tumors—there are few large series studying them. The existing series do not present patients treated in a uniform manner from either a surgical or chemotherapeutic point of view. Therefore, changes in therapy of ovarian sarcomas are usually made on the basis of literature on nonovarian sarcomas, and formulating an ideal management plan for the patient with either early or advanced ovarian sarcoma is not yet possible. Over 300 cases have been reported in the world literature, the largest series being those of Hanjani (201 cases), Azoury (43 cases), and the Gynecologic Oncology Group (30 cases). Series added to the literature since 1984 include Pfeiffer from Denmark (13 cases), Dictor from Sweden (22 cases), Prendiville from England (20 cases), and Barakat from Memorial Sloan-Kettering in New York (31 cases).

Overall survival with ovarian sarcoma has been poor, particularly when metastatic disease is found at the time of surgery. Most patients are dead of disease within 2 years of diagnosis, although long-term survivors have been reported in every series. Virtually all recent literature on diagnosis and management of ovarian sarcomas has focused on advances in chemotherapy, and some authors have attempted to address the issue of whether debulking surgery is of any value before chemotherapy.

Etiology

Sarcomas of the ovary may occur in any age group, although the majority (50% or more) of patients are postmenopausal and of low parity. Due to the rarity of ovarian sarcomas, insufficient epidemiologic data are available to determine whether prior pelvic radiation therapy is a risk factor for development, as it is for uterine sarcomas. No other known risk factors have been identified, although ovarian sarcomas have been reported to arise in foci of ovarian endometriosis. This association remains speculative at best.

Diagnosis and Natural History

There are no specific signs or symptoms unique to ovarian sarcomas. Because rapid growth is the rule with these tumors, most will present as a "classic" advanced abdominopelvic malignancy—that is, with ascites, an omental cake, and diffuse studding of peritoneal surfaces. Direct extension from tumor on the surface of the ovary is the most common mechanism of spread, although lymphatic and hematogenous spread also both undoubtedly occur.

PRESENTING SYMPTOMS

Presenting symptoms are usually nonspecific and similar to those that accompany metastatic epithelial ovarian cancers: bloating, abdominal discomfort, vague pain, or increasing abdominal girth. Most patients will be symptomatic for 4 months or less. Patients have normal Papanicolaou smears and regular menses; most postmenopausal patients will not have postmenopausal bleeding. Hormonal activity of these tumors is a rare event.

PHYSICAL EXAMINATION

Physical examination reveals an abdominal or pelvic mass in 80% or more of patients. Intravenous pyelogram and barium enema often reveal a "mass effect," and computed tomography (CT) scan of the pelvis and abdomen often will confirm the presence of a mass, ascites, omental cake, or peritoneal studding. A pleural effusion may occur with advanced disease, but parenchymal lung metastases are not common. Partial small-bowel obstruction may be evident by abdominal x-ray of the abdomen, CT scan, and physical examination in patients with extensive intraabdominal disease.

Staging

Staging for ovarian sarcomas is the same as for all other ovarian malignancies—that is, surgical, based on intraoperative findings. The current FIGO staging system and staging procedures required for patients with disease that appears to be confined to the ovary are described in Chap. 1.

Most series of ovarian sarcoma patients include many patients who have not been thoroughly staged; nevertheless, the vast majority (75% or more) will have gross extraovarian spread at initial surgery. Few data are available on the incidence of subclinical retroperitoneal nodal, omental, and diaphragmatic metastases in patients with disease confined to the ovary (FIGO stage I), as has been shown with ovarian epithelial malignancies. Occult spread in patients with clinical stage I ovarian sarcoma must be common,

Table 3-1. Distribution of ovarian sarcoma by stage

	Incidence (%)			
Study	*I*	*II*	*III*	*IV*
Hanjani et al.	18	17	65	
Morrow et al.	0	20	77	3
Anderson et al.	36		64	
Pfeiffer et al.	15	15	70	0
Dictor	18	23	50	9
Prendiville et al.	0	10	70	20
Barakat et al.	23	3	48	26

however, as most of these patients will die of metastatic disease following total abdominal hysterectomy and bilateral salpingo-oophorectomy (TAH/BSO), unless they receive postoperative therapy. The sole exception to this rule are patients with "low-grade" ovarian sarcomas, who may be cured by surgery alone. Table 3-1 illustrates the stage distribution of ovarian sarcoma.

Pathology

There is no formal, universally accepted classification of ovarian sarcomas, perhaps because the histogenesis of these tumors is still being debated. Nevertheless, several key points may be made about classification of ovarian sarcomas:

1. Ovarian sarcomas may be roughly divided in terms of behavior—that is, "low-grade" sarcomas or (more commonly) "high-grade" sarcomas.
2. Ovarian sarcomas that occur during puberty usually arise in dermoids (mature cystic teratomas) or in immature teratomas.
3. The diagnosis of "low-grade" versus "high-grade" sarcoma may be extremely difficult to make on frozen section analysis of tissue; if in doubt, the surgeon should complete surgical staging for disease that appears to be grossly confined to the ovary.
4. From a practical point of view, the type of high-grade ovarian sarcoma is of little independent prognostic significance as all will behave aggressively.

The malignant potential of an ovarian sarcoma (or its grade) is most often determined by the mitotic index of the tumor—that is, the number of mitoses per 10 high-power fields (HPFs). Counts greater than or equal to 10 mitoses per 10 HPFs, particularly when accompanied by infiltrative growth patterns and bizarre, pleomorphic cell architecture with significant atypia, are pathognomonic of high-grade ovarian sarcoma.

Two classification systems for ovarian sarcoma, one based on grade and one based on whether the sarcoma is pure or mixed (i.e., with both sarcomatous and epithelial elements), are listed in Tables 3-2 and 3-3, respectively.

Table 3-2. Classification of ovarian sarcoma by grade

- Low-grade
  - Adenosarcoma
  - Endolymphatic stromal myosis of the ovary
- High-grade
  - Mixed mesodermal (müllerian) tumor (heterologous)
  - Mixed mesodermal (müllerian) tumor (homologous or carcinosarcoma)
  - Leiomyosarcoma
  - Endometrioid stromal sarcoma
  - Teratoid sarcoma (arising in teratoma)
  - Undifferentiated sarcoma
  - Primary ovarian lymphoma

Table 3-3. Classification of ovarian sarcoma by histology

- Pure sarcomas (mesenchymal elements only)
  - Homologous (müllerian only)
    - Leiomyosarcoma
    - Endolymphatic stromal myosis (low-grade endometrial stromal)
    - High-grade endometrial stromal sarcoma
  - Heterologous
    - Angiosarcoma
    - Lymphangiosarcoma
    - Hemangiopericytoma
    - Rhabdomyosarcoma
    - Chondrosarcoma
    - Osteogenic sarcoma
    - Fibrosarcoma
    - Neurofibrosarcoma
- Mixed sarcomas (have epithelial elements)
- Mixed mesodermal (müllerian) tumors
  - Low-grade (adenosarcoma)
    - Homologous
    - Heterologous
  - High-grade
    - Homologous (carcinosarcoma)
    - Heterologous (mixed mesodermal)
- Sarcomas, undifferentiated
- Malignant lymphomas

LOW-GRADE OVARIAN SARCOMAS

Low-grade ovarian sarcomas are usually confined to the ovary at the time of diagnosis. Recurrences are uncommon after surgery, and long-term survival is the rule. Resection of recurrent disease also may result in long-term survival.

Adenosarcoma

Adenosarcoma was first described by Clement and Scully in 1978 as a low-grade variant of the malignant mixed mesodermal tumor.

Adenosarcoma contains benign epithelial (glandular) elements combined with low-grade sarcomatous stromal components.

Endolymphatic Stromal Myosis of the Ovary

Endolymphatic stromal myosis of the ovary was first described in 1960 and reviewed by Silverberg and Fernandez in 1981. Fewer than a dozen cases have been reported in the Western literature. This tumor probably arises in foci of ovarian endometriosis and may respond to progestational agents. Despite its "low-grade" nature, patient death from recurrent disease has been reported.

HIGH-GRADE OVARIAN SARCOMAS

High-grade ovarian sarcomas generally exhibit aggressive biological behavior, with metastatic disease present in most cases at the time of diagnosis and a high mortality rate when any extraovarian spread is present.

Teratoid Sarcomas

Teratoid sarcomas consist of sarcomatous tissue arising from the mesenchymal component of a preexisting teratoma or accompanying a teratocarcinoma. The type of sarcomatous tissue may vary. Seventy percent of patients are children or adolescents. As a rule, these tumors tend to pursue an aggressive clinical course.

Mixed Mesodermal (Müllerian) Tumors

Mixed mesodermal (müllerian) tumors contain elements of both adenocarcinoma and sarcoma (hence "mixed"). When the sarcomatous elements are stromal (e.g., bone, cartilage, or skeletal muscle not normally found in the ovary), the tumor is considered heterologous. When the sarcomatous elements are mesenchymal tissues normally in the ovary, the tumor is considered homologous (also known as carcinosarcoma). These tumors are characterized by aggressive growth and are most common during the sixth and seventh decades of life. They are the most common type of ovarian sarcoma overall.

Leiomyosarcomas

Leiomyosarcomas arise from smooth muscle elements normally found in the hilus of the ovary.

Fibrosarcomas

Fibrosarcomas may be considered of high malignancy potential when four or more mitoses per 10 HPFs are present. They occasionally occur during the second or third decade of life but more commonly are seen in postmenopausal women. They are comprised of a benign ovarian fibroma and a sarcoma.

Endometrioid Stromal Sarcomas

Endometrioid stromal sarcomas are most common in the fourth and fifth decades. In 9 of 23 cases reported, uterine sarcoma was present or later developed. Ten or more mitoses per 10 HPFs are needed to establish the diagnosis.

Ovarian Lymphomas

Ovarian lymphomas are rare; though both Hodgkin's and non-Hodgkin's lymphomas may occur, the former is rarer still.

Burkitt's lymphoma may involve the ovaries in 50% or more of patients. A small number of cases of primary plasmacytoma of the ovary have been reported.

Treatment

Surgery is the mainstay of treatment of ovarian sarcoma (regardless of grade or histology) in order to definitely establish the diagnosis, stage patients properly when disease appears to be confined to the ovary, and debulk patients with metastatic disease.

TYPE OF SURGERY

Except for the rare patient with low-grade sarcoma clinically confined to the ovary for whom preservation of hormonal production (contralateral ovary) and fertility (uterus) are important considerations, surgery should consist of TAH/BSO plus either staging for localized disease or debulking of metastatic disease. Unlike patients with germ cell tumors who rarely have bilateral ovarian or uterine involvement, except for the patient with dysgerminoma, there are few data to allow the clinician to proceed with unilateral oophorectomy only. Moreover, lack of effective, established adjuvant chemotherapy for ovarian sarcomas (again, unlike germ cell tumors) restricts the surgical options available to these patients.

SURGICAL PRINCIPLES

The ovary or ovaries should be resected, as well as obvious metastatic disease if present, and sent for frozen section analysis.

High-Grade Tumor Clinically Confined to the Ovary

TAH/BSO, washings, omentectomy, appendectomy, multiple biopsies, and retroperitoneal node sampling should be performed.

High-Grade Tumor with Any Extraovarian Spread

TAH/BSO, omentectomy, appendectomy, retroperitoneal node removal, and debulking of metastases should be performed.

Low-Grade Ovarian Sarcoma in Any Patient Desiring Preservation of Childbearing Capacity

Unilateral oophorectomy with full surgical staging (in the event the diagnosis is changed and to rule out rare metastases), TAH/BSO, and staging if childbearing is completed should be performed.

Factors Affecting Survival

STAGE OF DISEASE

The stage of disease is by far the most important factor affecting survival. Barakat et al. noted a mean survival of 104 months for eight patients with stage I or II disease versus 9.5 months in 23 patients with stage III or IV disease. Dictor similarly noted a significant survival advantage for stage I or II disease.

RESIDUAL DISEASE STATUS

There is no proof yet that the extent of debulking surgery is of prognostic importance, unlike the case of patients with ovarian epithelial cancers. In Barakat's series, prognosis was not altered in patients with stage II–IV disease regardless of whether they had no residual disease at the conclusion of cytoreductive surgery or large-volume residual disease. Other authors in series with smaller numbers of long-term survivors have commented on the possible role optimal (<2 cm) debulking surgery may have played in outcome. The issue will likely require a large cooperative study with patients operated and treated postoperatively in a uniform manner to settle the issue.

HISTOLOGIC TYPE

Low-grade ovarian sarcomas have superior survival rates compared to high-grade ovarian sarcomas. Within the high-grade category, there is no conclusive proof that the histologic type of ovarian sarcoma is significant.

Postoperative Therapy

There is no definitive proof that adjuvant therapy will improve prognosis for stage I high-grade ovarian sarcoma over surgery alone, as is suggested by some of the literature on uterine sarcoma, but the number of cases studied is too few to answer the question. The poor results with all forms of therapy for patients with advanced disease have not enabled clinicians to establish a "track record" on the best therapy for these patients. Table 3-4 outlines a summary of survival data.

Postoperative Therapy

All patients with high-grade ovarian sarcoma require postoperative therapy regardless of surgical stage. No standard therapy for ovarian sarcoma exists; current regimens invariably are developed from the nonovarian sarcoma literature. Some general comments may be made about therapy for ovarian sarcoma, however.

RADIATION THERAPY

Radiation therapy appears to offer little in the way of therapeutic efficacy.

1. As with uterine sarcoma, pelvic radiation might decrease the pelvic recurrence rate but would not be expected to improve survival rates, and the minimum effective dose to control microscopic disease in the upper abdomen (5,000 cGy) would exceed the tolerance of the small intestine.
2. Virtually all research has focused on the development of more effective chemotherapeutic regimens.
3. Although theoretically appealing, the combination of multiagent chemotherapy with abdominopelvic radiation therapy has

received little attention since first reported by Carlson and Day in 1983. This is perhaps because of the severe toxicity of this regimen; current regimens that are more dose-intensive will only amplify this problem.

CHEMOTHERAPY

The chemotherapies (Table 3-5) used for treatment of all gynecologic sarcomas may now be divided into the older regimens that were adriamycin-based and the newer regimens that center around cisplatin and ifosfamide. Though use of the latter two drugs has result-

Table 3-4. Survival of patients with ovarian sarcoma by stage

			Stage survival (%)			
Author/years	*No. of cases*	*Histology*	*I*	*II*	*III*	*IV*
Hanjani et al.						
1-year	201	MMT	44	20	19	—
5-year			32	7	0	—
Anderson et al.						—
2-year	14	Sarcoma	100	100	17	—
5-year			30	50	0	—
Barakat et al.						
5-year	31	MMT	30	—	17	—

MMT = mixed mesodermal (müllerian) tumor.

Table 3-5. Response rates of ovarian mixed mesodermal tumors to different chemotherapeutic regimens

Author	*Year*	*No. of patients*	*Regimen*	*Response (%)*
Older regimens				
Lele	1980	9	VAC	22%
Carlson	1983	12	VAC + RT	33%
Morrow	1984	13	VAC	31%
Newer regimens				
Anderson	1986	10	PAC or PA	100% including 4 complete responses, 4 sustained remissions
Wheelock	1987	6	PAC	17%
Plaxe	1990	13	PA	85%
Baker	1991	11	PA-DTIC	40%
Pfeiffer	1991	6	PAC	50%
Barakat	1992	21	PA	71%

VAC = vincristine, actinomycin-D, cyclophosphamide; RT = radiation therapy; DTIC = dacarbazine; PAC = cisplatin, Adriamycin, cyclophosphamide; PA = cisplatin, Adriamycin.

ed in a higher response rate for patients with metastatic ovarian sarcomas, the overall 5-year survival data have *not* shown any significant improvement, although investigators in the United States and abroad both report long-term survival of patients with advanced disease. It is hoped that continued investigation of new agents and drug combinations in patients with soft-tissue sarcomas will allow for further improvement in overall survival of patients' aggressive malignancies. Large cooperative clinical trials will be necessary due to the rarity of these tumors.

Selected Readings

Anderson WA et al. Platinum-based combination chemotherapy for malignant mixed mesodermal tumors of the ovary. *Gynecol Oncol* 32:319, 1989.

Azoury RS, Woodruff JD. Primary ovarian sarcomas: Report of 43 cases from the Emil Novak Ovarian Tumor Registry. *Obstet Gynecol* 37:920, 1971.

Baker TR, Piver MS, Caglar H, Piedmonte M. Prospective trial of cisplatin, adriamycin and dacarbazine in metastatic mixed mesodermal sarcomas of the uterus and ovary. *Am J Clin Oncol* 14:246, 1991.

Barakat R et al. Mixed mesodermal tumor of the ovary: Analysis of prognostic factors in 31 cases. *Obstet Gynecol* 80:660, 1992.

Carlson JA Jr. et al. Mixed mesodermal sarcoma of the ovary: treatment with combination radiation therapy and chemotherapy. *Cancer* 52:1473, 1983.

Clement PR, Scully RE. Extrauterine mesodermal (mullerian) adenosarcoma: A clinicopathologic analysis of 5 cases. *Am J Clin Pathol* 69:276, 1978.

Cooper P. Mixed mesodermal tumor and clear cell carcinoma arising in ovarian endometriosis. *Cancer* 42:2827, 1978.

Dictor M. Malignant mixed mesodermal tumor of the ovary: A report of 22 cases. *Obstet Gynecol* 65:720, 1985.

Hanjani P et al. Malignant mixed mesodermal tumors and carcinosarcoma of the ovary: Report of eight cases and review of the literature. *Obstet Gynecol Surv* 38:537, 1983.

Lele SB, Piver MS, Barlow JJ. Chemotherapy in management of mixed mesodermal tumors of the ovary. *Gynecol Oncol* 10:298, 1980.

Morrow CP et al. A clinical and pathologic study of 30 cases of malignant mixed mullerian epithelial and mesenchymal tumors. A Gynecologic Oncology Group study. *Gynecol Oncol* 18:278, 1984.

Pfeiffer P, Hardt-Madsen M, Rex S, Bertelsen K. Malignant mixed mullerian tumors of the ovary. Report of 13 cases. *Acta Obstet Gynecol Scand* 70:79, 1991.

Plaxe SC et al. Clinical features of advanced ovarian mixed mesodermal tumors and treatment with doxorubicin and cisplatin-based chemotherapy. *Gynecol Oncol* 37:244, 1990.

Prat J, Scully RE. Cellular fibromas and fibrosarcomas of the ovary: a comparative clinicopathologic analysis of seventeen cases. *Cancer* 47:2663, 1981.

Prendiville J, Murphy D, Rennison J et al. Carcinosarcoma of the ovary treated over a ten-year period at the Christie Hospital. *Int J Gynecol Cancer* 4:200, 1994.

Silverberg SG, Fernandez FN. Endolymphatic stromal myosis of the ovary: A report of three cases and literature review. *Gynecol Oncol* 12:129, 1981.

Simon SR, Wang SE, Uhl M, Shackney S. Complete response of carcinosarcoma of the ovary to therapy with doxorubicin, ifosfamide, and dacarbazine. *Gynecol Oncol* 41:161, 1991.

Wheelock J, Hancock K, Smith K. Cisplatin, doxorubicin, and cyclophosphamide (PAC) in the treatment of mixed mesodermal tumor of the ovary. *Cancer Treat Rep* 71:1275, 1987.

Young RH, Prat J, Scully RE. Endometrioid stromal sarcomas of the ovary: A clinicopathologic analysis of 23 cases. *Cancer* 53:1143, 1984.

4

Sex Cord–Stromal Ovarian Tumors

M. Steven Piver

Classification of Sex Cord–Stromal Tumors

Sex cord–stromal tumors represent 8% of all ovarian tumors and are the third most common type of ovarian tumor after epithelial and germ cell tumors. These tumors arise from the specialized gonadal stroma (sex cords) or from the nonspecific mesenchyme of the genital ridge itself. Because the embryonic gonad has both male and female potential, the sex cords in this stroma may each give rise to either a male or a female sex cord–stromal tumor, or both. Thus, they include ovarian tumors that contain granulosa cells, theca cells, and their luteinized derivatives, as well as Sertoli cells, Leydig cells, and fibroblasts that arise from the gonadal stroma. Ovarian tumors derived from this tissue may thus differentiate toward the ovary (granulosa cell tumor), the testes (Sertoli-Leydig cell tumor), or both (gynandroblastoma). This plural potentiality is reflected in the current World Health Organization (WHO) classifications of sex cord–stromal tumors (Table 4-1).

Unlike epithelial cancer, in which 70% of patients present with stage III–IV disease, sex cord-stromal tumors present in stage I in 70% of patients.

Adult Granulosa Cell Tumors

GENERAL CONSIDERATIONS

Adult granulosa cell tumors are sex cord–stromal tumors composed of granulosa cells with or without theca cells, fibroblasts, or both. Commonly, these tumors contain both cell elements but should be referred to as adult granulosa cell tumors. The terms *theca cell tumor* and *thecoma* should be reserved for tumors that contain theca cells only.

INCIDENCE

The adult granulosa cell tumor is the most common type of malignant sex cord–stromal tumor and, after the ovarian fibroma, the second most common of all sex cord–stromal tumors. The adult granulosa cell tumor represents 1–2% of all ovarian tumors, 5% of all ovarian cancers, and 95% of all granulosa cell tumors. It is the most common estrogenic ovarian tumor, although very rarely it can be androgenic. Although the peak incidence for adult granulosa cell tumors is between 50 and 55 years of age, they can occur in children, though rarely.

CLINICAL PRESENTATION

Since adult granulosa cell tumors primarily occur in postmenopausal women, postmenopausal bleeding is the most common symptom in this age group. Premenopausal women present with irregular uterine

Table 4-1. World Health Organization classification of sex cord–stromal tumors

I. Granulosa–stromal cell tumors
   A. Granulosa cell tumor
      1. Adult type
      2. Juvenile type
   B. Tumors in the thecoma/fibroma group
      1. Thecoma
         a. Typical
         b. Luteinized
      2. Fibroma-fibrosarcoma
         a. Fibroma
         b. Cellular fibroma
         c. Fibrosarcoma
      3. Stromal tumor with minor sex cord elements
      4. Sclerosing stromal tumor
      5. Unclassified
II. Sertoli–stromal cell tumors
   A. Sertoli cell tumor
   B. Leydig cell tumor
   C. Sertoli-Leydig cell tumor
      1. Well-differentiated
      2. Of intermediate differentiation
      3. Poorly differentiated
      4. With heterologous elements
      5. Retiform
      6. Mixed
III. Gynandroblastoma
IV. Sex cord tumor with annular tubules
V. Unclassified

bleeding, but occasionally may present with amenorrhea. In addition to abnormal uterine bleeding, many patients present with abdominal pain and on physical examination have a pelvic or a pelvic and abdominal mass. Because 10% of these tumors rupture before surgery, patients may present with acute abdominal findings secondary to hemoperitoneum. Endometrial biopsy may be consistent with endometrial hyperplasia in 20% from excess estrogen stimulation, while 5–10% of patients will ultimately develop endometrial carcinoma. Most granulosa cell tumors produce estradiol. Inhibin, a glycoprotein, is composed of alpha and beta subunits secreted by the granulosa cell tumors of the ovary. Lappohn et al. were the first to report elevated serum inhibin levels before clinical signs of recurrence of granulosa cell tumors and that inhibin levels reflected response to therapy. In addition, inhibin levels were normal in women with granulosa cell tumors free of disease. Ninety percent of patients present at stage I, and 90% are unilateral (stage IA) at the time of diagnosis.

TREATMENT

Surgery

Unilateral oophorectomy is the treatment of choice for young women with surgical stage I who desire preservation of fertility. All other patients with stage IA disease should have total abdominal hysterectomy and bilateral salpingo-oophorectomy (TAH/BSO) and appropri-

Table 4-2. Cisplatin, vinblastine, and bleomycin regimen for metastatic granulosa cell tumors

Author/year	*No. of patients*	*% response (no.)*	*% complete response (no.)*	*Duration of complete response (mos)*
Colombo/1986	11	82 (9)	55 (6)	7+ to 36+
Pecorelli/1988	13	92 (12)	54 (7)	4 to 27+
Zambetti/1990	7	58 (4)	43 (3)	7+ to 26+
Total	31	81 (25)	52 (16)	

Table 4-3. Adult versus juvenile granulosa cell tumor

Adult form	*Juvenile form*
1% prepubertal	50% prepubertal
Usually after age 30	Rarely after age 30
Mature follicles and Call-Exner bodies common	Immature follicles with secretion; Call-Exner bodies rare
Nuclei pale, commonly grooved	Nuclei dark, rarely grooved
Luteinization infrequent	Luteinization frequent

ate surgical staging. In carefully staged patients, there is no need for adjuvant therapy.

Chemotherapy

The most active cytotoxic regimen for recurrent or metastatic granulosa cell tumor consists of cisplatin, vinblastine, and bleomycin (PVB). Of the 31 patients in the three largest series reported, the overall response rate was 81% and the complete response rate was 52% (Table 4-2). Although follow-up in many cases is short, many of the complete responses appear to be durable. Although clearly an active regimen, PVB should be used with caution since there were a minimum of three chemotherapy-related toxicity deaths among the 31 patients.

Juvenile Granulosa Cell Tumors

GENERAL CONSIDERATIONS

Juvenile granulosa cell tumor (JGT), a subtype of granulosa cell tumor, is distinct histologically and clinically from the adult tumor (Table 4-3). Forty-four percent occur in the first decade, 80% by the second decade, and 97% by the third decade. JGT rarely has been associated with Maffucci's syndrome (enchondromatoses and hemangiomas) and Ollier's disease (enchoindromatoses).

CLINICAL PRESENTATION

In those cases occurring before puberty, most patients present with isosexual precocious puberty with breast development and growth of pubic and axillary hair. They frequently present with nonspecific abdominal pain and increasing abdominal girth, the latter secondary to rupture and hemoperitoneum (6%). In a report of 125 cases of JGT, only 2% were bilateral, and the authors reported only four cases that had spread beyond the ovary (stage II [3], stage III [1]). Similar to AGT, high serum levels of inhibin have been reported.

TREATMENT

Since JGTs occur in the very young and 95% are unilateral, unilateral salpingo-oophorectomy with preservation of the uterus and contralateral tube and ovary should be performed. Because of the possible problems with subsequent infertility by scarring of the contralateral normal ovary, biopsy is usually not performed. However, Young et al. reported involvement of the contralateral ovary within 1 year in an additional 2% of their stage IA patients. Although the results of systemic chemotherapy for recurrent JGT have been disappointing, there have been two long-term remissions using methotrexate, actinomycin-D, and cyclophosphamide (MAC).

PROGNOSIS

JGTs are primarily characterized by a benign clinical course, but a small percentage do recur and may be fatal. In the report by Young et al., survival for patients with stage IA without excretions was 99%; for stage IA with excretions, 90%; and for stage IC (ascites or positive peritoneal cytology), 80%. Although prognosis is related to stage, there was no distinct relationship between abnormal DNA content of the tumor and survival in patients with early- or advanced-stage JGT.

Thecoma and Fibroma Tumors

THECOMA

General Considerations

Thecomas, like fibromas, arise from the ovarian stroma and are composed exclusively of theca cells. In a report by Bjorkholm and Silversward, the average age of the patient was 59, and 84% of patients were postmenopausal. However, 10% did occur in patients below the age of 30. Postmenopausal bleeding was the most common presenting symptom and of these, 21% had a concomitant endometrial adenocarcinoma.

Treatment

In the young patient, unilateral salpingo-oophorectomy without surgical staging is the treatment of choice. Dilatation and curettage should be performed to rule out a coexisting endometrial cancer. In all other patients, TAH/BSO should be performed. If, on frozen section, there are significant nuclear atypia and a high mitotic count, surgical staging as for epithelial ovarian cancer should be performed. The management for metastatic malignant thecoma would be similar to that for ovarian fibrosarcoma.

Prognosis

Thecomas almost invariably have a benign clinical course and very rarely behave in a malignant manner. There is controversy about the diagnosis of a malignant thecoma, which requires nuclear atypia and high mitotic count.

LUTEINIZED THECOMAS

Luteinized thecomas are composed of steroid-type cells consistent with luteinized theca and stromal cells. Fifty percent are estrogenic, 39% nonfunctional, and 11% androgenic. Although they most commonly occur in postmenopausal women, unlike thecomas, 30% occur in patients below the age of 30. They invariably have a benign course, but rare malignant luteinized thecomas have been reported.

FIBROMAS

General Considerations

Fibromas are the most common benign solid ovarian tumor and the most common sex cord–stromal tumor of the ovary. With few exceptions, they behave in a benign manner. They represent 4% of all ovarian tumors. Unlike thecomas, they are not hormonally active. They occur primarily after the age of 40. Ninety percent are unilateral. Fibromas have been associated with two distinct syndromes:

1. Meigs' syndrome: Occurs in 1% of fibromas and consists of ovarian fibroma, ascites, and a right pleural effusion. With resection of the ovarian fibroma, the ascites and pleural effusion regress.
2. Basal cell nevus syndrome: Autosomal dominant condition that occurs in young women and is characterized by bilateral ovarian fibromas, basal cell nevi, skeletal abnormalities, and keratocytes of the jaw.

Treatment

Treatment for ovarian fibromas is similar to that for thecomas. If on frozen section there are greater than three mitoses per 10 high-power fields (HPFs), surgical staging should be carried out similar to that for epithelial ovarian cancer.

Prognosis

Although fibromas are almost invariably benign, some may behave with a malignant course. Fibromas characteristically have no mitoses per 10 HPFs. However, those with one to three mitoses per 10 HPFs are referred to as *cellular fibromas,* which behave in a low-grade malignant fashion. Those with greater than three mitoses per 10 HPFs are designated *fibrosarcoma*. The cellular fibroma and fibrosarcoma account for less than 1% of all ovarian fibromas.

SCLEROSING STROMAL TUMORS

General Considerations

Sclerosing stromal tumors are a distinct form of the thecoma/fibroma group of ovarian tumors. The average patient age is 27, and over 80% occur during the second and third decades. Unlike thecomas, they rarely present with symptoms of hyperestrogenism (abnormal uterine bleeding or endometrial hyperplasia) and even more rarely present with androgenic manifestations. They are all unilateral and benign.

Treatment

In the young woman, unilateral salpingo-oophorectomy without surgical staging should be performed. All other patients should have TAH/BSO.

Sertoli Stromal Cell Tumors

SERTOLI-LEYDIG CELL TUMORS

General Considerations

Sertoli-Leydig cell tumors account for less than 0.5% of all ovarian tumors. The average patient age is 25, and only 10% are over age 50.

There are five categories of Sertoli-Leydig tumors: (1) well-differentiated, (2) intermediate differentiation, (3) poorly differentiated with heterologous elements, (4) with heterologous elements, and (5) with retiform pattern. The heterologous type may have cartilage or striated muscle. One-third of the cases of Sertoli-Leydig cell tumors are androgenic and present with virilization, consisting of oligomenorrhea followed by amenorrhea. Subsequently, there is atrophy of the breasts and loss of the female body habitus, followed by hirsutism, balding, and clitoral enlargement. Although estrogenic signs are rare, if present they consist of irregular uterine bleeding in premenopausal women and postmenopausal bleeding. The remaining two-thirds of patients with Sertoli-Leydig cell tumors have no hormonal manifestations and present with abdominal pain or increasing abdominal girth.

Although the average patient age is 25, the well-differentiated Sertoli-Leydig cell tumors primarily appear after age 40, as compared to under 25 for those with intermediate poorly differentiated tumors.

Steroid synthesis has been reported in Sertoli-Leydig cell tumors. De la Cuesta et al. reported high concentrations of androgenic hormones and precursors from the delta-4 steroid pathway (7-OH progesterone, testosterone, and androstenedione). Ninety-seven percent are limited to the ovary, with approximately 2–3% having spread beyond the ovary, primarily to the pelvis. At surgery, 2% are bilateral, 80% are limited to one ovary (stage IA), and 12% are stage IC by either rupture or excretions on the external surface. Sertoli-Leydig cell tumors have been associated with elevated serum levels of alpha-fetoprotein.

Treatment

Surgery

Unilateral salpingo-oophorectomy is the treatment of choice in the young. If, on frozen section, one can make the diagnosis of poor differentiation or there are heterologous elements, both associated with a greater malignancy potential, surgical staging as for epithelial ovarian cancer should be carried out. The uterus, contralateral tube, and ovary should be preserved. For all other women, TAH/BSO and surgical staging as discussed above should be performed.

Chemotherapy

For those patients presenting with metastatic Sertoli-Leydig cell tumors, PVB similar to that given for granulosa cell tumors is an active regimen.

Prognosis

Prognosis is related to stage and grade of the tumor. In the report by Young and Scully, none of the well-differentiated tumors, 11% of those with intermediate differentiation, 59% of the poorly differentiated, and 19% of those with heterologous elements behaved in a malignant manner. The presence of retiform pattern may adversely affect prognosis, with 25% of the reported stage I retiform tumors having a malignant course compared to only 10% of tumors with a similar grade without retiform.

SERTOLI CELL TUMORS

Sertoli cell tumors account for 4% of sertoli stromal cell tumors and may result in isosexual pseudoprecocity. All are stage IA and, if poorly differentiated, may recur and may be fatal.

Leydig Cell Tumors

Leydig or hilus cell tumors are rare sex cord–stromal tumors. They arise primarily in the hilus of the ovary from hilar Leydig cells and are thus referred to as *hilus cell tumors*. There are no malignant hilus cell tumors. Rarely, they are located in the ovarian stroma and are referred to as *stromal Leydig cell tumors*, nonhilar type. They occur primarily in postmenopausal women, and 80% have manifestations of hyperandrogen secretion, with resultant virilization. Rarely, estrogen manifestations may be present. They are unilateral. The stromal Leydig cell tumor is composed of neoplastic theca cell proliferation with clusters of steroid-type cells. The crystaloid of Reinke within the steroid-type cells identifies them as stromal Leydig cells. To date there have only been seven cases of stromal Leydig cell tumors. They occur in postmenopausal women, are usually androgenic, and are benign.

Sex Cord Tumors with Annular Tubules

Sex cord tumors with annular tubules (SCTAT) are characterized by simple and complex annular tubules. It has been reported that SCTAT can produce estradiol and progesterone as well as inhibin. *Müllerian-inhibiting substance*, a glycoprotein hormone produced by the fetal Sertoli cells, correlated with the degree of tumor burden throughout the course of a patient with SCTAT. SCTAT tumors vary clinically and pathologically on whether Peutz-Jeghers syndrome (PJS) is present or not. SCTAT is associated with PJS in approximately one-third of patients characterized by oral mucocutaneous melanin pigmentation and gastrointestinal polyposis. In patients without PJS, 40% have symptoms of hyperestrogen and some have produced progesterone. Patients with PJS and SCTAT usually present with bilateral ovarian involvement (65%) in comparison to only 5% in patients with SCTAT without PJS. SCTAT in association with PJS has to date no malignant potential. However, 15% have an associated malignant adenoma of the cervix. In contrast, 20% of patients with SCTAT without PJS have metastasis at the initial surgery.

Lipid Cell Tumors

Lipid cell tumors are derived from ovarian stroma and account for less than 0.1% of all ovarian tumors. Lipid or lipoid cell tumors occur primarily in premenopausal women and are unilateral tumors. They are characterized by high urinary 17 ketosteroids and normal urinary 17-hydroxysteroid levels, as well as elevated serum testosterone and androstenedione levels. They have also resulted in Cushing's syndrome. Approximately 20% behave in a malignant manner. Chemotherapy has not been effective.

Gynandroblastoma

Gynandroblastoma is a rare tumor with a recognizable Sertoli-Leydig cell and granulosa cell elements. Feminization and virilization may occur because of the ovarian and testicular elements within the tumor. They are characteristically benign, although mortality from gynandroblastoma has been reported.

Selected Readings

Bjorkholm E, Silversward C. Prognostic factors in granulosa cell tumor. *Gynecol Oncol* 11:261, 1981.

Bohm J, Roder-Weber M, Hofler H. Bilateral stromal leydig cell tumor of the ovary: Case report and literature review. *Pathol Res Pract* 187:348, 1991.

Colombo N, Sessa C, Landoni F et al. Cisplatin, vinblastine, and bleomycin combination chemotherapy in metastatic granulosa cell tumor of the ovary. *Obstet Gynecol* 67:265, 1986.

de la Cuesta RS, Rock JA, Homsi R et al. Analysis of steroid production of a Sertoli-Leydig cell tumor. *Gynecol Oncol* 52:276, 1994.

Donovan JT, Otis CN, Powell JL et al. Cushing's syndrome secondary to malignant lipoid cell tumor of the ovary. *Gynecol Oncol* 50:249, 1993.

Kurman RJ, Goebelsmann U, Taylor CR. Steroid localisation in granulosa-theca tumours of the ovary. *Cancer* 43:2377, 1979.

Lappohn RE, Burger HG, Bouma J et al. Inhibin as a marker for granulosa cell tumors. *N Engl J Med* 321:790, 1989.

Paraskevas M, Scully RE. Hilus cell tumor of the ovary: A clinicopathological analysis of 12 Reinke-crystal–positive and 9 crystal-negative cases. *Int J Gynecol Pathol* 8:299, 1989.

Pecorelli S, Wagener P, Bonazzi C et al. Cisplatin, vinblastine, and bleomycin combination chemotherapy in recurrent or advanced granulosa cell tumor of the ovary. An EORTC Gynecologic Cancer Cooperative Group Study. *Proceed Am Soc Clin Oncol* 7:147, 1988.

Prat J, Scully RE. Cellular fibromas and fibrosarcomas of the ovary: A comparative clinicopathologic analysis of seventeen cases. *Cancer* 47:2663, 1979.

Roth LM, Sternberg WH. Ovarian stromal tumors containing Leydig cells. II. Pure Leydig cell tumor, non-hilar type. *Cancer* 32:952, 1973.

Young RH, Dickersin GR, Scully RE. Juvenile granulosa cell tumors: A clinicopathologic analysis of 125 cases. *Am J Surg Pathol* 8:575, 1984.

Young RH, Prat J, Scully RE. Ovarian Sertoli-Leydig tumors with heterologous elements. I. Gastrointestinal epithelium and carcinoid. A clinicopathologic analysis of 36 cases. *Cancer* 50:2448, 1982.

Young RH, Scully RE. Ovarian Sertoli cell tumors. A report of ten cases. *Int J Gynecol Pathol* 2:349, 1984.

Young RH, Scully RE. Ovarian Sertoli-Leydig cell tumors with a retiform pattern: A problem in histopathologic diagnosis. A report of 25 cases. *Am J Surg Pathol* 7:755, 1983.

Young RH, Scully RE. Ovarian Sertoli-Leydig cell tumors. A clinicopathological analysis of 207 cases. *Am J Surg Pathol* 9:543–569, 1985.

Young RH, Scully RE. Ovarian sex cord–stromal tumors. Recent progress. *Int J Gynecol Pathol* 1:101, 1982.

Young RH, Welch WR, Dickersin GR et al. Ovarian sex cord tumor with annular tubules: Review of 74 cases including 27 with Peutz-Jegher syndrome and four with adenoma malignum of the cervix. *Cancer* 50:1384, 1982.

Zaloudek C and Morris HJ. Sertoli-Leydig cell tumors of the ovary. *Am J Surg Pathol* 8:405, 1984.

Zambetti M, Escobedo A, Pilotti S et al. Cis-platinum/vinblastine/bleomycin combination chemotherapy in advanced or recurrent granulosa cell tumors of the ovary. *Gynecol Oncol* 36:317, 1990.

Zhang J, Young RH, Arseneau J et al. Ovarian stromal tumors containing lutein or Leydig cells (luteinized thecomas and stromal Leydig cell tumors). A clinicopathological analysis of fifty cases. *Int J Gynecol Pathol* 1:270, 1982.

5

Fallopian Tube Cancer

Peter G. Rose

Primary malignant tumors of the fallopian tube are the least common of all the gynecologic cancers. They have precluded prospective randomized trials and thus hindered our knowledge of this disease. Our current understanding of fallopian tube cancer is based on relatively small, retrospective, single-institution series. To date only two cooperative retrospective series with more than 100 patients have been reported.

Primary Adenocarcinoma

INCIDENCE

Fallopian tube cancer is the least common gynecologic cancer. Its frequency ranges from 0.3% to 1.0% of all gynecologic cancers according to various series. The majority of cases are seen in patients 40–60 years of age, with a mean age of 55, although it has been reported to occur as early as 18 years of age. This age at diagnosis is closer to the median reported for ovarian cancer (58 years) than that reported for endometrial cancer (61 years).

ETIOLOGY

The etiology of fallopian tube cancer remains unknown. A history of infertility is common, with a 40% incidence of nulliparity in one series of 47 patients. Chronic inflammation and tuberculous salpingitis have been suggested as possible predisposing factors. Chronic inflammation often coexists with a fallopian tube carcinoma. However, it is doubtful that this is a causative factor since chronic salpingitis usually involves both tubes and the inflammatory response is limited to the tube involved with the carcinoma. Secondly, tubal carcinoma occurs in postmenopausal women, a group with a low prevalence of chronic salpingitis. In Sedlis' review, the rate of pelvic tuberculosis was not higher than in the general population. The rarity of this malignancy makes any of these relatively common conditions unlikely etiologic factors.

PATHOLOGY

The rarity of fallopian tube cancer is in part related to the convention of attributing tubal carcinoma involving the ovary or endometrium as an ovarian or endometrial primary tumor, respectively.

Macroscopic Appearance

The tube is usually enlarged by the growth of the intraluminal tumor and appears fusiform. In approximately 50% of cases the fimbriated end of the tube is occluded with the development of pyosalpinx or hematosalpinx. On opening the tube, the lumen is found to be occupied by a solid mass, frequently with hemorrhagic and necrotic areas. The tumor may arise from any portion of the tube, but it most often originates in the ampullary portion. Fallopian tube cancer affects the right and left tubes with similar frequency and is bilateral in 10–26% of cases. In early stages, this bilaterality may represent an independent occurrence in both tubes, if the intervening endometrium is free of cancer. With more advanced cases, the tumor penetrates the tubal serosa and may involve the ovaries and uterus or other pelvic or abdominal organs.

Histology

The most frequent histologic type is adenocarcinoma, similar to the ovarian serous variety. Less common histologic types include clear-cell, endometrioid, adenosquamous, squamous cell carcinoma, sarcoma, choriocarcinoma, and malignant teratoma. The histologic differential diagnosis of primary malignant tumors of the fallopian tube should include a wide variety of benign tumors and the possibility of metastasis from other primary sites.

Various criteria to determine the definite diagnosis of primary fallopian tube carcinoma have been suggested. In 1949, Finn and Javert proposed the following gross criteria:

1. The tubes, at least in the distal portion, are abnormal. The fimbriated ends may be dilated and occluded, resembling chronic salpingitis.
2. There is a papillary growth in the endosalpinx.
3. The uterus and ovaries are either grossly normal or affected by a lesion other than cancer.

Finn and Javert also proposed the following microscopic criteria:

1. The epithelium of the endosalpinx is replaced in whole or in part by adenocarcinoma, and the histologic character of the cells resembles the epithelium of the endosalpinx.
2. The endometrium and ovaries are normal or contain a malignant lesion that, by its size, distribution, and histologic appearance, is secondary to a tubal primary tumor.
3. Tuberculosis has been clearly excluded.

In 1950, Hu et al. proposed additional criteria:

1. Grossly, the main tumor is in the tube.
2. Microscopically, chiefly the mucosa should be involved and should show a papillary pattern.
3. If the tubal wall is found to be involved to a great extent, the transition between benign and malignant tubal epithelium should be demonstrable.

More recently, gynecologic pathologists have thoroughly evaluated fallopian tubes removed at exploration for abdominal carcinomatosis. The transformation of in situ to invasive carcinoma in the tube has been identified and considered diagnostic of primary fallopian tube malignancy. Numerous studies of fallopian tube cancer also noted multifocal upper genital tract tumors. In one study from Roswell Park Cancer Institute, 37% of patients had multiple primary tumors occurring in the ovary (31%), uterus (11%), and cervix (3%). The concept of field neoplastic change of müllerian epithelium was proposed to explain the existence of multiple upper genital tract neoplasias. Bannatyne et al. reported seven cases of in situ or invasive tubal carcinoma after reviewing 251 cases of epithelial ovarian cancer. These authors stress that careful sectioning of the tube may identify tubal neoplasia in 5–10% of ovarian tumors. In the Roswell Park series, among 1,592 ovarian cancers pathologically evaluated over the study period, tubal neoplasia was present in 1.3% of cases. Adenocarcinoma in situ has been described as an entity, and some authors do not distinguish it from adenomatous hyperplasia; it is usually focal and contains abnormal mitotic figures and nuclear pleomorphism with large nucleoli. Rarely, squamous carcinoma in situ has been reported as an extension of cervical neoplasia.

Hu et al. divided fallopian tumors into three histologic classifications: grade I, papillary lesions; grade II, papillary-alveolar lesions; and grade III, alveolar-medullary lesions. Most pathologists no longer use this system, and the grade of the tumor is classified as well-, moderately, or poorly differentiated.

CLINICAL FEATURES

Symptoms and Signs

The most common presenting symptom is vaginal bleeding, seen in about 50% of patients. Other symptoms include abdominal pain and watery discharge. The abdominal pain is classically colicky in nature, due to the peristaltic activity of the fallopian tube. A dull, constant pain may occur due to chronic distention of the tubal wall and serosa. The vaginal discharge typically occurs as a gush of blood-stained fluid that may be associated with the colicky pain. Latzko described the classic syndrome of "hydrops tubae profluens" in 1916. It is characterized by an adnexal mass and colicky lower abdominal pain that is relieved by the discharge of copious serous fluid from the vagina. Although said to be pathognomonic, it is uncommonly encountered. The most common finding on physical examination is an elongated pelvic mass. Ascites may be present. Rarely, watery vaginal discharge or bleeding after hysterectomy has resulted in a diagnosis of fallopian tube carcinoma.

Diagnosis

The preoperative diagnosis of fallopian tube cancer is seldom made before surgery. In one review of 780 patients, only 10 (1.3%) were diagnosed preoperatively. Because of the rarity of the condition, the presence of a pelvic mass in a perimenopausal or postmenopausal woman usually suggests a primary ovarian neoplasm. Positive Papanicolaou smears have been reported in approximately 10% of cases. Patients with recurrent postmenopausal vaginal bleeding or an abnormal Papanicolaou smear (and for whom cervical and endometrial cancer have been ruled out by negative dilatation and curettage) should be suspected of having a tubal carcinoma. Laparoscopy may be helpful if the diagnosis is suspected and no pelvic mass is found by less-invasive methods.

Diagnostic Tests

Pelvic imaging studies usually demonstrate an adnexal mass that is cystic, complex, or solid in character. No specific pattern has been defined that could differentiate a tubal neoplasm from hydro- or pyosalpinx. In addition, this finding is usually interpreted to be an ovarian neoplasm, which is much more common. Computed tomography or magnetic resonance imaging may be helpful for evaluating spread to other intraabdominal or retroperitoneal structures. The detection of increased levels of the antigenic determinant CA125 has been described in patients with primary disease and with recurrent carcinoma. Positron emission tomography with fluorine-18-2-deoxyglucose has been reported to correlate with findings of recurrent disease.

Differential Diagnosis

Rarely does fallopian tube carcinoma enter the differential diagnosis of pelvic masses preoperatively. Intraoperatively, it should be distinguished from benign conditions that enlarge and affect the fallopian tubes such as endometriosis, ectopic pregnancy, hydrosalpinx, and tubo-ovarian abscess.

SPREAD PATTERN

The disease reaches the peritoneal cavity and its viscera through the tubal fimbria or through transmural invasion of the tubal wall. The mode of metastasis, according to most clinical studies, is intraperitoneal via the tubal ostia. Sedlis found the most frequent site of metastasis to be the peritoneum, followed by the ovaries and the uterus. The frequency of nodal metastasis in tubal cancer cannot be accurately determined since an evaluation for nodal involvement has not been done routinely by most authors. Tamimi et al. reported a 33% frequency of para-aortic nodal metastasis in their series of 15 patients. Nodal metastasis was present in two patients who had no other evidence of disease. This potential for nodal metastasis may explain the poor survival rate even when disease is apparently limited to the tube. Schray et al. found nodal involvement in 35% of their patients.

STAGING

Because of the clinical, therapeutic, and prognostic similarities to ovarian cancer, applying the ovarian staging system to tubal carcinoma has been proposed. Until recently, the International Federation of Gynecologists and Obstetricians (FIGO) did not have a staging classification for fallopian tube carcinoma. Although this entity represents a small fraction of all gynecologic cancers, the FIGO Committee thought a staging system should be established. The rules decided on are to a large extent similar to those for ovarian cancer staging. In 1991, FIGO accepted an official staging system for fallopian tube cancer (Table 5-1). In a review of 558 patients, 33%, 33%, and 33% were stage I, II, or II and IV, respectively. This is a more favorable statistic than for ovarian carcinoma, in which 70% of patients have stage III and IV disease. Peters et al. analyzed stage I patients and found a 50% depth of tubal muscularis invasion the only significant prognostic variable. However, other authors have not shown the depth of tubal invasion to be prognostic. Asmussen et al. reported two of two patients who died despite having disease limited to the tubal mucosa. Although tubal invasion is important, other factors must also be operative.

TREATMENT

Surgery

Surgical therapy for fallopian tube cancer should be the same as it is for ovarian cancer. In cases grossly confined to the tube, a careful staging procedure should be performed that includes peritoneal washings and systematic inspection and palpation of the peritoneal surfaces. Omentectomy, bilateral pelvic and para-aortic lymphadenectomy, and peritoneal biopsies should be performed. A limited number of patients with stage I disease have been treated with surgery alone without evidence of recurrence. One study examining routine lymphadenectomy found no cases of nodal metastasis in a small series of patients with disease grossly confined to the adnexa. Positive peritoneal washings carry prognostic significance, with a 5-year survival rate of 20% versus

Table 5-1. FIGO fallopian tube cancer staging*

Stage 0	Carcinoma in situ (limited to tubal mucosa).
Stage I	Growth limited to the fallopian tubes.
Stage IA	Growth is limited to one tube with extension into the submucosa and/or muscularis but not penetrating the serosal surface; no ascites.
Stage IB	Growth is limited to both tubes with extension into the submucosa and/or muscularis but not penetrating the serosal surface; no ascites.
Stage IC	Tumor either stage IA or IB with tumor extension through or onto the tubal serosa, or with ascites present containing malignant cells or with positive peritoneal washings.
Stage II	Growth involving one or both fallopian tubes with pelvic extension.
Stage IIA	Extension and/or metastasis to the uterus and/or ovaries.
Stage IIB	Extension to other pelvic tissues.
Stage IIC	Tumor either stage IIA or IIB and with ascites present containing malignant cells or with positive peritoneal washings.
Stage III	Tumor involves one or both fallopian tubes with peritoneal implants outside of the pelvis and/or positive retroperitoneal or inguinal nodes. Superficial liver metastases equals stage III. Tumor appears limited to the true pelvis but with histologically proven malignant extension to the small bowel or omentum.
Stage IIIA	Tumor is grossly limited to the true pelvis with negative nodes but with histologically confirmed microscopic seeding of abdominal peritoneal surfaces.
Stage IIIB	Tumor involving one or both tubes with histologically confirmed implants of abdominal peritoneal surfaces, none exceeding 2 cm in diameter. Lymph nodes are negative.
Stage IIIC	Abdominal implants greater than 2 cm in diameter and/or positive retroperitoneal or inguinal nodes.
Stage IV	Growth involving one or both fallopian tubes with distant metastases. If pleural effusion is present, there must be positive cytology to be stage IV. Parenchymal liver metastases equals stage IV.

*Staging for fallopian tube is by the surgical pathologic system. Operative findings designating stage are determined before tumor debulking.

67% for cases with negative peritoneal washings. If extratubal spread is found at the time of surgery, a maximal tumor-reductive effort should be performed with the main objective of leaving minimal (<1 cm) residual disease. Significant improvement in survival for patients with residual tumors less than 1 cm compared to those with larger residual tumors has been demonstrated. Barakat et al. noted an 83% 5-year survival rate for patients with stage II, III, or IV disease with no residual disease versus 29% with gross residual disease.

Radiotherapy

The efficacy of radiation therapy for tubal carcinoma is difficult to determine from the current literature due to the lack of uniformity in staging criteria, treatment fields, dosage, fraction size, and type of radiation used. The use of radiation therapy directed solely to the pelvis is of doubtful benefit because of the disease's potential for intraperitoneal dissemination. As in ovarian cancer, the entire peritoneal cavity may be at risk, and curability is limited by our inability to deliver therapeutic doses to the entire abdomen.

Chemotherapy

Indications

Because of the rarity of fallopian tube cancer, no controlled clinical trials have been performed. The role of adjuvant therapy for early-stage disease has not been defined.

Hormonal Therapy

The tubal epithelium is hormonally sensitive; however, the efficacy of hormonal therapy is not supported in the literature. Both estrogen and progesterone receptors have been identified in fallopian tube carcinomas. However, numerous authors have reported no response to hormonal therapy. Although responses were noted with cytotoxic regimens that included progesterone, the role of progesterone in these regimens is unclear.

Single-Agent Chemotherapy

A variety of alkylating agents including nitrogen mustard, thiotepa, chlorambucil, cyclophosphamide, and melphalan have been used for fallopian tube carcinoma. More recently, favorable responses have been seen with cisplatin used as a single agent.

Combination

Although the use of cisplatin-based combination chemotherapy for fallopian tube cancers has been reported since 1980, the cumulative experience is limited (Table 5-2). The overall response rate is 60%, with a 48% complete response rate. Peters et al. reported 46 patients evaluable for chemotherapy response. The response rate for 12 patients receiving cisplatin-containing multiagent chemotherapy was 81%, 75% of which were complete responses. This was significantly different than the response rates seen with multiagent chemotherapy (29%) or single-agent therapy (9%) without cisplatin. However, response rates for regimens without cisplatin may be low because they were used often for recurrent disease and after radiation. Barakat et al. reported 38 patients treated with cisplatinum, doxorubicin, and cyclophosphamide (N = 24) or cisplatinum and cyclophosphamide (N = 14). No difference in survival was noted.

RESPONSE TO THERAPY

Like ovarian cancer, in the absence of clinically evident or progressive disease, disease status is difficult to assess. Response to therapy and recurrence have correlated with CA125 levels.

Second-Look Surgery

The results of second-look laparotomy have been shown to be of prognostic importance in ovarian cancer. Overall, 65% of patients undergoing the procedure have no evidence of disease. The likelihood of having a negative second-look is related to the amount of residual tumor after initial surgery. Nodal evaluation is essential,

Table 5-2. Cisplatin-based therapy for fallopian tube carcinoma

Author	*N*	*PR*	*CR*	*Total*
Jacobs et al.	9	—	4	4
Maxon et al.	12	2	9	11
Peters et al.	16	1	12	13
Rose et al.	14	1	2	3
Morris et al.	9*	4	1	5
Muntz et al.	7	2	3	5
Barakat et al.	26	—	11	11
Pectasides et al.	11	2	8	10
Total	104	12	50	62

*Evaluated at second-look laparotomy.

and para-aortic nodal metastasis have been detected as the only evidence of persistent disease at second-look laparotomy. Survival for the patients who were pathologically disease-free was significantly different than for those who were clinically disease-free. Second-look laparoscopy is a less invasive means to determine disease status and, if positive, may be useful. However, the procedure is less sensitive and, if negative, should be confirmed by second-look laparotomy.

SURVIVAL AND RECURRENCE

The most important prognostic factor that correlates with survival is stage of the disease. Most authors have found significantly different survival rates between patients with disease confined to the pelvis and those with disease beyond the pelvis. Survival figures range from 40% to 60% for localized disease (stages I and II) and from 0% to 16% for more advanced disease (stages III and IV). In a multicenter retrospective study of 68 patients with stage I and II fallopian tube carcinomas, patients with grade 1 tumors had a significantly longer survival rate than patients with grade 2 or 3 tumors. Approximately 20% of patients who have a negative second-look laparotomy develop recurrent disease. In many cases, recurrences after negative second-look laparotomy have been at distant sites, such as the supraclavicular nodes, lungs, brain, kidney, and axilla.

Sarcomas

Malignant mixed mesodermal tumors of the fallopian tube are uncommon, with slightly more than 50 cases reported. However, they comprise a greater percentage of fallopian tube cancers than does ovarian sarcoma compared to ovarian carcinoma. The mean age at presentation, clinical features, stage at presentation, and spread pattern do not appear different from the more commonly encountered adenocarcinoma. An equal number of homologous and heterologous fallopian tube tumors have been reported. The diagnosis is not suspected or established until the final pathology report is completed. The prognosis of sarcoma patients is poor: Most patients survive less than 2 years, although long-term survival has been reported. Muntz et al. reported improved survival when the disease is confined to the muscularis. Carlson et al. reviewed 35 cases with sufficient treatment and follow-up data. Nine patients (26%) were disease-free after 36 months. In each case disease was limited to the pelvis, all disease was resected, and postoperative treatment was used (chemotherapy and radiation therapy, N = 5; chemotherapy alone, N = 2; and radiation therapy alone, N = 2). As in ovarian carcinoma, negative second-look laparotomy has been associated with long-term survival.

Trophoblastic Tumors

Tubal molar pregnancy occurs in 1 per 5,333 ectopic gestations or one per every 1.6 million normal intrauterine pregnancies. Primary choriocarcinoma of the tube is an even rarer entity and may be gestational or nongestational. Choriocarcinoma involving the tube should be distinguished from a primary intrauterine tumor or a malignant ovarian germ cell tumor. Preoperatively, the diagnosis mimics an ectopic pregnancy. A study from the New England Trophoblastic Disease Center reported 16 cases of tubal gestational trophoblastic disease (GTD). Tubal GTD accounted for 0.8% of GTD cases managed at the referral center. The frequency of partial moles, complete moles, and choriocarcinoma was similar: 31%, 31%, and 38%, respectively. None of the patients presented with symptoms of hyperemesis, toxemia, theca lutein cysts, hyperthyroidism, respiratory insufficiency, or markedly elevated human chorionic gonadotropin (hCG) (>30,000 U/ml). The surgical approach may be conservative (i.e., unilateral adnexectomy). All of the partial and four of the five complete molar pregnancies reported by the New England Trophoblastic Disease Center responded to partial or complete salpingo-oophorectomy. One patient with a complete molar pregnancy developed metastatic disease requiring chemotherapy. Pregnancy after conservative therapy consisting of unilateral salpingo-oophorectomy and chemotherapy has been reported.

Chemotherapy is an essential component in the management of tubal choriocarcinoma. Ober and Maier reviewed 76 cases of tubal choriocarcinoma. Forty-six of 59 patients treated in the prechemotherapy era died in contrast to one of 17 diagnosed in the postchemotherapy era. Treatment should be monitored by serum hCG titers. Nongestational choriocarcinoma has a poorer prognosis. Nongestational choriocarcinoma can be diagnosed only if germ cell elements other than choriocarcinoma are present.

Metastatic Tumors

Approximately 80% of tubal malignancies are metastatic from other sites, most commonly from the ovary and endometrium. Extragenital primary cancers metastasizing to the tube are much rarer, and other sites include the breast and gastrointestinal tract. With metastatic disease to the tube, the mucosa is intact. There is serosal involvement or nests of metastatic deposits are seen in the lymphatics underneath the epithelium.

Selected Readings

Asmussen M, Kaern J, Kjoerstad K et al. Primary adenocarcinoma localized to the fallopian tubes: Report on 33 cases. *Gynecol Oncol* 30:183, 1988.

Bannatyne P, Russell P. Early adenocarcinoma of the fallopian tubes. *Diagn Gynecol Obstet* 3:49, 1981.

Barakat RR, Rubin SC, Saigo PE et al. Cisplatin-based combination chemotherapy in carcinoma of the fallopian tube. *Gynecol Oncol* 42:156, 1991.

Barakat RR, Rubin SC, Saigo PE et al. Second-look laparotomy in carcinoma of the fallopian tube. *Obstet Gynecol* 82:748, 1993.

Carlson JA, Ackerman BL, Wheeler JE. Malignant mixed muellerian tumor of the fallopian tube. *Cancer* 71:187, 1993.

Finn WJ, Javert CT. Primary and metastatic cancer of the fallopian tube. *Cancer* 2:803, 1949.

Hu CY, Taymor ML, Hertig AT. Primary carcinoma of the fallopian tube. *Am J Obstet Gynecol* 59:58, 1950.

Jacobs AJ, McMurray EH, Parham J et al. Treatment of carcinoma of the fallopian tube using cisplatin, doxorubicin, and cyclophosphamide. *Am J Clin Oncol* 9:436, 1986.

Jones OV Primary carcinoma of the uterine tube. *Obstet Gynecol* 26:122, 1965.

Kein M, Rosen A, Lahousen M et al. Radical lymphadenectomy in the primary carcinoma of the fallopian tube. *Arch Gynecol Obstet* 253:21, 1993.

Latzko W. Linkseitiges Tubenkarzinom rechtsietige karzinomatose tubo-ovarian cyste. *Zentralbl Gynakol* 40:599, 1916.

Markman M, Zaino R, Busowski J, Barakat R. Carcinoma of the Fallopian Tube. In WJ Hoskins, CA Perez, RC Young (eds), *The Principles and Practice of Gynecologic Oncology*. Philadelphia: Lippincott, 1992. P 790.

Maxon WZ, Stehman FB, Ulbright TM et al. Primary carcinoma of the fallopian tube: Evidence for activity of cisplatin combination therapy. *Gynecol Oncol* 26:305, 1987.

Morris M, Gershenson DM, Burke TW et al. Treatment of fallopian tube carcinoma with cisplatin, doxorubicin and cyclophosphamide. *Obstet Gynecol* 70:1020, 1990.

Muntz HG, Rutgers JL, Tarraza HM et al. Carcinosarcomas and mixed muellerian tumors of the fallopian tube. *Gynecol Oncol* 34:109, 1989.

Muntz HG, Tarraza HM, Goff BA et al. Combination chemotherapy for advanced adenocarcinoma of the fallopian tube. *Gynecol Oncol* 40:268, 1991.

Muto MG, Lage JM, Berkowitz RS et al. Gestational trophoblastic disease of the fallopian tube. *J Reprod Med* 36:57, 1991.

Ober WB, Maier RC. Gestational choriocarcinoma of the fallopian tube. *Diagn Gynecol Obstet* 3:213, 1981.

Pectasides D, Barbounis V, Sintila A et al. Treatment of fallopian tube carcinoma with cisplatin-containing chemotherapy. *Am J Clin Oncol* 17:68, 1994.

Peters III WA, Andersen WA, Hopkins MP. Results of chemotherapy in advanced carcinoma of the fallopian tube. *Cancer* 63:836, 1989.

Peters WA, Andersen WA, Hopkins MP et al. Prognostic features of carcinoma of the fallopian tube. *Obstet Gynecol* 71:757, 1988.

Rose PG, Piver MS, Tsukada Y: Fallopian tube cancer—the Roswell Park Experience. *Cancer* 66:2661, 1990.

Rosen A, Klein M, Lahousen M et al. Primary carcinoma of the fallopian tube—a retrospective analysis of 115 patients. *Br J Cancer* 68:605, 1993.

Rosen AC, Sevelda P, Klein M et al. A comparative analysis of management and prognosis in stage I and II fallopian tube carcinoma and epithelial ovarian cancer. *Br J Cancer* 69:577, 1994.

Schray MF, Podratz KC, Malkasian GD. Fallopian tube cancer: The role of radiation therapy. *J Radiother Oncol* 10:267, 1987.

Sedlis A. Primary carcinoma of the fallopian tube. *Obstet Gynecol Surv* 16:209, 1961.

Tamimi HK, Figge DC. Adenocarcinoma of the uterine tube: Potential for lymph node metastases. *Am J Obstet Gynecol* 141:132, 1981.

Weber AM, Hewett WF, Gajewski WH et al. Malignant mixed muellerian tumors of the fallopian tube. *Gynecol Oncol* 50:239, 1993.

II
Cervix Cancer

6

Preinvasive Lesions of the Cervix: Diagnosis and Management

Ronald E. Hempling

The widespread use of cervical exfoliated cytologic screening has resulted in a 70% decline in the mortality from cervix cancer observed in the United States in the last 50 years. Moreover, the study of exfoliative cytology has helped elucidate the natural history of cervix cancer, which, for the most part, demonstrates an orderly, histologic documentable progression from a site of origin in normal endocervical epithelium through worsening stages of dysplasia (mild, moderate, and severe) to an in situ lesion and eventually invasive cancer. Equally important has been the repeated observation that the progression of the disease may be halted, frequently permanently, by excision or destruction of the abnormal area or areas. An understanding of the natural history of preinvasive lesions of the cervix, as well as their appropriate identification and management, is crucial if the heretofore described decline in mortality is to be maintained.

Nomenclature

The terminology used in the description of preinvasive epithelial lesions of the cervix has undergone substantial revision in the last 25 years (Table 6-1). The original standard description used the term *dysplasia*. This term referred to a spectrum of change in the surface epithelium that ranged from minor abnormalities in squamous metaplastic epithelium to near complete replacement of the epithelial layer of a given specimen or segments of the cervix by immature, neoplastic cells.

The term *mild dysplasia* described the condition in which undifferentiated cells (atypical cells with hyperchromatic nuclei and increased nuclear-cytoplasmic ratio demonstrating an increased mitotic index) occupy approximately the lower one-third of the epithelium. *Moderate dysplasia* described the finding that such cells replace two-thirds of the thickness of the normal epithelium, and *severe dysplasia* described the condition in which all but one or two of the most superficial cell layers of the cervical epithelium are replaced by undifferentiated cells. When the entire surface epithelium is replaced by such cells, the diagnosis of carcinoma in situ is made. All degrees of dysplasia are preinvasive; that is, the basement membrane (stromal-epithelial junction) remains intact. In the 1970s the term *cervical intraepithelial neoplasia* was introduced. Studies showed that the natural history of mild and moderate dysplasia was significantly different from that of severe dysplasia and carcinoma in situ and, furthermore, that the distinction between severe dysplasia and carcinoma in situ was artificial and of no clinical significance. Accordingly, the terms *dysplasia* and *carcinoma in situ* were replaced by the term cervical intraepithelial neoplasia (CIN) grades I–III, with grade I being equivalent to mild dysplasia, grade II to moderate dysplasia, and grade III including the two categories of severe dysplasia and carcinoma in situ.

Table 6-1. The 1988 Bethesda System for reporting cervical/vaginal cytologic diagnosis

Pap class	*Pap disease classification*	*CIN classification*	*Bethesda classification*
I: Benign	Benign	None	Atypical cells of undetermined significance
II: Atypical benign	Atypical cells are present but not dysplastic. Atypia is due to inflammatory koilocytosis atypia (mild)	None	Does not describe otherwise defined inflammatory, preneoplastic or neoplastic cellular changes
III: Suspicious	Cells consistent with dysplasia (1) mild (2) moderate	CIN I, CIN II	LGSIL ± cellular changes compatible with HPV
IV: Strongly suspicious for malignancy	Abnormal cells consistent with severe dysplasia or carcinoma in situ	CIN III	HGSIL ± cellular changes compatible with HPV
V: Conclusive for malignancy	Abnormal cells consistent with invasive cancer	None	Squamous cell carcinoma

CIN = cervical intraepithelial neoplasia; LGSIL = low-grade squamous intraepithelial lesion; HGSIL = high-grade squamous intraepithelial lesion; HPV = human papillomavirus.
Source: MS Piver, RE Hempling, KA Craig. Neoplasms of the Cervix. In JF Holland, E Frei, RC Bast et al. (eds), *Cancer Medicine* (3rd ed). Philadelphia: Lea & Febiger, 1993. Pp 1631–1646.

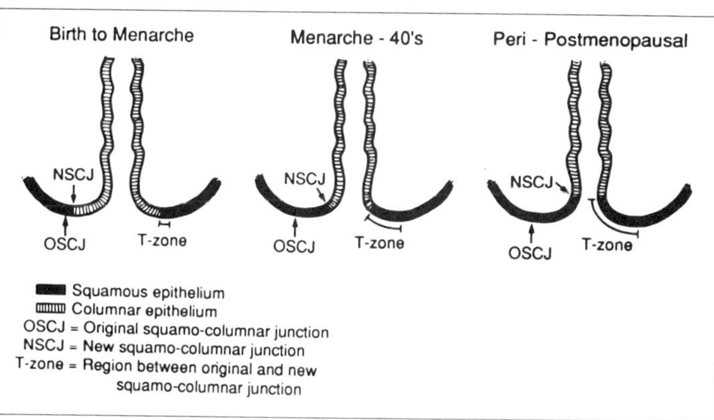

Fig. 6-1. The transformation zone. (From TC Wright Jr, RM Richart. Pathogenesis and Diagnosis of Preinvasive Lesions of the Lower Genital Tract. In WJ Hoskins, CA Perez, RC Young [eds], *Principles and Practice of Gynecologic Oncology*. Philadelphia: Lippincott, 1992. Pp 509–536.)

Recently there has been further modification in the terminology used to describe the histopathologic and cytopathologic changes observed in preinvasive lesions of the cervix. This change was based on an improved understanding of the role played by human papillomavirus (HPV) in the development of preinvasive lesions of the cervix, as well as invasive cancer. This system introduced the terms *low-grade squamous intraepithelial lesion* (LGSIL) and *high-grade squamous intraepithelial lesion* (HGSIL). The former term had approximately the same meaning as mild dysplasia and CIN I, whereas the latter included both moderate dysplasia (CIN II) and severe dysplasia/carcinoma in situ (CIN III). When cytopathologic or histopathologic evidence of HPV was observed, the diagnosis was modified to include these changes.

The most recent classification system has engendered no small amount of controversy. While its supporters contend that it simplifies the classification and treatment of precursor lesions, its critics maintain that the natural history of moderate dysplasia (CIN II) and severe dysplasia (CIN III) are not the same and that the diagnosis of HGSIL will result in unnecessary surgical manipulation of the cervix.

Regardless of the system used, communication between pathologist and clinician is imperative when any diagnosis is not clear.

Localization and Cellular Characteristics

SQUAMOCOLUMNAR JUNCTION

Prior to the fifth gestational month, the vagina and exocervix are covered by columnar epithelium, which is then replaced by squamous epithelium. The junction between the squamous epithelium of the exocervix and the columnar epithelium originating from the endocervical glands is referred to as the *squamocolumnar junction* (Fig. 6-1). During adolescence and during the first pregnancy, squamous epithelium (referred to as *metaplastic squamous epithelium*) replaces the columnar epithelium by metaplasia to form a new squamocolumnar junction that is progressively closer to the external os of the cervix. This metaplastic process is enhanced in the presence of an acidic environment in the vagina and under the influence of estrogen and progesterone. The area between the old and new squamocolumnar junction is referred to as the *transformation zone* and appears to be the site of origin of the majority of dysplastic and neoplastic cervical lesions. It is in this region that the carcinogens thought to be responsible for the development of cervical neoplasia appear to have their most significant impact.

CELLULAR CHANGES AND GROWTH FACTOR RECEPTORS

Mitotic Activity

In the normal squamous epithelium that covers the cervix, mitotic activity is confined to the parabasal layer. Mitotic activity in more superficial layers characterizes preinvasive precursors and, indeed, correlates with the degree of abnormality—that is, mitoses found in the upper third of the cervical epithelium are found in HGSILs. Moreover, ploidy analysis indicates that both diploid and aneuploid mitotic figures are observable and that aneuploid figures with greater mitotic activity demonstrate a greater proclivity to progress.

Koilocyte

Cells demonstrating perinuclear clearing and nuclear atypia are termed *koilocyte*. While electron microscopic studies and in situ hybridization techniques have demonstrated that koilocytes may indicate the cytopathic effect of HPV, perinuclear halos have been described in specimens obtained from patients with *Trichomonas vaginalis*, *Gardnerella vaginali*, and *Candida* species.

Epidemiology

INCIDENCE

It is estimated that 200,000 cases of cervical dysplasia are diagnosed in the United States each year. The majority of cases of CIN III are diagnosed in patients age 20–34 years with the peak incidence of 100/100,000 women years observed in the 25- to 29-year age group. The significance of the peak age at diagnosis of CIN III lies in its comparison to the peak age adjusted incidence of invasive cervical carcinoma, which occurs in the late fourth and early fifth decade of life. This near decade in difference in the peak age at diagnosis may be attributable to a latent period between the progression from preinvasive to invasive forms of cervical cancer. However, it has been estimated that 5% of CIN III lesions will progress to invasion in less than 3 years. Moreover, there is no reliable means of determining which lesions will progress or, more important, at what stage in the path to progression a given lesion is at the time of diagnosis.

Interestingly, while the age-adjusted incidence of cervical cancer for white women (7.9/100,000) is nearly half that of black women (12.8/100,000) or Hispanic women (15.8/100,000), the difference in age-adjusted incidence of in situ disease between the three groups differs by only slightly more than 5% (whites, 36.8/100,000; blacks,

Table 6-2. Risk factors for cervical intraepithelial neoplasia and cervix cancer

Early sexual activity (before age 17)
Multiple sexual partners
Male sexual partner has multiple partners
Human papillomavirus infection of the cervix
Smoking
Human immunodeficiency virus

30.4/100,000; and Hispanics, 33.1/100,000). This finding may reflect more access to therapy for diagnosis of in situ lesions than a proclivity for progression.

CLINICAL PROFILE RISK FACTORS

Numerous epidemiologic studies lend support to the nearly 200-year-old contention that cervix cancer and, therefore its precursor lesions, bear the characteristics of a sexually transmitted disease. The rarity of the disease among celibate nuns and higher incidence among prostitutes indicate that sexual activity, including age at first intercourse and number of partners, play an important role in the development of this disease. Case-control studies demonstrate a fivefold risk for the development of cervix cancer among women with multiple pregnancies (more than 10), multiple sexual partners, and a husband who has had multiple sexual partners (Table 6-2).

Schiffman and coworkers evaluated the relative risk for the development of CIN in a case-control study performed in Portland, Oregon. A twofold or greater relative risk for the development of CIN in HPV-negative women was observed among patients with six or more sexual partners, age at first intercourse of 16 years or earlier, a history of oral contraceptive use, three or more live births, and low socioeconomic status. While a slight increase in risk for patients who smoke cigarettes was observed, the risk was of a lesser significance than that reported by other researchers who have determined that smoking is an independent risk factor for the development of CIN. Similarly, although contraceptive use appears to be an independent risk factor for the development of cervix cancer in this study, the data are not compelling. Conversely, other studies did demonstrate an increased risk for the development of CIN among contraceptive users who were also HPV-16–positive.

Infectious Agents

While, as mentioned, cervix cancer and its preinvasive precursor lesions bear many of the hallmarks of a sexually transmitted disease, studies that have attempted to associate known venereal pathogens with these lesions have, until recently, failed to establish a causal relationship.

Herpes Simplex Virus

In the 1960s and 1970s, herpes simplex virus type II appeared to be a likely candidate for causation. The frequency with which the disease was detected was significantly greater among patients with cervix cancer than among control groups. However, while segments of the herpes virus genome have been detected in human cervix cancer, the frequency with which this occurs is far too low to prove a causative association. Additionally, prospective case-control studies failed to demonstrate an increased risk for the development of cervix cancer among herpes simplex virus–positive patients. In summary, while not causative, there may be some evidence that herpes simplex viruses serve as one of many cofactors in the development of cervix cancer.

Human Papillomavirus

Within the last 15 years, a growing body of evidence has accumulated to indicate that HPV is the venereally transmitted agent that serves as an important cofactor in the development of cervix cancer and its precursors. Over 60 different strains of this double-stranded DNA virus have been characterized, and at least 20 of these have been found in the human genital tract.

EPIDEMIOLOGY. While initial epidemiologic studies failed to demonstrate a clear association between HPV infection and cervical neoplasia, subsequent studies presented compelling evidence for such an association. A study that compared 759 patients with cervix cancer to 1,467 controls detected HPV-16/18 in 62% of patients with cervix cancer and 32% of controls. The presence of such DNA increased the risk of developing cervix cancer from 2.1 for a negative assay to 9.1 for a positive assay, even after controlling for all other risk factors.

Several studies have specifically addressed the significance of HPV presence for the development of precursor lesions. From a review of eight studies conducted between 1982 and 1989, a data base was created of 2,627 patients who had been evaluated for the presence of HPV infection and associated cervical abnormalities. Of 791 patients with confirmed cervical disease, 377 had LGSIL (CIN I), 261 had HGSIL (CIN II-III), and 153 had invasive cancers. HPV DNA was detected in 627 of these patients (79.3%). This detection rate was significantly ($p < .001$) higher than the rate observed among patients with atypia of uncertain significance (23.7%) or among 1,566 patients with no evidence of atypia or neoplasia (6.4%). Moreover, while 70% of LGSILs, 88% of HGSILs, and 90% of invasive cancers were assay-positive for HPV DNA, the different types of HPV DNA within each lesion group varied substantially. HPV-6/11 accounted for 24% of all positive patients with LGSIL but only 3% of patients with HGSIL, while HPV-16 was found in 24% of patients with LGSIL and 54% of patients with HGSIL. These data allowed for stratification of HPV types into low-risk (HPV-6/11, -42, -43, -44), intermediate-risk (HPV-31, -33, -35, -51, -52), and high-risk (HPV-16, -18, -45, -46) based on the calculation of the relative risk of association of a given viral type with a given lesion (Table 6-3). These data indicate that the association of HPV infection and cervical neoplasia is strong and type-specific, that LGSIL is associated with a heterogeneous group of HPV types, and that the widely held belief that HPV-6/11 is responsible for the majority of such lesions may be untrue. Additionally, it was observed that HPV-16 was numerically the most important viral type detected and was associated with nearly half of all HGSILs, but was also detected in 16% of LGSILs and 15% of apparently healthy women.

Cohort studies have demonstrated that patients with any HPV infection were 11 times more likely (95% confidence interval 3.7–31.0; attributable risk 78%) to have CIN II or III than those without HPV infection. When adjusted for other known risk factors for CIN, there was no substantive change in these calculations. Much of this excess risk was attributable to HPV-16/18. Among patients with documented HPV-16/18 infection, the relative risk was

Table 6-3. Classification of human papillomavirus types by risk of neoplasia and cancer

High-risk types
16
18
45
56
Intermediate-risk types
31
33
35
51
52
58
Low-risk types
6
11
42
43
44

Source: KD Hatch. Preinvasive cervical neoplasia. *Semin Oncol* 21:12–16, 1994.

11% (95% confidence interval 4.6-26.0; attributable risk 52%), while for any other virus type the relative risk was less than 3.5% and attributable risk less than 13%.

A large case-control study attempted to evaluate the role of HPV in coordination with other known risk factors for the development of CIN. Using unconditional logistic regression analysis, adjustment for HPV-positive DNA between cases and controls left only parity (>three live births) as a significant independent risk factor for the development of CIN. Among HPV-positive women, there was no evidence that sexual activity, education, income, or smoking remained associated with the development of precursor lesions.

While these data strongly support a crucial, perhaps causal, role for HPV in the development of cervix cancer and its precursor lesions, they fail to completely reconcile the near 100-fold difference in age-specific incidence of HPV-positive DNA patients (9,000–80,000/100,000 women years) and the development of CIN III (10–100/100,000 women years) reported by the Working Group on Preinvasive Cervical Neoplasia and Population Based Cancer Registries. Clearly, cofactors must be operant.

MOLECULAR GENETICS OF HPV-INDUCED TRANSFORMATION. Characterization and analysis of the genome of HPV has led to an understanding of the transformational activity of the virus. The 7800 base pair DNA is functionally divided into early (E) or late (L) based on protein products that appear either early or late in the course of viral replication. The most significant areas in the genome, with respect to transformation, appear to be the E2, E6, and E7 open reading frames (ORFs). The E2ORF appears to encode a growth regulatory substance that suppresses the activity of proteins encoded by the E6/E7ORF.

The exact mechanism by which transformation of host cells by HPV DNA occurs is not completely understood. However, two events appear to be crucial for transformation to occur. These events are the loss of the function of the E2ORF and the incorporation of transcriptionally active HPV DNA into the host DNA. It has been theorized that these two events result in the expression of proteins encoded by the E6 and E7 ORFs. Proteins encoded by these two ORFs appear to be interactive with the antioncogenic function of the retinoblastoma gene and the p53 gene. Interestingly, studies have demonstrated that the E6 protein of the high-risk HPV-16 DNA binds strongly to the p53 oncogene. Conversely, low-risk HPV-6/11 DNA may remain episomal and its E6-E7 products bind either weakly or not at all to host cell suppressor gene proteins.

Human Immunodeficiency Virus

An association between human immunodeficiency virus (HIV) seropositivity and the development of cervical dysplasia/neoplasia is well established. Studies have demonstrated that the frequency of cervical dysplasia among HIV-positive women may be as high as 40%. Moreover, the severity of disease with respect to lesion grade, extent of disease, and recurrence following treatment have all been demonstrably higher among seropositive women than among seronegative women. The precise reason for this association is unclear. However, the most likely explanation lies in the combination of common behavioral risk factors and the predisposition to HPV infection. The combination of HPV infection and low CD4 helper/inducer T lymphocyte count appears to significantly affect the development and course of squamous intraepithelial lesions of the cervix.

Screening

POPULATION AND FREQUENCY

In 1988, the American Cancer Society, the American College of Obstetrics and Gynecology, and representatives of several health care specialties issued a consensus recommendation for cervical cytologic screening. This recommendation states that "all women who are or have been sexually active or have reached age 18 should undergo an annual Pap test and pelvic examination. After a woman has had three or more consecutive satisfactory annual examinations with normal findings, the Pap smear may be performed less frequently at the discretion of her physician." While it is generally agreed that this statement endorses annual cervical cytologic screening, several caveats are worthy of mention (Table 6-4).

Pap Smear Screening in the Elderly (More than 65 Years of Age)

Although no mention of an age at which to discontinue screening is made in the joint resolution regarding screening for cervical cancer, recent publications indicate that the cessation of screening in women older than 60 years of age is acceptable practice. However, other studies have demonstrated that patients older than 65 years of age account for 25% of the nearly 13,000 new cases of cervix cancer diagnosed each year and 40% of the 7,000 annual deaths attributable to cervix cancer. These studies also demonstrated savings of $5,907 and 3.7 years of life for every 100 Pap smears performed among a population of elderly, low-income women. Thus, in the face of this data there is no cogent reason that cervical cytology should

Table 6-4. Frequency for Papanicolaou (Pap) smears

Condition	*Age or time*
Initial screening	Age 18 or onset of sexual activity
Initial negative smear in high-risk individuals (onset of intercourse at an early age, multiple sexual partners, high-risk male sexual partner, human papillomavirus infection, smoking)	Annually
Initial negative Pap smear in low-risk individuals (celibate, both partners monogamous, reliable cytology laboratory)	Following three negative yearly smears, every 3 years
DES offspring	Age 14, onset of menstruation or initiation of sexual activity, every 6–12 months
Following hysterectomy for benign disease	Every 3 years
Following treatment for CIN or invasive cancer	Every 3 months for 2 years, every 6 months for 3 years, and yearly thereafter

DES = diethylstilbestrol; CIN = cervical intraepithelial neoplasia.

not be performed on a regular basis for women 65 years of age and older. Such a practice is mentioned here only to condemn it.

Low-Risk Populations

Implicit in the American Cancer Society recommendation is the existence of a group of patients whose risk for developing CIN or invasive cancer is low enough to warrant screening at intervals greater than 1 year. The aforementioned epidemiologic evidence would indicate that patients truly at low risk for the development of squamous intraepithelial lesions and cervix cancer (1) are celibate or, if sexually active, are monogamous with a monogamous partner; (2) are nonsmokers; (3) have had a reliably performed and interpreted, satisfactory, negative cervical cytology annually for the preceding 3 years; or (4) have undergone hysterectomy for benign disease. Moreover, the extent to which the interval between Pap smears should be lengthened in low-risk populations remains controversial. The 1980 recommendation of the American Cancer Society of 3 years was based on large population-based and case-control studies performed outside the United States. These data demonstrate only a 3% change in the reduction in cumulative incidence of cervix cancer in populations that were screened every 3 years. Several authors have stated that these data may not be directly applicable to populations in the United States and have demonstrated an increased risk for cervix cancer even when the interval is lengthened to 2 years.

If a change in the annual Pap smear dictum is to be considered for a given patient or group of patients who meet criteria for inclusion in a low-risk population, important caveats must be born in mind. First, the Pap smear is not a perfect test. Even in the best of hands, a 5% false-negative rate can be expected. In light of the findings that indicate that 5% of CIN III lesions will progress to invasive disease in less than 5 years, the implications of a false-negative examination become obvious if the next exam is to be performed 3 years hence. Second, the elimination of an annual cervical cytology does *not* imply the elimination of an annual bimanual examination.

At-Risk Populations

Absent those characteristics that would classify a patient as "low risk," annual cervical cytologic screening for disease-free patients should be the norm. More frequent screening is warranted for some patients. Recommendations for screening in such patients are outlined in Table 6-4 and are discussed in greater detail later in this chapter. Worthy of mention is the small group of patients who were exposed to diethylstilbestrol (DES) in utero. Such patients should have their first Pap smear and pelvic examination at menarche, by age 14 years, when they become sexually active, or in the face of the development of symptoms such as discharge, bleeding, or pain. Cytologic sampling of the cervix and all four quadrants of the vagina should be performed initially and every 6–12 months thereafter.

CERVICAL CYTOLOGY: LIMITATIONS AND PERFORMANCE

While cervical cytologic sampling demonstrates excellent specificity (proportion of disease-free patients who have a negative test), its sensitivity (proportion of patients with disease who have a positive test) has been shown repeatedly to be relatively low. False-negative rates of 8–50% have been reported. The recognition that the majority of neoplastic lesions of the cervix arise at the squamocolumnar junction and sampling of this area as opposed to sampling of only the vaginal pool has markedly decreased the false-negative rate. Most authorities would agree that currently the false-negative rate of cervical cytology approximates 20% but can be reduced to 5% or less when a technically satisfactory smear is interpreted by a competent cytopathologist.

The Pap Smear: Technical Considerations

A satisfactory cytologic specimen can be obtained if the following guidelines are observed.

Patient Preparation

1. Patients should be instructed not to douche for 24 hours prior to cytologic sampling.
2. Pap smears should not be obtained during menses.
3. Intravaginal medications should be discontinued for at least 1 week prior to cervical cytologic sampling.

Examination

1. The Pap smear should be obtained prior to the bimanual examination.
2. The entire cervix and portio should be visualized.
3. Minimal lubrication should be used.

Obtaining the Specimen

Cytologic sampling should precede obtaining specimens for the detection of sexually transmitted disease or treatment of the cervix with acetic acid prior to colposcopy (Fig. 6-2).

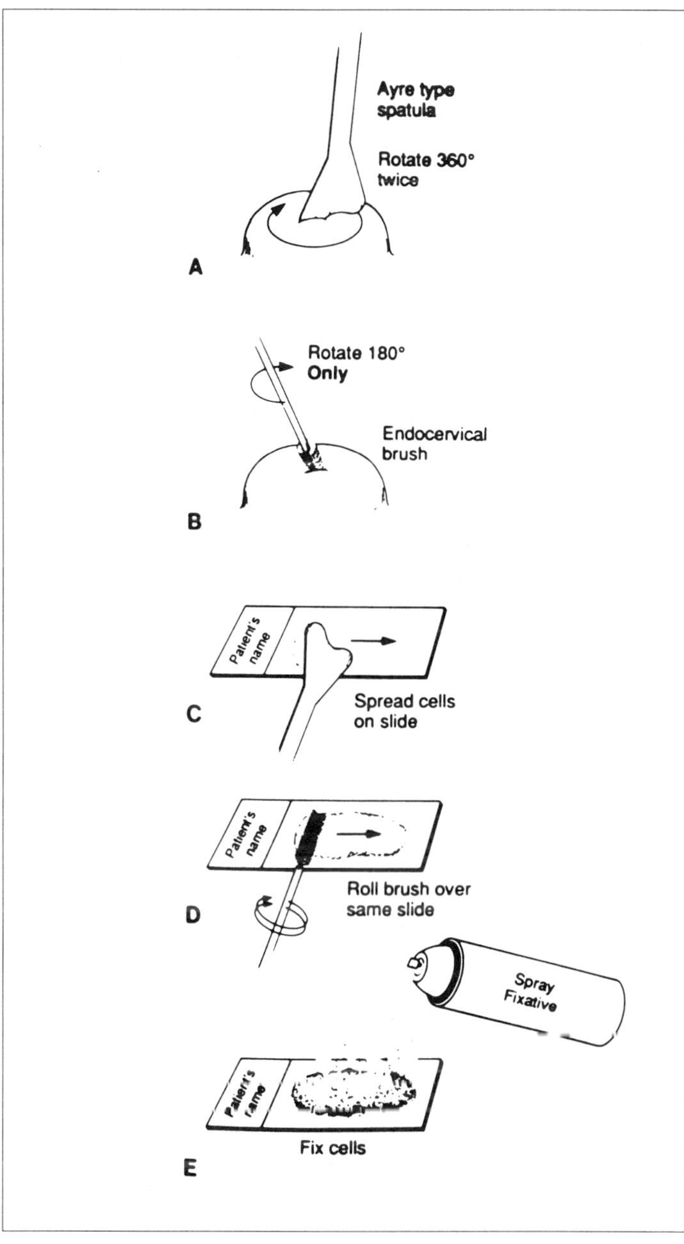

Fig. 6-2. Preferred procedure for obtaining a Pap smear. (From TC Wright Jr, RM Richart, Pathogenesis and Diagnosis of Preinvasive Lesions of the Lower Genital Tract. In WJ Hoskins, CA Perez, RC Young [eds], *Principles and Practice of Gynecologic Oncology*. Philadelphia: Lippincott, 1992. Pp 509–536.)

SAMPLING THE EXOCERVIX/PORTIO. The exocervix should be sampled first. A wooden Ayre-type spatula is placed on the cervix and rotated with firm but gentle pressure for a full 360 degrees. This specimen is then spread uniformly over a glass slide labeled with the patient's name, hospital number, and date.

SAMPLING THE ENDOCERVIX. Following the exocervical sample, the endocervix is sampled. The importance of sampling the endocervix cannot be understated. Studies have demonstrated a marked decrease in the false-negative rate of Pap smears when this technique is used.

Endocervical samples may be obtained by irrigation, by a saline-moistened cotton-tip applicator, or by an endocervical brush. Studies have indicated that the use of the endocervical brush results in a significant increase in the number of endocervical cells observed on cytologic smears. The endocervical brush is a collection device, not a curette. It is best used by gentle insertion into the endocervical canal and a single rotation of 180 degrees. Following this rotation, the brush is extracted and rolled over the face of the slide containing the exocervical sample. Vigorous brushing of the endocervical canal will result in bleeding, which may obscure cytologic evaluation as well as further inspection of the cervix. The risk of bleeding mandates that the procedure be used with care, if at all, in pregnant patients. In such patients, the moistened cotton-tipped applicator will suffice. However, a study of 300 pregnant patients demonstrated that the use of the cytobrush rather than a cotton-tipped applicator yielded a significant increase in adequate and abnormal smears with no adverse effect on pregnancy events observed among two groups so evaluated.

FIXATION. *Immediately after* the endocervical sample is obtained and rolled onto the slide, the specimen should be fixed. Time is of the essence, as air drying results in artifactual changes that hamper interpretation. If spray fixative is used, the container should be held at least 10 inches from the slide to avoid destruction of the cells by the propellant.

Management Decisions: Evaluation of the Abnormal Pap Smear

Crucial to the appropriate management of the patient with an abnormal cervical cytology are two precepts: (1) the Pap smear is a screening tool, not a diagnostic tool, and (2) definitive treatment must be based on histopathologic (biopsy) diagnosis.

THE NATURAL HISTORY OF INTRAEPITHELIAL LESIONS OF THE CERVIX

A wide variety of results have been reported by studies that have evaluated the natural history of CIN lesions with regard to regression, persistence, and/or progression (Table 6-5). Such differences are ascribable to differences in inclusion criteria and reflect the effect of invasive diagnostic modalities in the progression of disease. Studies of patients who have been followed by Pap smear and colposcopy only demonstrate that many dysplastic lesions progress and that the proportion of progressive lesions increases with the severity of disease (Table 6-5). Indeed, authorities agree that CIN III is a true cancer precursor and that most patients who do not undergo biopsy

Table 6-5. Natural history of squamous precursor lesions of the cervix

Author	*Diagnosis*	% *Negative*	% *Persistence*	% *Regression*
Hall	Slight dysplasia	62	24	13
	Moderate dysplasia	33	49	18
	Severe dysplasia	19	48	33
Nasiell	Slight dysplasia	62	22	30
	Moderate dysplasia	54	16	30
Baron	All dysplastic	6	28	66
Fox	All dysplastic	31	9	60
Koss	CIN I and II	39	15	42
	CIS	25	61	6
Syrjonen	CIN I	58	22	15
	CIN II	53	24	20
	CIN III	14	15	69

CIN = cervical intraepithelial neoplasia; CIS = carcinoma in situ.

or treatment will develop invasive cancer if they are followed long enough. While statistical support for this statement may not be readily apparent, there may be enough clinical experience to support the contention. Regardless, it is important to recall that while regression appears to be the norm for many CIN lesions, even low-grade lesions can demonstrate a progressive course. Thus, it is important to determine whether a lesion will progress at diagnosis.

DIAGNOSTIC MODALITIES

Colposcopy and Directed Biopsies

The appropriate management of cervical precursor lesions hinges on histopathologic confirmation of cytologic diagnosis and determination of the extent of disease. Over the last 25 years, examination of the cervix with magnification (colposcopy) has become an integral part of this evaluation.

The colposcope is a stereoscopic binocular low-power microscope. Colposcopic evaluation of the cervix is preceded by the application of dilute (4%) acetic acid to the cervix. This maneuver cleanses the cervix of mucus and debris and accentuates abnormal epithelium (acetowhite) and vascular changes that accompany neoplastic lesions. The vascular changes most frequently associated with HGSILs are punctation (end-on view of capillaries) and mosaicism (view of vessels running parallel to the surface).

The primary objectives of colposcopic examination are the following.

Determination of the Extent of Disease

Colposcopic evaluation of the cervix can help determine the size of the lesion, the area of the cervix involved, and whether the lesion can be seen in its entirety. Therapeutic strategies can be based on these findings.

Evaluation of the Transformation Zone

It should be recalled that the entire squamocolumnar junction is an area at risk for neoplastic lesions. Hence, its entire evaluation, in the face of cytologic abnormalities, is of crucial importance.

Directed Biopsy

Direct tissue sampling of areas of the cervix at highest probability of diagnosing the cytopathologically observed abnormality can be achieved by magnified examination of the cervix.

Numerous schemes have been described to report colposcopic findings. Perhaps the simplest of these describes the procedure by including whether it is (1) satisfactory (entire transformation zone visualized) or unsatisfactory (entire transformation zone not visualized); (2) whether the lesion is visualized in its entirety or not visualized in its entirety; and (3) a description of the vascular pattern of the lesion. While the expert colposcopist can frequently correlate colposcopic findings with histologic diagnosis, treatment strategies based on cytopathology and colposcopy in the absence of histologic confirmation should be discouraged in all but the rarest of circumstances.

Endocervical Curettage

Most authorities recommend that endocervical curettage be a routine part of the evaluation of the abnormal Pap smear even if the entire lesion is visible on colposcopic examination. Histologic confirmation of the absence of disease in the endocervical canal is crucial to the planning of definitive therapy (excisional versus ablative) or the maintenance of a conservative posture toward isolated lesions. Equally sanguine is the recommendation to avoid this operation in pregnant patients.

Cone Biopsy

The judicious use of colposcopy, colposcopically directed biopsies, and endocervical curettage in the evaluation of the abnormal Pap smear has led to a reduction in the need for diagnostic cervical conization. Nevertheless, this operation remains the final arbiter of determining the presence or absence of invasive disease when colposcopically directed biopsies and endocervical curettage yield equivocal results. Diagnostic conization should be performed if:

1. There is no colposcopically detectable lesion.
2. The entire lesion cannot be visualized.
3. The diagnosis of microinvasion is made by biopsy.
4. There is disagreement between cytology and colposcopically directed biopsy.
5. Adenocarcinoma in situ is diagnosed.
6. The results of endocervical curettage demonstrate disease.

EVALUATION OF INDIVIDUAL ABNORMALITIES

Figure 6-3 is demonstrative of a scheme that outlines the evaluation and treatment of cytologically detected cervical abnormalities.

Atypical Squamous Cells of Undetermined Significance

Regardless of the classification system, Pap smear interpretation has invariably included a description of cells that are neither clearly dysplastic nor clearly normal. Older classification systems define such cells as "atypical benign cells" or class II. The frequency with which such cells are reported ranges between 1.5% and 5.0%. Early recommendations for the management of such abnormalities were based on the premise that these cells represented inflammatory changes in response to infectious processes. Hence, the dictum of

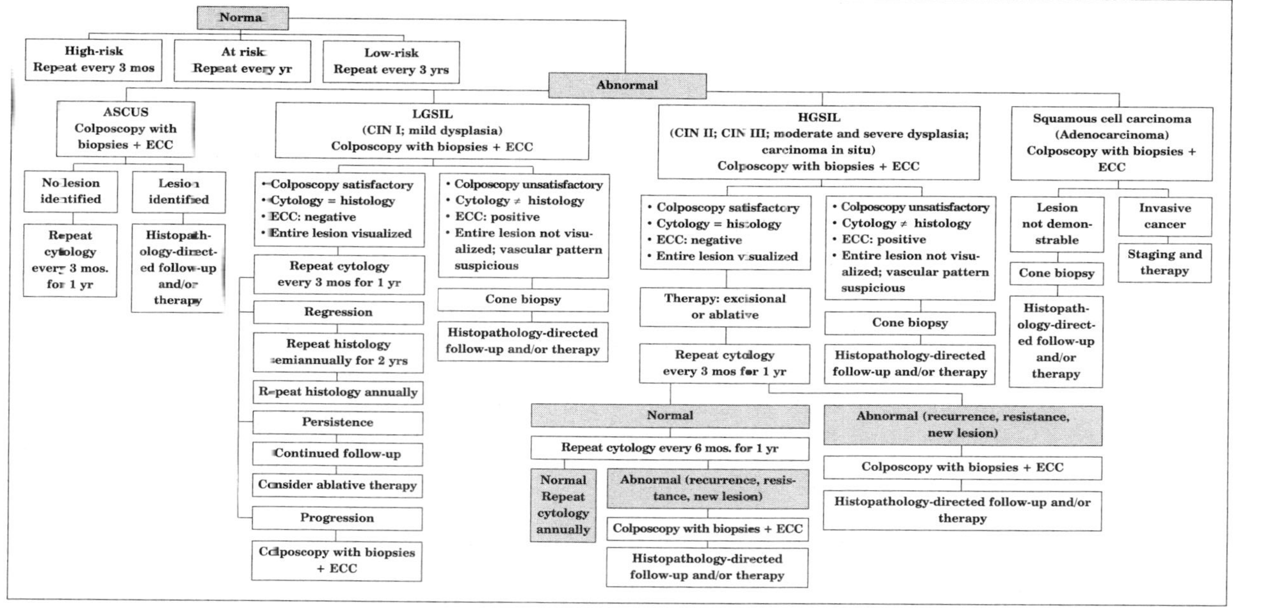

Fig. 6-3. Cervical cytologic evaluation. (ASCUS = atypical squamous cells of undetermined significance; ECC = endocervical curettage; LGSIL = low-grade squamous intraepithelial lesion; HGSIL = high-grade squamous intraepithelial lesion; CIN = cervical intraepithelial neoplasia.)

"treat and repeat" became the hallmark of evaluation for smears that demonstrated atypical but not clearly dysplastic cells. In fact, over the last 20 years, results from retrospective and prospective studies have clearly illustrated the danger of such a recommendation. Histopathologic evaluation of such patients demonstrates that 25–50% will have cervical dysplasia and approximately half of these will have high-grade lesions. One to three percent will have invasive cervical cancers.

In summary, it appears that a substantial enough proportion of patients with the diagnosis of atypical squamous cells of undetermined significance (ASCUS) on cervical cytologic examination harbor significant histopathologic abnormalities to warrant colposcopic evaluation and biopsy. The time-honored tradition of repeating atypical cytologies prior to definitive diagnostic procedures is mentioned here only to condemn it.

Low-Grade Squamous Intraepithelial Lesions

The evaluation of the patient with LGSIL (CIN I) on cervical cytology is remarkably controversial. The high regression rate and low progression rate of this lesion would lend support to the contention that nothing more than repeat cytologic evaluation at 4-month intervals constitutes adequate therapy. Nevertheless, it should be recalled that as many as 10% of patients with LGSILs may have HGSILs on further evaluation, and about 0.5% have been found to have invasive cancers. Accordingly, it would appear that colposcopy with biopsy and endocervical curettage is the most prudent evaluation for patients with LGSIL.

Equally controversial is the management of the LGSIL lesion. Proponents of conservative management with assiduous follow-up and resampling every 4 months point out that the risk of progression of LGSILs is extremely small and that excisional or ablative therapy with its incumbent, albeit small, risk of cervical injury is meddlesome for a lesion that carries a low oncogenic potential.

Authors who favor a more aggressive approach point out that there is no accurate way of measuring the oncogenic potential of a given LGSIL and that in a highly mobile society and particularly among patients in whom reliability for follow-up is questionable, ablative therapy provides insurance against progression regardless of the small risk of cervical injury.

Due to this controversy, some individualization of therapy appears prudent. While for the majority of patients, it would appear that histologic confirmation of LGSIL with assiduous follow-up—that is, repeat cytology every 4 months and institution of ablative therapy only in cases of progression or persistence for greater than 1 year—will obviate the misdiagnosis of an invasive lesion. A "see and treat" policy may be prudent if the patient is unable or unwilling to keep follow-up appointments. The use of the loop electrosurgical excision procedure (LEEP) in such circumstances has proved particularly efficacious (see the discussion below of treatment modalities).

High-Grade Squamous Intraepithelial Lesion (Moderate Dysplasia [CIN II] to Severe Dysplasia/Carcinoma in Situ [CIN III])

Few, if any, authorities would argue the need for colposcopy and directed biopsies as well as endocervical curettage among patients with HGSIL reported on cervical cytology. The purposes of this diagnostic regimen are to ensure the absence of an invasive lesion and to guide definitive therapy—that is, ablative versus excisional. If colposcopic evaluation is satisfactory (visualization of the entire transformation zone), cytology and biopsy of the most abnormal area that is colposcopically evaluable are in accord, the endocervical curettage demonstrates no abnormalities, and the entire lesion is visualized, the option of ablative therapy becomes viable. In the absence of any of the foregoing, cone biopsy must be performed to rule out invasive disease.

TREATMENT MODALITIES

Once the absence of invasive disease has been assured, a variety of therapeutic modalities is available for the treatment of precursor lesions of the cervix. The choice of modality depends on the nature of the lesion and the experience of the clinician.

Electrocautery

In the largest series reported to date, over 1,800 patients were treated with electrocoagulation diathermy with an overall eradication rate of 97%.

Cold Coagulation and Cryosurgery

The Somm cold coagulator has been used to treat a reported 1,600 patients. Despite the apparently shallow depth of destruction, a success rate of 95% following a single treatment has been reported. However, six invasive lesions (two microinvasive and four frankly invasive carcinomas) were subsequently discovered in treated patients.

Cryosurgery uses a refrigerant, usually N_2O, that cools a shaped probe to a temperature of approximately –50°C. To ensure adequate freezing, a double-freeze technique composed of a 3-minute freeze, a 5-minute thaw, and a second 3-minute freeze with an ice ball extending 4–5 mm beyond the edge of the probe is used.

While success rates of 90% or more are reported in CIN I and CIN II lesions, a 15–20% decrease in the success rate is observed following a single treatment for CIN III lesions. Initial observations demonstrated a significant increase in failure rates for cryotherapy among patients whose lesions occupied greater than two quadrants of the cervix. More recent studies have reported a 38% failure rate among patients whose lesions were greater than 30 mm in diameter, but only a 5% failure rate for lesions less than 30 mm in diameter. These observations may be explicable when one considers the finding that the thermal damage inflicted by cryotherapy extends to 5–6 mm, while the maximum depth of CIN-involved glands in a small but not insignificant percentage of cases reached 7.83 mm. Yet another disadvantage of cryotherapy is that the healing process following treatment results in the recession of the squamocolumnar junction into the endocervical canal. As a result, re-evaluation by colposcopy and cytology become increasingly difficult.

CO_2 Laser Surgery

The term *laser* is an acronym for *l*ight *a*mplification by *s*timulated *e*mission of *r*adiation. A laser is a device that produces a highly directional coherent (single-wave) light beam that can be focused to a very small spot. The CO_2 laser that provides light in a 10.6 μm range is the most widely used in the treatment of precursor lesions of the cervix. Because this wavelength is in the far infrared range and hence invisible, a supplementary helium-neon laser is used to provide an aiming beam. The energy of the laser is highly absorbed by intracellular water, with resultant conversion to steam and encumbant tissue vaporization. The laser is usually mounted on a colposcope and manipulated by controls that offer excellent precision in guiding the direction of the beam. The spot size of the beam and laser wattage afford a range of power densities that permit either vaporization of broad areas of tissue or scalpel-like incisions. Perhaps the most attractive aspect of the use of lasers in the treatment of CIN is that the abnormal area or areas can be accurately delineated and the volume of tissue ablated or excised can be accurately measured.

Technique

Colposcopic examination is performed and the abnormal areas on the cervix are identified. Such areas, which usually include the entire transformation zone, are then circumscribed by using the laser with an intermittent mode. Excision or ablation is then performed with the laser set at a power output of 20–25 watts and a spot size of 1.5–2.0 mm, yielding a power density of 800–1400 watts/cm^2. Excision or ablation includes a 3- to 4-mm margin of normal exocervical tissue and is carried to a *measured depth* of at least 7 mm in order to include endocervical glands.

Results

Results from recent studies demonstrate cure rates of near 95% or greater for all degrees of dysplasia. Persistence and recurrence rates described in large series are less than 5%.

Studies that have compared the use of laser surgery to cryotherapy in the treatment of CIN lesions have resulted in controversial findings. While several authorities have reported no difference in cure rates between the two modalities, others have demonstrated that while cure rates for CIN I and CIN II lesions are identical for the two modalities, the failure rate for CIN III lesions among patients treated with cryotherapy approaches 30%, while for patients with CIN III lesions treated with laser surgery the failure rate is only 5%. Further analysis of these rates indicated that for lesions of less than 30 mm in diameter, the failure rates for the two techniques were nearly identical at 5%. However, for lesions greater than 30 mm in size, the failure rate following cryotherapy was 38% compared to only 8% following laser surgery.

Loop Electrosurgical Excision Procedure

Concerns over the inadvertent ablative therapy of invasive cervical cancers have rekindled interest in excisional therapy for CIN lesions. Recently researchers have developed a low-voltage electrodiathermy loop that has the advantages of ablative therapy and provides submittable tissue for histopathologic evaluation.

Equipment

The LEEP wire is thin (0.2 mm in diameter), sterilized, insulated, stainless steel. LEEP wires are available in various sizes. The wire is heated by any one of a number of sophisticated electrosurgical generators that permit the optimal blend of cutting and coagulation current to be applied, thereby minimizing blood loss. As in the operating room, the use of such equipment mandates that the patient be grounded. A vacuum system evacuates the plume generated from the procedure.

Technique

The cervix is visualized and evaluated by colposcopy, and the abnormal areas and transformation zone are identified. Local anesthesia is administered. Vasopressin may be used to decrease blood loss. The generator wattage and blend are selected. A loop of appropriate size to encompass the lesion is selected and inserted into the cervical tissue approximately 5 mm lateral to the edge of the lesion and impressed to a depth of 5–7 mm. The loop is then drawn slowly across the lesion parallel to the surface of the cervix. The average cutting time is only a few seconds. Bleeding is usually minimal and may be controlled with electrocautery or chemical cautery. A second or third pass may be required if the entire lesion is not removed with the first excision.

Results

Collected series from the United Kingdom totalling over 2,000 patients demonstrated a success rate of approximately 95% for all grades of CIN, with the majority of patients having undergone a single treatment. Similar results have been reported in the United States. Success rates of 96% for CIN I lesions, 88% for CIN II lesions, and 94% for CIN III lesions have been reported.

Concerns and Disadvantages

The ease with which the LEEP procedure can be performed and its low complication rate (bleeding, 1–2%; cervical stenosis, <1%) have led several authors to recommend a "see and treat" policy for CIN lesions. This recommendation eliminates the steps of cervical biopsy and endocervical curettage in the evaluation of abnormal cervical cytology. Proponents of this regimen point out that the expert colposcopist can readily identify and easily correlate dysplastic changes without biopsy confirmation and thus definitively treat the patient with savings of the dollars and time required for biopsy confirmation. Opponents point out that the level of expertise required for such judgment is not universal and that a substantial number of low-grade lesions with high spontaneous regression rates will undergo unnecessary excisional procedures.

Cone Biopsy

Because of the widespread use of colposcopically directed biopsy, it has been estimated that only about 10% of patients currently referred for evaluation of abnormal cytology will eventually require cervical conization. Current indications for cone biopsy include (1) a positive endocervical curettage (indicating disease in the endocervical canal, the exact extent of which is unclear); (2) a cytologic assessment that indicates an abnormality not consistent with tissue diagnosis; (3) a situation in which the entire transformation zone is not visualized by colposcopy; (4) a cervical biopsy that is consistent with microinvasion; and (5) a cervical biopsy that detects in situ adenocarcinoma.

Technique

The size and depth of the cone biopsy are determined by the preoperative colposcopic evaluation and the use of Schiller's iodine solution. Preliminary suture ligation of the cervical branches of the uterine artery as well as the use of vasopressin have traditionally been recommended to decrease bleeding from the cone bed. While traditionally performed with scalpel and scissors, the CO_2 laser has gained wide popularity as an excisional tool for the performance of cone biopsy. Studies have demonstrated a significant decrease in both blood loss and late complications (infection and cervical stenosis) when the CO_2 laser is used for cervical conization as opposed to traditional methods. Distortion of the endocervical margin of the cone biopsy when performed by CO_2 laser has been reported but may be averted by excising the apex of the specimen with a scalpel.

Complications

Most large series describe complications that require intervention in about 15% of cases. The most common complication is hemorrhage, both immediate and delayed. Cervical stenosis occurs in 1–5% of cases.

The effect on future fertility and premature birth rate of cone biopsy is controversial. Several studies have demonstrated a significant increase in early pregnancy wastage, while others have failed to do so.

Results of Therapy

Whether performed with scalpel or CO_2 laser, large studies have reported that the cure rate for CIN III lesions treated with cervical conization ranges between 87% and 97%.

Of concern is the patient whose cone biopsy demonstrates disease extending to the margin of resection. The frequency with which this event is reported ranges from 5% to 40%, and the management of such patients remains somewhat controversial. Citing studies that have demonstrated residual disease in up to 50% of patients who underwent hysterectomy following cone biopsy with positive margins, some authorities have recommended further surgical evaluation for such patients. However, others have demonstrated that abnormal cytology following cone biopsy appears to be a more useful indicator of disease persistence than positive resection margins. Overall, while it would appear that the patient with a positive margin on cone biopsy is at increased risk for persistence or recurrence of disease, assiduous follow-up with cytology, colposcopy, and histologic sampling should obviate the need for further surgery in the majority of such patients.

Hysterectomy

Hysterectomy continues to provide a viable option for the definitive therapy of HGSILs. However, in light of the excellent cure rates observed with less radical treatment modalities, hysterectomy should rarely, if ever, be prescribed as definitive therapy in the absence of other indications for surgery. Such indications include (1) the presence of other gynecologic disorders that require surgical correction, such as symptomatic leiomyomata, pelvic relaxation, or persistent adnexal disease; (2) the desire for surgical sterilization in a patient for whom failure rates with tubal interruption procedures are unacceptable; (3) a patient's unwillingness or inability to comply with instructions for assiduous follow-up after cone biopsy, particularly if a positive margin is noted; (4) persistent or recurrent disease following conservative therapy; and (5) patient anxiety regarding the efficacy of conservative therapy.

Cervical Intraepithelial Neoplasia in Pregnancy

Studies have demonstrated that patients diagnosed with LGSIL or HGSIL in pregnancy can be successfully managed by frequent cervical cytologic examination and colposcopically directed biopsy. Conization should only be performed if cytology or biopsy indicate microinvasive disease or frank invasion cannot be ruled out by other means. If the results of conization fail to demonstrate invasive cancer, the patient may continue her pregnancy, as can the patient with microinvasive disease (<3 mm of invasion). Assiduous follow-up after delivery is mandatory.

Adenocarcinoma In Situ of the Cervix

The relative increase in invasive cervical adenocarcinomas as compared to their squamous counterparts has renewed interest in glandular precursor lesions and their management.

CYTOLOGIC DETECTION

The natural history of adenocarcinoma in situ of the cervix (ACIS) is not clearly understood. The lesion is thought to arise in the endocervical canal, making its detection in the absence of a thorough endocervical cytologic sample less likely. Even in the face of endocervical sampling, reports of the accuracy of detecting intraepithelial glandular (CIGN) lesions vary from 50% to 91%, with the majority of series reporting rates more closely approximating the former figure. Difficulties in correctly diagnosing CIGN lesions on cytologic specimens may well arise from a lack of uniformity in morphologic criteria and the finding that as many as 50% of CIGN lesions will be accompanied by squamous lesions that are more readily recognizable and more frequently diagnosed.

COLPOSCOPY

Unlike squamous precursor lesions, in which colposcopically detectable vascular patterns herald the presence of abnormalities, glandular precursors do not routinely lend themselves to colposcopic evaluation. Possible explanations for this discrepancy may lie in the endocervical location of the lesion beyond the range of the colposcope.

HISTOLOGIC CONFIRMATION

While several authors have maintained that ACIS is a disease multifocal in origin and is characterized by skip lesions in the endocervical canal, other authors have failed to confirm this finding. Nevertheless, concerns over the possible multifocality of the disease and the potential sites in which it may arise have led many authors to recommend a cervical cone biopsy in all patients with ACIS as the best means of determining the extent of disease. In light of the unresolved issue of multifocality in skip lesions, this recommendation appears to be prudent.

TREATMENT

Definitive therapy for ACIS remains controversial. Several authors recommend hysterectomy as the only safe, definitive therapy for the disease. These authors cite studies that demonstrate residual disease in the majority of hysterectomy specimens examined following cone biopsy for ACIS. Furthermore, they hold that the possible multifocality of the disease may belie its presence even in the patient who has negative cone margins. Additionally, the absence of predictable colposcopic and cytologic assurances of the absence of disease, as seen in squamous lesions, makes adequate follow-up difficult.

On the other hand, several small series of patients with ACIS who had tumor-free margins on conization have been followed for up to 5 years without evidence of recurrence. These studies are supported by the work of other authors who contend that conization with tumor-free margins serves as adequate therapy for ACIS. These authors contend that the disease is rarely multifocal and frequently located within 25 mm of the cervical os (18 of 19 cases). Moreover, in collected series of hysterectomy specimens following conization with tumor-free margins, residual disease is rare. While assiduous follow-up with frequent endocervical sampling is required, it would appear that for a select group of patients intent on maintaining fertility, cervical conization may be adequate therapy for ACIS with cone margins free of disease.

Conversely, there appears to be unanimity of opinion regarding the management of patients with positive cone margins. Over one-half of such patients will demonstrate residual disease in the hysterectomy specimen. While some authors indicate that repeat conization to exclude the possibility of invasive disease offers the option of continued conservative management, it would appear that hysterectomy in such patients is the more prudent choice.

Selected Readings

Baggish MS, Dorsey JH, Adelson M. A ten year experience treating cervical intraepithelial neoplasia with the CO_2 laser. *Am J Obstet Gynecol* 161:60, 1989.

Baron BA, Richart RM. A statistical model of the natural history of cervical carcinoma. II. Estimates of the transition time from dysplasia to carcinoma in situ. *J Natl Cancer Inst* 45:1025, 1970.

Bertrand M, Lickrish GM, Colgan TJ. The anatomic distribution of cervical adenocarcinoma in situ: Implications for treatment. *Am J Obstet Gynecol* 157:21, 1987.

Boyce JG, Fruchter RG, Romanzi L et al. The fallacy of the screening interval for cervical smears. *Obstet Gynecol* 76:627, 1990.

Brand E, Berek JS, Hacker NF. Controversies in the management of cervical adenocarcinoma. *Obstet Gynecol* 71:261, 1988.

Buller RE, Jones HW III. Pregnancy following cervical conization. *Am J Obstet Gynecol* 142:506, 1982.

Buxton EJ, Luesley DM, Wade-Evans T et al. Residual disease after cone biopsy: completeness of excision and follow-up cytology as predictive factors. *Obstet Gynecol* 75:29, 1987.

Duncan ID. Place of "cold" coagulation at 100°C in the management of CIN [abstract]. Proceedings of the World Congress in Cervical Pathology and Colposcopy. São Paulo, 1987.

Dyson N, Howle PM, Mounger K et al. The human papillomavirus 16E7 oncoprotein is able to bind to the retinoblastoma gene product. *Science* 243:934, 1989.

Ferenczy A. A comparison of cryo- and carbon dioxide laser therapy for cervical intraepithelial neoplasia. *Obstet Gynecol* 66:793, 1985.

Fink DJ. Changes in American Cancer Society checkup guidelines for the detection of cervical cancer. *CA* 38:127, 1988.

Fox CH. Biologic behavior of dysplasia and carcinoma in situ. *Am J Obstet Gynecol* 99:960, 1967.

Hall JE, Walton L. Dysplasia of the cervix: A prospective study of 206 cases. *Am J Obstet Gynecol* 100:662, 1968.

Koss LG, Stewart FW, Foote FW et al. Some histologic aspects of behavior of epidermoid carcinoma in situ and related lesions of the uterine cervix. *Cancer* 16:1160, 1963.

Lorincz AT, Reid R, Jenson AB et al. Human papillomavirus infection of the cervix: Relative risk associations of 15 common anogenital types. *Obstet Gynecol* 79:328, 1992.

Mandelblatt JS, Fahs MC. The cost-effectiveness of cervical cancer screening for low income elderly women. *JAMA* 259:2409, 1988.

Nasiell K, Nasiell M, Vaclavinkova V et al. Behavior of moderate cervical dysplasia during long-term follow-up. *Obstet Gynecol* 61:609, 1983.

Nasiell K, Roger V, Nasiell M et al. Behavior of mild cervical dysplasia during long-term follow-up. *Obstet Gynecol* 67:665, 1986.

NCI Workshop. The 1988 Bethesda System for reporting cervical/vaginal cytologic diagnosis. *JAMA* 262:931, 1989.

Ostor AG, Pagano R, Davoren RAM et al. Adenocarcinoma in situ of the cervix. *Int J Gynecol Pathol* 3:179, 1984.

Pater MM, Hughes GA, Hyslop DE et al. Glucocorticoid dependent oncogenic transformation by type 16, but not type 11 human papillomavirus DNA. *Nature* 335:82, 1988.

Pearson S, Whitaker J, Ireland D et al. Invasive carcinoma of the cervix after laser treatment. *Br J Obstet Gynecol* 96:486, 1989.

Reeves WC, Brinton LA, Mauance G et al. Human papillomavirus infection and cervical cancer in Latin America. *N Engl J Med* 320:1437, 1989.

Richart RM, Wright TC. Controversies in the management of low-grade cervical intraepithelial neoplasia. *Cancer* 71:1413, 1993.

Schafer A, Friedmann W, Mielke M et al. The increased frequency of cervical dysplasia/neoplasia in women infected with human immunodeficiency virus is related to the degree of immunosuppression. *Am J Obstet Gynecol* 164:593, 1991.

Schiffman MH, Bauer HM, Hoover RN et al. Epidemiologic evidence showing that human papillomavirus infection causes most cervical intraepithelial neoplasia. *J Natl Cancer Inst* 85:958, 1993.

Syrjonen K, Kataja V, Yliskoski M et al. Natural history of cervical human papillomavirus lesions does not substantiate the biologic relevance of the Bethesda system. *Obstet Gynecol* 79:675, 1992.

Ward P, Coleman DV, Malcolm DB. Regulatory mechanisms of the papillomavirus. *Genetics* 5:97, 1989.

Weisbrot IM, Stabinsky C, Davis AM. Adenocarcinoma in situ of the uterine cervix. *Cancer* 29:1179, 1972.

Werness BA, Levine AJ, Howle PM. Association of human papillomavirus type 16 and 18 E6 proteins with p53. *Science* 248:76, 1990.

Wright TC, Gagnon S, Richart R et al. Treatment of cervical intraepithelial neoplasia using the loop electrosurgical excision procedure. *Obstet Gynecol* 79:173, 1992.

Zur Hausen H. Herpes simplex virus in human genital cancer. *Int Rev Exp Pathol* 25:307, 1983.

Zur Hausen H. Human genital cancer: Synergism between two virus infections or synergism between a virus infection and initiative agents? *Lancet* 2:489, 1982.

7

Cervical Cancer

Ronald E. Hempling

Cervical cancer is the second most common cancer among women worldwide. Approximately 450,000 new cases are diagnosed each year, and nearly 200,000 deaths are attributable to the disease.

In the United States, cervix cancer is the third most common gynecologic malignancy, accounting for approximately one-fifth of all such cancers. In 1994, approximately 15,000 new cases were diagnosed and approximately 4,600 women died of the disease. While the age-adjusted incidence in mortality of cervix cancer has declined nearly 70% in the last half-century, resulting in an overall incidence of 8.7/100,000 and mortality of 3.0/100,000, a continued disparity in the incidence and mortality is observed when white and nonwhite populations are compared. The incidence of the disease among nonwhite women is 14.3/100,000, while among white women it is 7.9/100,000. Similarly, age-adjusted mortality among nonwhite women is 6.9/100,000, while age-adjusted mortality among white women is 2.6/100,000.

Detection and treatment of preinvasive cervical lesions accounts in large measure for the decline in mortality from cervix cancer among American women today.

Patient Profile: Risk Factors and Symptoms

RISK FACTORS

Risk factors are discussed in detail in Chap. 6 and enumerated in Table 6-2.

SYMPTOMS

The peak age at diagnosis of cervix cancer is between 45 and 50 years. The most common presenting complaint is abnormal vaginal bleeding. Such bleeding may take the form of intermenstrual bleeding, postcoital bleeding, or bleeding after douching. Not infrequently, the patient has a thin, serosanguinous, persistent, foul-smelling discharge.

Patients who present with advanced disease may complain of pelvic pressure or pain. Invasion of the perineural lymphatics may result in pain that is sciatic in distribution. Disruption of normal bowel or bladder function and leg edema are more common complaints of patients with advanced disease.

Evaluation and Staging

PHYSICAL FINDINGS

The physical findings on examination of the patient with cervix cancer are stage-dependent. They may range from cachexia, bilateral lower extremity edema, and supraclavicular adenopathy in the patient with advanced disease, to a patient with no abnormal findings in the case of a patient with occult lesions confined to the cervix.

Table 7-1. FIGO staging of carcinoma of the cervix

Stage	*Criteria*
I	Carcinoma is strictly confined to the cervix (extension to the corpus should be disregarded).
IA	Preclinical carcinomas of the cervix (i.e., those diagnosed only by microscopy).
IAi	Minimal microscopically evident stromal invasion.
IAii	Lesions detected microscopically that can be measured. The upper limit of the measurement should not show a depth of invasion of more than 5 mm taken from the base of the epithelium, either surface or glandular, from which it originates; and a second dimension, the horizontal spread, must not exceed 7 mm. Larger lesions should be staged as IB.
IB	Lesions of greater dimensions than stage IAii regardless of whether seen clinically. Preformed space involvement should not alter the staging but should be specifically recorded so as to determine if it should affect treatment decisions in the future.
IIA	Extends to the upper two-thirds of the vagina.
IIB	Extends to the paracervical tissue.
IIIA	Extends to the lower one-third of the vagina.
IIIB	Pelvic sidewall extension or ureteral obstruction on intravenous pyelogram.
IVA	Bladder or rectal mucosal involvement.
IVB	Distant metastasis.

The gross appearance of the lesion depends on whether the tumor is exophytic (the most common form of cervical malignancy), endophytic, or ulcerative. Exophytic lesions are friable and bleed easily. In some cases, the malignancy may develop entirely within the endocervical canal. In such cases, the portio may appear normal, but palpation demonstrates a firm, indurated, ballooned or barrel-shaped cervix.

DIAGNOSIS

While exfoliative cytology may indicate a cervical abnormality, any suspicious lesion, regardless of cytologic diagnosis, should be biopsied.

STAGING

Clinical Staging

Guidelines for the staging of cervix cancer are established by the International Federation of Obstetricians and Gynecologists (FIGO) (Table 7-1).

The FIGO stage of a given cervical cancer is determined in large measure by physical examination. At examination, meticulous attention should be paid to known sites of extrapelvic dissemination—that is, supraclavicular areas and the abdomen as well as complete pelvic examination. It is important to palpate the entire vagina to determine if the disease is confined to the cervix (IB), extends to the upper two-thirds of the vagina (IIA), or the lower one-third of the vagina (IIIA). Extension of the tumor into the parametria (IIB) or to the pelvic sidewall (IIIB) is best determined by rectovaginal examination (Figs. 7-1 and 7-2).

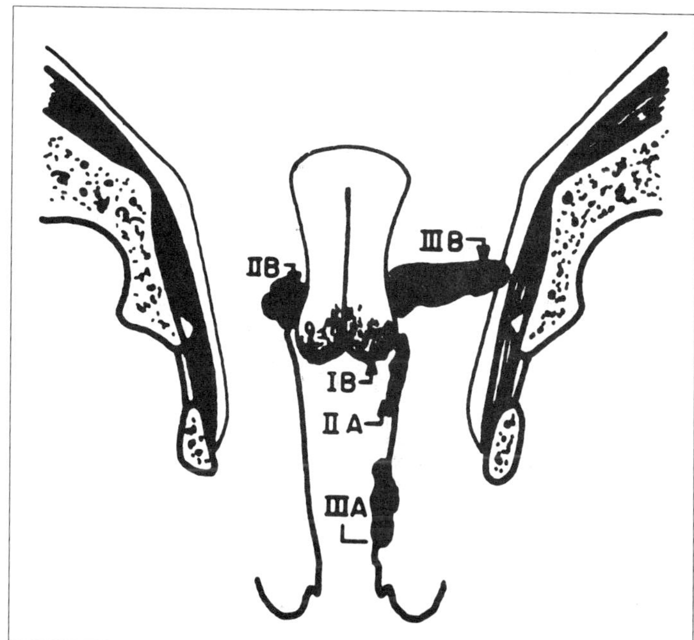

Fig. 7-1. FIGO stages IB to IIIB (stage IA is a microinvasive lesion and so is not shown here).

Determining the Extent of Disease

In addition to physical examination, FIGO allows complete blood count, liver function studies, chest x-ray, intravenous pyelography, cystoscopy, and sigmoidoscopy as additional studies in determining the extent of disease.

PYELOGRAPHY, CYSTOSCOPY, AND SIGMOIDOSCOPY. Studies have evaluated the routine use of pyelography, cystoscopy, and sigmoidoscopy in patients with cervical cancer. The routine use of these modalities in early-stage patients proved of little value.

OTHER IMAGING MODALITIES. Computerized tomography, lymphangiography, and magnetic resonance imaging have all been used in the evaluation of patients with cervical cancer. These techniques, however, appear to lack the reproducible sensitivity and specificity that would warrant their routine use for determining the extent of disease.

Surgical Staging

Absent substages of stage I cervical carcinoma, the disease remains one that is still staged based on nonsurgical findings, despite authoritative studies that have demonstrated that the discrepancy between clinical and surgical assessment of disease ranges between 20% and 40%.

Of crucial significance in such patients is the presence of disease remote from standard pelvic treatment portals—for example, in the para-aortic nodes. During the 1970s, researchers determined that 16%, 28%, and 33% of patients with stage II, stage III, and stage IV cervix cancer, respectively, had metastasis to the para-aortic nodes. Failure to deliver therapy to these areas is probably one of the major

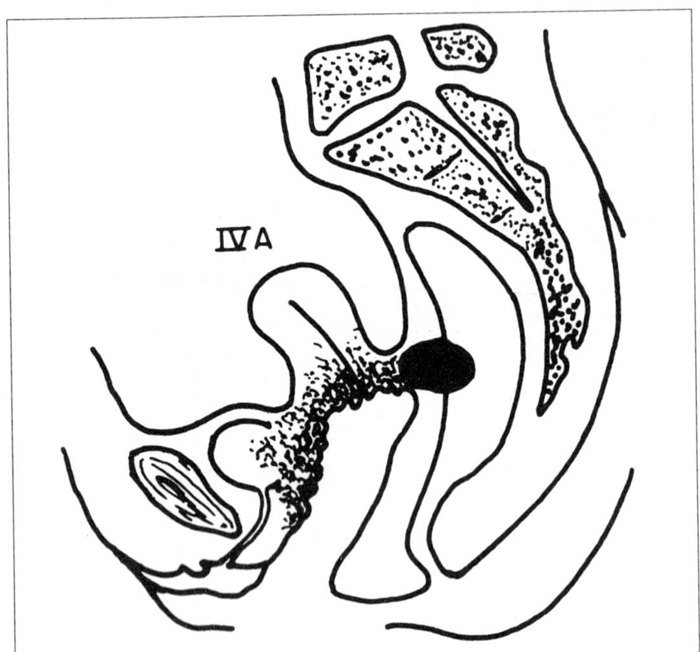

Fig. 7-2. FIGO stage IVA with involvement of the bladder mucosa or rectal mucosa.

reasons that 5-year survival for stage IIB–IVA cervix cancer has not improved during the last 40 years (Table 7-2).

Two techniques for operative assessment of nodal involvement by cervical cancer have been proposed: transperitoneal and retroperitoneal. The transperitoneal approach is associated with a prohibitively serious complication rate of 25–60% when extended-field radiation is mandated by surgical findings. An extraperitoneal approach to the iliac and aortic nodes that uses a J-shaped incision in the left lateral anterior abdominal wall has resulted in a marked reduction in enteric complications. A frequency of less than 5% is reported.

The surgical staging of cervical carcinoma remains controversial. While several authors contend that the use of extended-field radiation alone or in combination with chemotherapy may have a saluatory effect on survival, others maintain that the usefulness of extended-field radiation is limited by the coexistence of intraperitoneal disease in a substantial number of patients who have metastasis to the para-aortic nodes.

Peritoneal Cytology

Peritoneal washings obtained for cytology at the time of surgery for cervix cancer have not been found to have prognostic value.

Additional Tests

Tumor Markers

SQUAMOUS CELL CARCINOMA ANTIGEN. Squamous cell carcinoma antigen, a subfraction of the tumor-associated antigen TA4, is a

Table 7-2. Para-aortic node metastasis with stage II, III, and IV cervical cancer

	I		*II*		*III*		*IV*	
Study	*No.*	*%*	*No.*	*%*	*No.*	*%*	*No.*	*%*
Sudarsanam et al. (1978)	155	7	43	16	19	15	3	0
Buchsbaum (1979)	16	25	19	5	104	32	10	40
Nelson et al. (1977)	—	—	63	14	39	38	2	0
Rutledge (1975)	21	—	50	14	41	34	1	0
Piver (1977)	—	—	44	13	49	36	7	57
Hughes et al. (1980)	140	4	80	17	96	23	23	43
Berman et al. (1984)	158	5	265	16	180	25	17	17
Ballon et al. (1981)	22	23	48	18	23	17	—	—
Welander et al. (1981)	—	—	63	20	38	26	12	13
Delgado (1978)	18	0	—	—	—	—	—	—
	530	6	675	16	589	28	75	33

Source: Adapted from MS Piver. Current Management of Lymph Node Metastasis in Early and Locally Advanced Cervical Cancer. In FN Rutledge, RS Freedman, DM Gershenson (eds), *Diagnosis and Treatment Strategies for Gynecologic Cancer*. Houston: University of Texas Press, 1987 Pp 251 264.

4800-kd protein. Elevated levels of squamous cell carcinoma antigen are observed in over half of patients with primary cervical cancers and nearly 75% of patients with recurrent disease.

Several authors have reported that serial measurements of squamous cell carcinoma antigen correlate reasonably well with response to therapy, and elevated levels may precede clinical detection of recurrent tumor by several months.

CARCINOEMBRYONIC ANTIGEN. While more frequently observed among patients with adenocarcinoma of the cervix, the usefulness of the carcinoembryonic antigen in monitoring response to therapy and detecting recurrence has not been extensively evaluated.

Oncogene Expression

Studies have demonstrated an association between c-*myc* and H-*ras* overexpression among patients with cervix cancer. Increased amplification of c-*myc* is observed in all stages of disease, but more prominent overexpression is seen in advanced stages. Moreover, expression of either oncogene appears to have prognostic significance.

Cytometric Analysis

The results of the study of the prognostic value of flow cytometric analysis of cervix cancer have lacked uniformity. A significant improvement in prognosis for patients with DNA indices of less than 1.5 has been described in several studies, but other researchers have failed to confirm these findings.

Survival

The overall survival rate for patients with cervix cancer is stage-dependent. Stage I is subdivided into stage IA (microinvasive) and IB (frankly invasive). The 5-year survival rate decreases progressively from stage I through stage IV: IA, 98–100%; IB, 85–90%; II, 65%; III, 35%; and IV, 15%. This decrease is due in part to the increasing incidence of pelvic and para-aortic lymph node metastasis observed with increasing stage.

Patterns of Dissemination

Direct extension and pelvic nodal metastasis form the primary modes of dissemination. Spread to the common iliac and aortic nodes, as well as blood-borne and intraperitoneal metastasis, occur late in the course of the disease.

Microinvasive Carcinoma of the Cervix

DEFINITION: DEPTH OF INVASION

The diagnosis and management of microinvasive carcinoma of the cervix remains controversial. At its inception, the concept of microinvasive carcinoma of the cervix is the identification of a disease entity that carries with it little or no risk of extrauterine spread and may be successfully treated by nonradical modalities. In 1974, the Society of Gynecologic Oncologists (SGO) defined a microinvasive cervical carcinoma as a lesion that invades the cervical stroma of 3 mm or less below the base of the overlying epithelium and does not invade the lymphatic vascular spaces (LVSs). This definition gained wide acceptance. The 1989 *Technical Bulletin of the American College of Obstetricians and Gynecologists* modified the definition to include a lack of detectable confluency (fusion of advancing tongues of tumor). In 1985, the FIGO Cancer Committee changed its definition of stage IA cervical cancer by subdividing microinvasive carcinoma into stage IAi and IAii. The stage IAi lesions are described as those with minimal microscopically evident stromal invasion, and stage IAii lesions are described as having a depth of invasion of 5 mm or less taken from the base of the epithelial stromal junction or glandular epithelium from which the lesion originates and a horizontal spread that must not exceed 7 mm. Vascular or lymphatic space involvement did not alter staging. Concern over the inclusion of stage IAii lesions (≤ 5 mm invasion) has led to both retrospective and prospective evaluations of the potential for undertreatment of lesions at this stage of disease. Among 464 patients in 10 collected series in which invasion of the stroma was 3 mm or less, only one (0.21%) patient was found to have nodal metastasis. In contrast, of 132 patients in whom tumor invasion was measured at depths of 3.1–5.0 mm, nine patients (6.8%) had pelvic lymph node metastasis. The difference between these two proportions was highly significant ($p<.0005$) (Table 7-3).

Subsequent studies have described pelvic lymph node metastasis in 5–7% of patients with 3–5 mm of invasion, but only 0.5% of those with less than 3 mm of invasion.

The foregoing data indicate a significant risk of extrauterine disease among patients with greater than 3 mm of stromal invasion. Accordingly, such patients should not be considered candidates for conservative therapy.

Table 7-3. Frequency of lymph node metastasis based on invasion depth*

Study	*Depth of invasion <3.0 mm*		*Depth of invasion 3.0–5.0 mm*	
	No. of patients	*No. of patients with positive nodes*	*No. of patients*	*No. of patients with postive nodes*
Smith Foushee et al. (1969)	16	0	13	1
Roche and Norris (1975)	9	0	21	0
Leman et al. (1976)	32	0	3	0
Seski et al. (1977)	37	0	0	0
Taki et al. (1979)	55	0	0	0
Yajima and Noda (1977)	90	0	0	0
Hasumi et al. (1980)	106	1	29	4
Van Nagell et al. (1982)	52	0	32	3
Creasman et al. (1985)	24	0	8	0
Simon et al. (1986)	43	0	26	1
TOTAL	464	1 (0.21%)	132	9 (6.8%)

*Chi-square $p < .0005$.
Source: Adapted from MS Piver, PG Rose, MF Freedman. Changes in FIGO staging [letter]. *Am J Obstet Gynecol* 158:678, 1988.

LYMPHATIC SPACE INVOLVEMENT AND CONFLUENCY

Both lymphatic space involvement and confluency must be absent if the lesion is to meet criteria outlined by the SGO for the diagnosis of microinvasion. Inferential evidence of an increased risk of lymph node metastasis in the face of either of these findings had led most gynecologic oncologists to recommend radical therapy if either is diagnosed.

DIAGNOSIS AND TREATMENT

Diagnosis

While colposcopically directed biopsy and endocervical curettage are essential steps in evaluation, a biopsy that demonstrates microinvasion must be confirmed by cervical conization to ensure the absence of histologic features that might alter therapy.

Management Decision: Radical Versus Conservative

Studies that have compared simple hysterectomy to radical radiation or radical surgery for patients with microinvasive squamous cell carcinoma of the cervix have demonstrated no evidence of a significant increase in risk of recurrence or death from cervical cancer among patients treated with conservative therapy. Recent reports that describe a low incidence of residual disease in hysterectomy specimens following cone biopsy with negative margins substantiate the contention that in highly motivated patients who have a strong desire for maintaining fertility, cone biopsy may serve as adequate therapy.

Stage IB Cervical Cancer

Seventy percent of cervix cancers are clinically confined to the cervix at initial presentation. Two apparently equal efficacious modes of therapy for the treatment of such lesions are available: radical hysterectomy and pelvic lymphadenectomy and radical pelvic radiotherapy.

SURGICAL TREATMENT

Types of Hysterectomy

In a report by Piver, Rutledge, and Smith five types of hysterectomy for the treatment of cervical cancer were described. These classes of hysterectomy and their respective indications are outlined in Table 7-4 and Figs. 7-3 and 7-4.

Class I, II, and III hysterectomies are the most commonly performed. When pelvic lymphadenectomy is performed, all nodes from the common, external, and internal iliac vessels as well as the obturator fossa must be removed. The obturator lymph nodes are among the primary node group and are the most frequently involved by cervical cancer.

Postoperative Complications

In a review of nearly 7,000 patients treated by radical hysterectomy over the last 40 years, pulmonary embolism was noted in less than 1% of patients. Protracted bladder dysfunction occurred in 4% of

Table 7-4. Five classes of hysterectomy

Class	*Description*	*Indication*
I	TeLinde modification: Removal of all cervical tissue without dissecting into the cervix itself. Exposure of vasculature achieved by incision of pubovesical ligament with resultant lateral deflection of the ureter.	HGSIL (CIN III) Microinvasive (≤ 3-mm invasion) carcinoma
II	Moderately extended hysterectomy: Uterosacral and cardinal ligaments divided midway between attachment to sacrum and pelvic sidewall, respectively; upper one-third of vagina is removed.	Microinvasive carcinoma of cervix >3–≤ 5-mm invasion Uncertain cone margins
III	Meigs: Uterosacral and cardinal ligaments are divided at their attachment to sacrum and pelvic sidewall, respectively. Upper half of the vagina is removed. Pelvic lymphadenectomy is a routine part of the operation.	Selected stage IB–IIA lesions of the cervix
IV	Class III hysterectomy plus removal of *all* periureteral tissue; more extensive excision of paravaginal tissue; superior vesical artery is sacrificed.	Anterior: central recurrence where conservation of bladder is feasible
V	Class IV hysterectomy plus resection of involved distal ureter or portion of bladder.	Central recurrence involving portions of distal ureter or bladder

HGSIL = high-grade squamous intraepithelial lesion; CIN = cervical intraepithelial neoplasia.

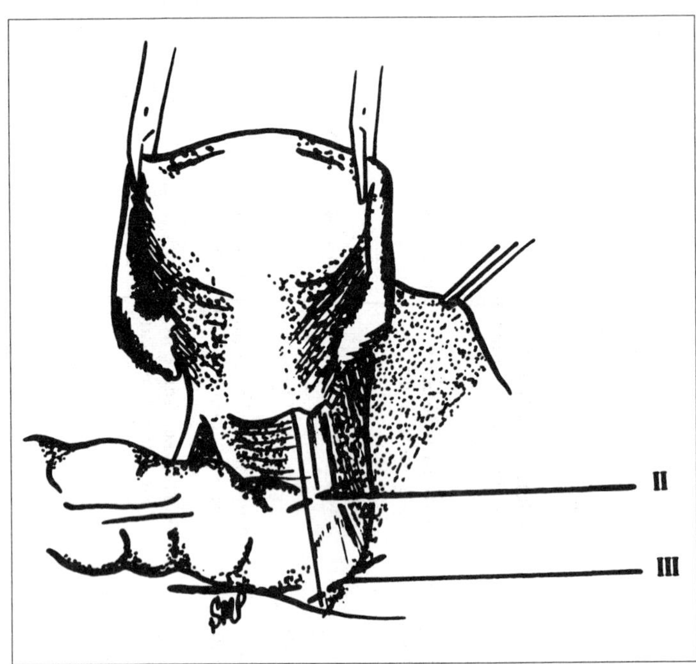

Fig. 7-3. With a class II hysterectomy, the uterosacral ligaments are divided midway between the uterus and their sacral attachments. With the class III operation, the uterosacral ligaments are excised at their sacral attachments.

cases. The rate of ureterovaginal and/or vesicovaginal fistula formation has decreased substantially over the last 40 years and now approximates 2.5%. Similarly, the incidence of lymphocyst formation has declined to about 2.5% following the advent of closed suction drainage. Operative mortality associated with the procedure is less than 1%.

RADIATION THERAPY

Treatment

Briefly, treatment is usually accomplished by a combination of teletherapy using supervoltage or megavoltage photons that deliver 5,040 cGy in 28 fractions to a standard pelvic port. Teletherapy is routinely followed by one or two brachytherapy applications that deliver an additional 7,000 cGy to the parametrial tissue with a resultant overall tumor dose of 10,000–12,000 cGy.

Complications of Therapy

Serious urinary tract complications, including fistula formation, occurred in about 2% of patients treated with radiation therapy. Serious gastrointestinal complications are reported in 3.3%. Curative doses of radiation therapy will result in ovarian ablation in virtually all patients and severe vaginal stenosis in over 50% of patients.

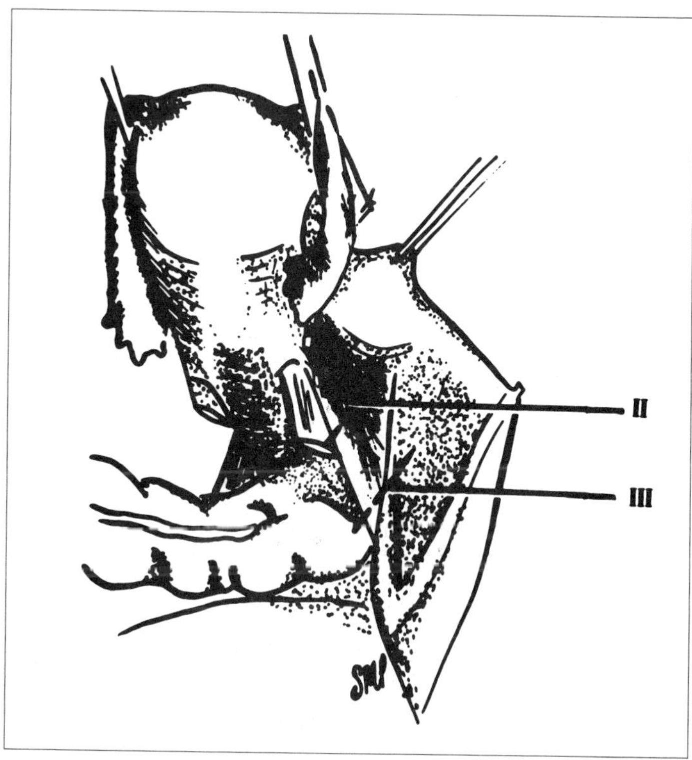

Fig. 7-4. Medial one-half of the cardinal ligament is removed with a class II hysterectomy. With a class III operation, the cardinal ligament is removed at the pelvic sidewall.

OUTCOME OF THERAPY

A recent literature review evaluated survival among 2,741 patients from 15 collected series who underwent surgical therapy for stage IB-IIA cervical cancer over the last 40 years. Overall survival was 83%, but a marked improvement in survival was noted in patients operated on before 1970 (73.6%) and those operated on in more recent years (87.9%). Nearly identical survivorship has been reported for similar-stage patients treated with radiation therapy. Several large series have described 5-year survival for stage I cervical cancer of 85–92%.

CHOICE OF THERAPY

The traditional reason for the choice of radical surgery over radiation in the treatment of localized cervix cancer has centered around patient age and the preservation of ovarian function. Recent studies have demonstrated that the risk for ovarian metastasis is less than 1% for patients with squamous carcinoma and 1.7% for patients with adenocarcinomas.

Neither age nor obesity will contraindicate surgery as therapy for stage I cervix cancer. Patients with significant adnexal disease,

Table 7-5. Size of cervical lesions and pelvic lymph node metastasis in stage IB cervical cancer

	Piver and Chung (1957–1967)			*Gynecologic Oncology Group (1981–1984)*		
Lesions	*No. of patients*	*No. with metastasis*	*%*	*No. of Patients*	*No. with metastasis*	*%*
≤ 3 cm	94	20	21.1	325	50	15.4
>3 cm	51	19	37.2	152	35	23.0
Total	145	39	26.0	477	85	17.8

Source: MS Piver, RE Hempling, KA Craig. Neoplasms of the Cervix. In JF Holland, E Frei, RC Bast, Jr et al. (eds), *Cancer Medicine* (3rd ed). Philadelphia: Lea & Febiger, 1993. Pp. 1631–1646.

inflammatory bowel disease, or prior radiation therapy may not be candidates for curative radiation.

Arguably the most significant factor in determining the success of the operation is lesion size. Stage IB cervical carcinoma lesions range in size from less than 1 cm to more than 6 cm. The recognition in the early 1970s that the excellent 5-year survival rate in patients with stage I cervix cancer was not universal led researchers to evaluate clinical parameters that were associated with improved outcome. Exemplary of these findings was a retrospective analysis of 145 women with stage IB cervix cancer treated with radical hysterectomy and bilateral pelvic lymphadenectomy. This study demonstrated that a cervical lesion size of 3 cm or less at clinical presentation and the absence of metastasis in the resected pelvic lymph nodes were significantly associated with 5-year survival rates approaching 90%. Indeed, the near 30% decline in 5-year survival rates among patients with lesion size greater than 3 cm was ascribed to the nearly 16% increase in positive pelvic lymph nodes observed among these patients (Table 7-5). More recent data have been reported from prospective analyses of patients with stage I cervix cancer performed by the Gynecologic Oncology Group (GOG). The first of these reports described 477 women with clinically appreciable stage I cervix cancer treated by radical surgery. Among patients with lesions of 3 cm or less, the frequency of lymph node metastasis was 15.4%, whereas among patients with lesions larger than 3 cm, 23% had positive nodes. A more recent evaluation of this population of patients noted a significant (p <.001) difference in 3-year disease-free interval among patients with lesions of 3 cm or less (85.5%) as opposed to those with lesions greater than 3 cm (68.4%).

The disappointing results for patients with cervical lesions measuring more than 3 cm in size treated by radical surgery suggest that radiation therapy is the treatment of choice for patients with stage IB cervical carcinoma whose lesions are more than 3 cm in size.

Among patients who are not surgical candidates but have lesions 3 cm or less, survival rates equalling those obtained by surgery can be achieved with radiation therapy. In a prospective study, patients with lesions of 3 cm or less who were not medically suited for surgery were compared to patients with similar lesion size treated by surgery. The 5-year survival rate for patients treated by radiation was 92–94%; for those treated by surgery it was 87.5–100%. These values do not differ significantly.

POSTOPERATIVE TREATMENT OF LYMPH NODE METASTASIS IN STAGE IB CERVICAL CANCER

Recent studies that have evaluated patients with surgically treated stage I cervical cancer have identified four risk factors that are significantly associated with lymph node metastasis. These factors are (1) depth of invasion ($p = .0001$); (2) capillary lymphatic space invasion ($p = .0001$); (3) tumor grade ($p = .01$); and (4) gross versus occult primary lesion. Multivariate analysis confirmed capillary space involvement, depth of invasion, parametrial involvement, and patient age as independent variables.

In hopes of improving survival, several authors have recommended the use of adjuvant pelvic teletherapy for patients with positive pelvic lymph nodes at surgery. In a collaborative GOG trial, the results of adjuvant teletherapy in 195 patients with stage IB squamous cell carcinoma of the cervix with positive pelvic nodes were evaluated. While the treated group demonstrated a decrease in local recurrence rate (84% versus 50%), the 5-year survival rate for patients who received pelvic radiation was 60% and for those who were untreated, it was 59%. While this study failed to demonstrate a survival advantage for treated patients, it suffers from a lack of uniformity in treatment regimens and that over half the patients in the treated group received 5,500 cGy or less of whole-pelvis radiation.

Better results have been reported by a small series of 52 patients with stage IB and IIA cervical cancer who had pelvic lymph node metastasis and were treated with either 4,000 cGy or 5,500–6,000 cGy of adjuvant pelvic teletherapy. Among those who received a lower dose, the 5-year survival was 53%. This rate did not differ from the 49% 5-year survival for untreated patients. However, the 5-year survival rate increased to 85% among women who received 5,500–6,000 cGy postoperative pelvic teletherapy.

Most retrospective studies that address the issue of adjuvant pelvic teletherapy for patients with pelvic lymph node metastasis and stage IB cervical cancer are biased because patients with more extensive nodal metastasis are more likely to be treated than those with one or two positive nodes. In hopes of obviating such a bias, 60 matched pairs of irradiated and nonirradiated patients according to stage, lesion size, and number and location of positive nodes were evaluated. Patients received a median dose of 5,000 cGy and 75% of the patients received a dose of 5,000 cGy or more. No significant difference was found between absolute 5-year survival for the surgery group (72%) and the surgery plus radiation group (64%).

Stage II, III, or IVA Cervical Cancer

Radiation therapy is the treatment modality of choice for patients with stage II, III, or IVA cervical cancer. The 5 year survival rate for such patients has remained essentially unchanged in the last four decades, primarily due to a failure to recognize and treat disease remote from the pelvis (i.e., in the para-aortic nodes) and the limited tolerance of normal tissues to higher doses of radiation.

Table 7-6. Survival rates for treated cervical cancer patients with positive para-aortic nodes

Study	*Year*	*No. of patients*	*Survival (%)*	*Follow-up*
Nelson	1977	1/8	13.0	4 yrs
Wharton	1977	3/24	12.5	2 yrs or more
Buchsbaum	1979	5/21	25.0	6 yrs
Hughes	1980	3/22	13.6	5 yrs
Piver	1981	3/31	9.6	5 yrs
Welander	1981	8/31	25.8	27–106 mos
Ballon	1981	4/18	23.0	5 yrs (actuarial)
Tewfik	1982	5/23	22.0	45–155 mos
Berman	1984	34/98	25.0	3 yrs (actuarial)
Brookland	1984	6/15	40.0	41–93 mos
Potish	1985	7/17	40.0	5 yrs (actuarial)
Lo Polla	1986	4/13	30.0	5 yrs
Blythe	1986	3/11	25.0	16–41 mos
Total		86/332	26.0	

Source: Adapted from WB Jones. Surgical approaches for advanced or recurrent cancer of the cervix. *Cancer* 60:2103, 1987.

SURGICAL STAGING AND CYTOREDUCTION

Surgical staging provides useful information for the planning of therapy. In a report of patients who received radiation therapy for cervical cancer following extraperitoneal staging, it was found that among patients with negative pelvic nodes, the 5-year relapse-free survival rate was 86%. While significantly better than that for patients with positive nodes, those with microscopically positive nodes and macroscopically resected nodes had nearly identical 5-year relapse-free survivals of 57% and 56%, respectively. Each of these was significantly (p <.001) better than patients who had non-resectable grossly involved pelvic nodes (0%).

Recently published data indicate that these observations may be extendable to patients with para-aortic lymph node metastasis treated with para-aortic radiation. None of the 19 patients with microscopic or small (<2 cm) disease had para-aortic failure as compared to 29% of patients with 2- to 5-cm disease and 70% of patients with greater than 5 cm disease. Moreover, 5-year survival rates were 50% for those patients with only microscopic disease, while no patient with greater than 5-cm disease survived 5 years (Table 7-6).

RADIATION THERAPY

Chemoradiation

As the maximum tolerated dose of radiation is now used to treat advanced cervix cancer, the evaluation of agents (radiosensitizers) that have the ability to potentiate the cytotoxic effect of radiation on cells has become an area of intense interest in the last three decades. Among the most important interactions between cytotoxic drugs and ionizing radiation are cell cycle specificity, cell synchronization to a radiosensitive phase of the cell cycle, impaired tumor repopulation, and inhibition of repair of sublethal injury.

Several agents, alone and in combination, have been evaluated as radiation sensitizers.

Hydroxyurea

Hydroxyurea is an S-phase cell cycle–specific inhibitor of DNA synthesis (inhibits ribonucleotide reductase) that reportedly acts as a radiation sensitizer by three mechanisms: (1) cell destruction in the relatively radioresistant S-phase of the cell cycle; (2) recruiting surviving cells at the G1/S interface, a relatively radiosensitive phase of the cycle; and (3) inhibiting repair of sublethal damage induced by radiation. Seven prospective randomized trials and one nonrandomized trial have been conducted in which hydroxyurea was used as a radiation sensitizer. All the randomized trials demonstrate improved progression-free survival for patients randomized to hydroxyurea versus placebo or misonidazole.

The trials that used hydroxyurea every third day during radiation and after radiation for a total of 28 courses over 12 weeks reported the best results compared to trials in which hydroxyurea was administered only twice weekly and only during radiation therapy.

Authorities have concluded that "while each of these [the above noted reports] studies by itself is open to some criticism, taken as an entity, they do suggest a role for hydroxyurea with radiation as standard therapy for patients with cervix cancer."

Cisplatin

The myelosuppression noted by some authors that accompanies the administration of hydroxyurea to patients receiving radiation has led other researchers to investigate less myelosuppressive agents. Chief among these is cisplatin. While the mechanism by which cisplatin may enhance radiation cytotoxicity is not completely clear, enhanced cytotoxicity by this cell cycle–nonspecific alkylating agent, as well as inhibition of repair of sublethal damage, appear to play prominent roles.

Small studies that have used cisplatin in combination with radiation therapy for patients with advanced cervix cancer have reported an approximate 20–30% improvement in response rates over radiation alone. However, the short follow-up of these patients, as well as the variability of the regimens used, preclude definitive conclusions.

Cisplatin Combinations as Radiation Sensitizers

Cisplatin plus 5-fluorouracil (5-FU) has been used concurrently with radiation therapy in several small studies among patients with advanced or recurrent cervical cancer. While complete response rates approaching 90% were reported, treatment-related complications were frequent and responses were not durable.

Non–Platinum-Containing Regimens

A sequential series of phase I/II studies that used standard or split-course pelvic teletherapy, a single brachytherapy application, and either 5-FU or 5-FU plus mitomycin-C in a total of 200 patients has been reported. Three-year actuarial pelvic control rates and actuarial survival by stage did not differ substantially from other reported series, and the use of the combination of 5-FU and mitomycin-C was associated with a significant ($p = .004$) increase in the incidence of serious radiation-induced complications.

NEOADJUVANT CHEMOTHERAPY

Randomized trials that have used cisplatin-based regimens before the treatment of advanced cervical cancer have been reported.

Survival rates in all three trials failed to demonstrate an advantage of neoadjuvant therapy over radiation alone.

NEW RADIATION MODALITIES

High-Dose Brachytherapy

High-dose brachytherapy offers the theoretical advantage of delivering 0.5–5.0 Gy per minute as opposed to 0.4–0.8 cGy per hour, which is the standard for low-dose brachytherapy. Proponents of the technique point out that its use obviates the need for anesthesia and hospitalization in the application of brachytherapy.

While survival and recurrence rates appear to be comparable to standard teletherapy and conventional low-dose brachytherapy, treatment regimens vary widely from institution to institution, and a disconcerting rate of late-occurring bowel and bladder injury has led some authors to question the efficacy of this technique.

Fast Neutron Therapy

Fast neutron therapy offers the theoretical advantage of a diminished dependency on oxygen for its cytotoxic effect and a diminished capacity of exposed cells to repair lethal damage. Studies in which californium 252 has been used in the treatment of patients with cervix cancer have failed, however, to demonstrate a significant advantage over standard therapy.

Recurrent Cervical Cancer

An estimated 35% of patients with cervix cancer will suffer recurrence of disease, the majority (80%) of which will occur within 2 years of initial therapy. The likelihood and time to recurrence appear to vary inversely with the stage of disease.

RECURRENCE FOLLOWING RADICAL SURGERY

Approximately 15% of patients treated for stage IB–IIA cervical cancer by radical surgery will suffer a recurrence of disease. Of these recurrences, approximately one-fourth will be local (at the apex of the vagina) and approximately one-fourth will be regional (in the pelvis or along the pelvic sidewall). The remaining 35–50% of recurrences are remote from the pelvis.

The surgical management of local recurrence following radical hysterectomy for stage IB–IIA cervical cancer, while feasible, is rarely reported and universally disappointing. The poor results from such procedures have led most authors to recommend radiotherapy for the treatment of local regional recurrence following surgery for stage IB–IIA cervical cancer. Unfortunately, the use of this modality has been less than uniformly successful. Salvage is reported in less than 35% of patients when radiation therapy is used.

SURGERY AND CHEMOTHERAPY FOR RECURRENCE FOLLOWING RADIATION THERAPY

Surgical Therapy

Surgical therapy for patients with recurrent cervical cancer following radiation therapy is an option limited to patients with central recurrence of disease. Only a small percentage of patients will therefore be eligible.

Patient Selection

The absence of disease remote from the histologically diagnosed central recurrence must be assured by physical examination, imaging studies, and laboratory evaluation. The triad of unilateral leg edema, sciatic pain, and ureteral obstruction in patients with recurrent cervix cancer is ominous and virtually pathognomonic of unresectable disease.

Choice of Procedure

RADICAL HYSTERECTOMY. The management of small-volume central recurrence following radiation therapy by radical hysterectomy has been reported by several authors. However, the prohibitive rate of serious postoperative complications (20–40%) has led to the abandonment of this procedure in all but the most highly selected patients.

PELVIC EXENTERATION. Total pelvic exenteration includes the radical resection of the uterus, urinary bladder, vagina, rectosigmoid colon, and anus. Exenterative operations may be either total (as described above), anterior (preservation of the rectosigmoid colon and anus), or posterior (preservation of the bladder), depending on the location of the recurrence. However, the high complication rate and the possible increased risk of incomplete resection combined with current reconstructive techniques have led most authorities to abandon all but the total pelvic exenteration.

At laparotomy, the most crucial event is the initial determination of resectability. Evaluation of the entire abdominal pelvic cavity must be carried out to ensure the absence of disease remote from the central recurrence or fixation of the parametrium to the pelvic sidewall. Nonresectable disease is reported in 20–50% of patients who undergo laparotomy. The most frequently noted reason for the determination of nonresectability was the finding of macroscopic peritoneal disease observed in 49 (44%) patients. Parametrial extension of disease accounted for discontinuation of the operation in 40% of patients, and the presence of nodal metastasis, either pelvic or para-aortic, was observed in 40% of patients.

Among patients with pelvic lymph node metastasis who undergo exenteration, 5-year survival ranges from 5% to 20%. The presence of pelvic lymph node metastasis should be considered a contraindication to surgery in all but the most highly selected patients.

Significant modifications in the original operative procedure described have lessened the operative morbidity and mortality as well as increased patient acceptance of the exenterative operation. The use of an isolated segment of ileum as a urinary conduit eliminated many of the complications associated with wet colostomy. The use of the sigmoid colon avoids the need for a small-bowel anastomosis but is associated with a higher incidence of hyperchloremic acidosis than is ileal urinary diversion.

The use of the transverse colon as a urinary conduit offers the advantage of using tissues remote from the standard radiation field and thus lessens the frequency of utero-enteric leaks. This theory is confirmed in a recent study in which the incidence of complications accompanying the construction of a transverse colon conduit in patients undergoing exenterative surgery (23%) was significantly ($p < .05$) lower than for those undergoing either ileal conduit (42%) or sigmoid conduit (61%).

Over the last decade there has been increasing interest in the use of continent urinary diversion among patients who undergo exenterative surgical procedures. Both ileum ascending colon and terminal ileum have been successfully used to create low-pressure, nonrefluxing, vesicostomies that are accompanied by relatively low complication rates and high continence rates.

Resection of the pelvic viscera leaves a large, denuded pelvic cavity. Adherence of small bowel to this area with subsequent obstruction, fistula formation, and/or perineal dehiscence has been a major source of morbidity and mortality for patients undergoing exenterative operations. Within the last 15 years, several authors have described a variety of methods to avoid intimate contact between the small bowel in this denuded area. The omentum creates a lid that effectively separates the bowel from the pelvic cavity and eventually descends to fill the pelvic defect. If the omentum is not large enough to create an adequate lid, the use of Vicryl mesh has been reported with satisfactory results.

In highly selected cases, supralevator exenterations have been performed. This procedure allows colorectal anastomosis facilitated by the end-to-end stapling device and obviates the need for permanent colostomy.

Vaginal reconstruction at the time of exenterative operation has been reported using a variety of techniques. The use of gracilis myocutaneous flaps, split-thickness skin graft placed in an omental cylinder, isolated segments of sigmoid colon, and femoral gluteal flaps has been reported.

While operative mortality from exenterative surgery has declined over the last 40 years, operative morbidity remains formidable. Twenty-five to 60% of patients will suffer significant postoperative complications. Infectious morbidity occurs in 10–50% of patients. Complications that require reoperation (small-bowel obstruction, fistula formation, or uteroenteric anastomotic leak or stricture) are reported in as many as 30% of patients. The mortality that accompanies reoperation varies among institutions from about 10% to over 50%.

Operative mortality in over 2,000 patients who underwent exenterative operations over the last 40 years is about 12% and cumulative 5-year survival in this group is 35.7%. Trends toward decreased mortality and improved survival are due in large measure to improved perioperative care and careful patient selection (Table 7-7).

Chemotherapy

Patients who develop recurrent cervix cancer following initial therapy that is amenable neither to radiation nor to surgery are treated with systemic chemotherapy. Thirty-eight cytotoxic agents have been evaluated in patients with advanced or recurrent squamous cell carcinoma of the cervix. Response rates for these patients are uniformly disappointing. It is theorized that the altered blood supply to the site of recurrence in the pelvis and the limited marrow reserve that results from radiation therapy may contribute to these poor response rates.

Cisplatin

Cisplatin is the most effective single agent used in the treatment of recurrent cervix cancer. The GOG has published three trials encompassing a total of 798 patients. In a review of the use of single-agent cisplatin in the treatment of recurrent squamous cell carcinoma of

Table 7-7. Operative mortality and 5-year survival following pelvic exenteration

Author	*Year*	*No. of patients*	*Operative mortality*	*5-year survival*
Douglas and Sweeny	1957	23	(1) 4.3%	(5) 22.0%
Parsons and Friedell	1964	112	(24) 21.4%	(24) 21.4%
Brunschwig	1965	535	(86) 15.0%	(108) 20.1%
Bricker	1967	153	(15) 10.0%	(53) 34.6%
Krieger and Embree	1969	35	(4) 11.0%	(13) 37.0%
Ketcham et al.	1970	162	(17) 7.4%	(62) 38.2%
Symmonds et al.	1975	198	(16) 8.0%	(64) 32.3%
Rutledge et al.	1977	296	(40) 13.5%	(99) 33.4%
Averette et al.	1984	92	(23) 23.9%	(37) 34.0%
Morely et al.	1989	100	(2) 2.0%	(61) 61.0%
Lawhead et al.	1989	65	(6) 9.2%	(15) 25.0%
Soper	1989	69	(5) 7.2%	(28) 40.5%
Shingleton	1989	143	(9) 6.3%	(71) 50.0%
Hatch et al.	1990	31	(0) 0.0%	(20) 68.0%
Total		2,008	(243) 12.1%	(707) 35.2%

Source: Adapted from PJ DiSaia, WT Creasman. *Clinical Gynecologic Oncology*. St. Louis: Mosby, 1993.

the cervix, it was concluded that the drug is more effective in patients who have not received prior chemotherapy, the response rate approximates 23% regardless of dose or schedule, and complete responses do occur with resultant improvement (approximately 5 months) in survival.

A provocative phase II trial of the combination of bleomycin, ifosfamide, and cisplatin (BIP) in 49 patients with recurrent cervical cancer has been reported. An overall response rate of 69% and complete response rate of 20% were reported. Toxicity was not prohibitive. The median duration of response was 8.4 months, and median survival was 10.2 months.

Maintaining that there were little data to substantiate the efficacy of bleomycin in the treatment of recurrent squamous cell carcinoma of the cervix and in hopes of avoiding pulmonary toxicity associated with the use of this drug, a collaborative trial of weekly cisplatin followed by cisplatin and ifosfamide in the treatment of 49 patients with recurrent squamous cell carcinoma of the cervix has been described. An overall response rate of 27.5% was observed and 20% of patients were complete responders. These data indicate that the addition of ifosfamide to cisplatin offered no significant added advantage in the treatment of recurrent cervix cancer.

Trials have evaluated the combination of 5-FU and cisplatin in the treatment of recurrent cervix cancer. The initial response rate of 50% has not been reduplicated in subsequent trials.

Ifosfamide, a structural analog of cyclophosphamide, has been evaluated as both a single agent and in combination regimens in the treatment of recurrent squamous cell carcinoma of the cervix. Phase III trials that have evaluated single-agent ifosfamide in patients with recurrent cervical cancer describe response rates of 15–30%.

Adenocarcinoma

ADENOCARCINOMA OF THE CERVIX

While in most earlier series adenocarcinoma of the cervix comprised only approximately 5% of invasive cervical lesions, recent studies describe an incidence rate of 10–20%. It is theorized that this increase is a reflection of the decreasing incidence of squamous cell carcinoma over the past few years.

The World Health Organization classified cervical adenocarcinoma into five subtypes: (1) endocervical adenocarcinoma, (2) endometrioid adenocarcinoma, (3) clear-cell carcinoma, (4) adenoid cystic carcinoma, and (5) adenosquamous carcinoma.

The average age of patients with adenocarcinoma of the cervix is similar to that for squamous cell carcinoma of the cervix. However, while squamous cell carcinoma is associated with human papillomavirus (HPV) infection, early age at first intercourse, multiple sexual partners, multiple pregnancies, cigarette smoking, and human immunodeficiency virus, patients with adenocarcinoma of the cervix appear to have risk factors similar to those associated with endometrial adenocarcinoma, including obesity, diabetes, hypertension, and nulliparity. Nevertheless, preliminary data indicate that HPV-16/18 may be detectable in over 50% of preinvasive glandular dysplastic lesions.

Controversy remains over whether adenocarcinoma of the cervix carries a significantly worse prognosis than squamous carcinoma of the cervix. In a study of 367 patients with cervical adenocarcinoma treated between 1965 and 1985, it was found that in lesions measuring less than 3 cm in diameter, the 5-year disease-free survival rate was 88% and the total pelvic failure rate, regardless of therapy, was 6%. Patients with lesions greater than 3 cm in diameter had a significant ($p < .002$) decrease in both 5-year disease-free survival (45–65%) and local control rates (23%).

It appears that among patients with adenocarcinoma of the cervix who have small (<3 cm) lesions, survival and pelvic control rates comparable to those achieved with squamous cell carcinoma are demonstrable with standard treatment modalities.

The lower survival and pelvic control rates observed among patients with bulky (≥ 6 cm) barrel-shaped (Fig. 7-5) cervical adenocarcinomas have led some authors to recommend adjuvant hysterectomy following radical radiation in hopes of decreasing the risk of recurrence and improving survival. In a study of 367 patients with cervical adenocarcinoma, no advantage was found in either survival or control rates in patients with stage IB or stage II cervical adenocarcinoma in whom adjuvant hysterectomy followed radiation therapy. A more extensive review of 371 patients with bulky cervical adenocarcinoma, 244 of whom were treated with radiation therapy alone and 117 of whom underwent adjuvant hysterectomy, found no significant advantage in local control rates for patients who underwent hysterectomy compared to those treated with radiation therapy alone, when treatment groups were adjusted for prognostic variables predictive of poor outcome. Ten-year survival and local control rates for patients treated with radiation therapy alone were 64% and 85%, respectively. Adjuvant hysterectomy improved these rates less than 5% in each incidence.

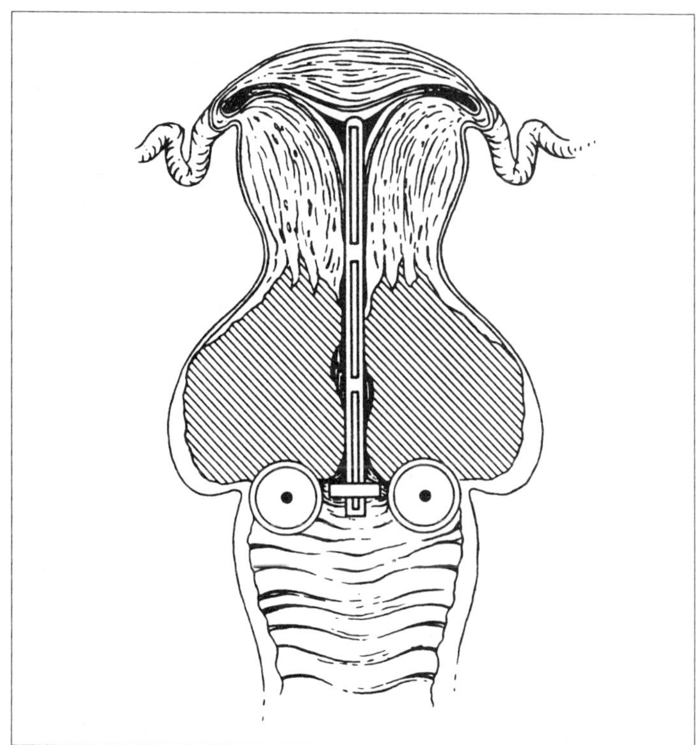

Fig. 7-5. Barrel-shaped carcinoma of the cervix.

The failure of adjuvant hysterectomy to improve survival in patients with bulky cervical adenocarcinoma is most likely due to the association of such lesions with metastasis remote from the standard treatment fields.

VARIANTS OF ADENOCARCINOMA OF THE CERVIX

Adenosquamous Carcinoma

Adenosquamous carcinoma accounts for 5–25% of all cervical adenocarcinomas. Although some authors have thought that survival rates are significantly worse for patients with this tumor than for those with adenocarcinoma, this observation is controversial. Treatment is similar, stage for stage, to that for other cervical cancers.

Glassy-Cell Carcinoma

Glassy-cell carcinoma is a poorly differentiated, rare form of adenosquamous carcinoma composed of cells with a ground-glass cytoplasm, distinct cellular borders, and prominent nuclear nucleoli. It is considered to be more aggressive than adenocarcinoma or adenosquamous carcinoma of the cervix, but its poor prognosis is likely related to the poor differentiation of the tumor rather than the glassy cell appearance. Whether a glassy cell carcinoma exists as a separate entity has been questioned.

Radical surgery plus adjuvant pelvic radiotherapy has demonstrated some efficacy in patients with stage I disease, but this report must be confirmed before standard therapy, the recommended therapy for patients with glassy cell carcinoma of the cervix, is abandoned.

Clear-Cell Adenocarcinoma

Clear-cell adenocarcinomas are characterized by the presence of varying combinations of clear and hobnail-shaped tumor cells arranged in solid masses and in papillary tubules. Many clear-cell adenocarcinomas have been detected in women exposed in utero to diethylstilbestrol. Treatment is similar to that for other cervical malignancies.

Adenoma Malignum

Adenoma malignum, which accounts for 1–3% of cervical adenocarcinomas, is also known as *minimal deviation adenocarcinoma* because the glands are well-differentiated and may even appear benign. However, this term is incorrect because these tumors are frequently deeply invasive and have a high frequency of early pelvic lymph node metastasis; moreover, unlike other carcinomas of the cervix, they more commonly spread intraperitoneally. Up to 5% of women with adenoma malignum have Peutz-Jeghers syndrome with buccal melanin and intestinal polyposis.

Adenoidcystic Carcinoma

Adenoidcystic carcinoma, a rare type of adenocarcinoma commonly identified in the respiratory tract, salivary glands, and breast is known as cylindroma, cylindromatous adenocarcinoma, or adenocystic carcinoma. Fewer than 75 cases of cervical tumors with adenoidcystic pattern have been reported. They are difficult to diagnose by light microscopy and are more easily diagnosed by electron microscopy. The overall prognosis is poor because such tumors have a higher incidence of lung and lymphatic metastasis than that seen with squamous cell carcinomas of the cervix. No satisfactory treatment has been proposed.

Suboptimal Treatment Scenarios

INVASIVE CANCER DIAGNOSED FOLLOWING SIMPLE HYSTERECTOMY

In the past, patients with suspected invasive cervical carcinoma detected at the time of standard hysterectomy were thought to have a poor prognosis. However, early studies documented that patients with only microscopic disease in the cervix, gross tumor in the cervical specimen with apparent tumor-free margins, or tumor cut through at the surgical margin but no known gross disease had an excellent 5-year survival rate ranging from 84% to 96% when treated in a timely fashion with radiation therapy. For patients with a postoperative biopsy positive for disease or who received treatment more than 6 months following initial surgery, the 5-year survival rate was only 47%. These findings are confirmed in a report that describes 122 patients who were treated with simple hysterectomy for invasive cervical cancer. Survival by groups as originally described in earlier reports was similar, and a significant improvement in 5-year disease-free survival was observed among patients with no gross disease at the initiation of therapy (75%) compared with those with gross disease at the time of initiation of therapy (39%).

Radical parametrectomy, upper vaginectomy, and bilateral pelvic lymph node dissection has been described in the treatment of patients with stage I cervical cancer who are originally treated with simple hysterectomy. Excellent 5-year survival is reported in carefully selected patients.

CARCINOMA OF THE CERVICAL STUMP

Stage for stage, carcinoma of the cervical stump is treated as cervical carcinoma of the intact uterus. When radiation therapy is used, however, the short cervix and the absence of the uterine cavity limits the amount of intracavitary cesium. It decreases the effective dose to the paracervical areas and thus requires higher-dose radiation than would normally be required for each stage. With the absence of the uterine fundus to protect loops of intestine from intracavitary cesium radiation and the not infrequent occurrence of fixation of the sigmoid colon by adhesions to the cervical stump, intestinal complications are higher than in patients receiving radiation of the intact uterus. However, 5-year survival rates are equal to those for cancer of the intact uterus. In the largest series reported (202 cases), the 5-year survival rates (no evidence of disease) were by stage: I, 91%; IIA, 77%; IIB, 54%; IIIB, 29%; and IV, 12.5%.

CERVICAL CANCER DURING PREGNANCY

Cervical cancer is an infrequent complication of pregnancy, with an average incidence rate of 1 per 2,020 pregnancies (0.45 per 1,000). This incidence varies according to whether the author also included cervical cancer diagnosed during the postpartum period and the length of the postpartum period, which in some series has been as long as 18 months. Ideally, the incidence includes only the diagnosis made during pregnancy.

Age, Symptoms, Type, and Survival

The average maternal age of 34 is approximately 14–16 years younger than the average age for invasive squamous cell carcinoma not associated with pregnancy. The most common symptom is abnormal vaginal bleeding, but approximately 20% of women are asymptomatic. More than 90% have squamous cell carcinoma and the remaindor adenocarcinoma. The 5-year survival rates, stage for stage, are equal to those in nonpregnant patients. Delivery by the vaginal or abdominal route does not adversely affect the 5-year survival rate

Conization

Before the advent of colposcopically directed biopsies, many patients underwent conization, with an average risk of abortion during the first trimester of 15–35% and bleeding that required transfusion in as many as 20–30%. With the advent of colposcopically directed biopsies, accuracy became nearly universal (99.5%) and the complication rate was reduced to only 0.6%. Conization of the cervix is usually reserved for patients with (1) a Pap smear suspicious of invasive cancer and (2) a transformation zone that is not fully visualized or (3) a colposcopically directed biopsy that demonstrated microinvasion. A wedge resection of the area of the transformation not seen may be performed rather than full conization. Endocervical curettage should be avoided.

Treatment

Before 24 weeks' gestation, invasive cervical cancer is treated, stage for stage, as in the nonpregnant patient, with the understanding that it will result in the death of the fetus. Patients with cervical cancer in its early stages can be treated by radical hysterectomy and pelvic lymphadenectomy or pelvic irradiation followed by intrauterine and vaginal cesium. Patients in the first trimester of pregnancy are treated by the latter method and 70% abort the fetus before receiving 4,000 cGy of radiation to the pelvis. However, during the second trimester of pregnancy, because abortion frequently does not occur, the fetus must be removed surgically before radiation therapy. When the cervical cancer is detected at the time of fetal viability, cesarean section is performed before initiation of therapy. Invasive cervical cancer detected early during the third trimester poses the most difficult decision for both physician and mother. Patients with cervical cancer diagnosed 4–8 weeks prior to fetal viability must be treated individually. Thus, the patient's concern for fetal survival must be weighed against the risk associated with delayed therapy. If expert neonatal care is available, delay beyond 30–34 weeks is probably not justified. Once one decides to wait until fetal viability, the lecithin/sphingomyelin ratio should be determined to ensure that there is fetal lung maturity prior to delivery.

Rare Tumors of the Cervix

VERRUCOUS CARCINOMA OF THE CERVIX

Verrucous carcinoma of the cervix is a variant of squamous cell carcinoma and rarely originates in the cervix. To date, fewer than 30 cases have been reported.

Diagnosis

This cancer, characterized by an exophytic wart-like growth that is difficult to differentiate from condyloma acuminatum and papillary squamous tumors of the cervix, exhibits a high degree of maturation and levels of nuclear atypia that often result in negative cervical cytology. Moreover, superficial biopsies frequently reveal only the benign characteristics of the tumor, and malignant diagnosis is made only by deep biopsies of the growth.

Treatment

Because wide local excision results in a high local recurrence rate and a high incidence of associated lymph node metastasis with the recurrence, a more rational approach of treatment would be a radical approach (radical hysterectomy for stages I and II) including resection of the lymph nodes. For patients with more locally advanced cervical cancer, radiation therapy should be used.

SMALL-CELL CANCERS OF THE CERVIX

Electron microscopy allows for identification of neurosecretory granules of the neuroendocrine carcinomas and special silver salt stains (argyrophilic stains) allow identification of carcinoid tumors and thus differentiate the different types of small-cell cervical cancers.

Neuroendocrine Carcinoma of the Cervix

Neuroendocrine carcinoma is a variant of small-cell carcinoma characterized by the presence of neurosecretory granules. They are characterized by early widespread metastasis. Local tumors are best treated by radiation therapy and require postoperative chemotherapy. The ideal systemic chemotherapy regimen for such patients has yet to be described, but encouraging results in a small group of patients treated with cisplatin, doxorubicin, and etoposide have been described.

Carcinoid Tumors of the Cervix

Carcinoids originating from the cervix are rare tumors of endocrine origin. They originate from argyrophil cells in the cervix. Approximately 25 cases have been reported, and none were associated with carcinoid syndrome. Except for rare stage I cases treated by surgery, few patients with carcinoid of the cervix have responded to treatment.

Oat Cell Carcinoma

Oat cell carcinoma is a rare, aggressive form of small-cell cancer with the appearance of bronchogenic oat cell carcinoma.

Small-Cell Carcinomas Without Neuroendocrine Granules or Argyrophilic Staining

Squamous cell carcinomas that contain basaloid features composed of small cells with the invading pattern of common squamous cell cancer of the cervix and not associated with neuroendocrine granules or argyrophilic staining should be treated as ordinary squamous cell carcinoma. These tumors are not as aggressive as the other three small-cell cancers.

CERVICAL SARCOMAS

Cervical sarcomas are rare tumors that originate in the cervix and include leiomyosarcomas, stromal cell sarcomas, rhabdomyosarcomas, adenosarcomas, and mixed müllerian sarcomas. Of the approximate 100 reported cases, no standard treatment has been followed and the prognosis has been uniformly poor irrespective of treatment.

MALIGNANT LYMPHOMAS OF THE CERVIX

Malignant lymphoma originating in the cervix is a rare entity that occurs in approximately one of every 730 cases of malignant lymphoma. Over the past 30 years, approximately 30 cases have been reported. Diagnosis is by biopsy of suspicious lesions even in the presence of normal cervical cytology, as cervical cytology was accurate in fewer than one-half of the reported cases. Pretherapy evaluation should include bipedal lymphangiography. Because these lesions are so highly radiocurable, there is little place for surgery in their treatment.

MALIGNANT MELANOMA OF THE CERVIX

Fewer than 15 cases of malignant melanoma of the cervix have been reported. Like other melanomas, the only survivors are those treated by surgery. To state that melanoma is arising primarily in the cervix, there should be melanocytes in the normal cervical epithelium and junctional changes demonstrated in the tumor. The prognosis is poor and only a few of the reported patients are known to be alive.

Selected Readings

Averette HE, Nguyen HN, Donato DM et al. Radical hysterectomy for invasive cervical cancer. A 25 year prospective experience with the Miami technique. *Cancer* 71:1422, 1993.

Buxton EJ, Meanwell CA, Hilton C et al. Combination bleomycin, ifosfamide, and cisplatin chemotherapy in cervical cancer. *J Natl Cancer Inst* 81:359, 1989.

Delgado G, Bundy BN, Fowler WC et al. A prospective surgical-pathological study of stage I squamous cell carcinoma of the cervix: A Gynecologic Oncology Group study. *Gynecol Oncol* 35:314, 1989.

Delgado G, Bundy B, Zaino R et al. Prospective surgical-pathological study of disease-free interval in patients with stage IB squamous cell carcinoma of the cervix: A Gynecologic Oncology Group study. *Gynecol Oncol* 38:352, 1990.

Eifel PJ, Morris MM, Oswald MJ et al. Adenocarcinoma of the uterine cervix. Prognosis and patterns of failure in 367 cases. *Cancer* 65:2507, 1990.

Greer BE, Easterling TR, Mclennan DA et al. Fetal and maternal considerations in the management of stage IB cervical cancer during pregnancy. *Gynecol Oncol* 34:61, 1989.

Himmelmann A, Holmberg E, Janson I et al. The effect of postoperative external radiotherapy on cervical carcinoma stage IB and IIA. *Gynecol Oncol* 22:73, 1985.

Jones WB. Surgical approaches for advanced or recurrent cancer of the cervix. *Cancer* 60:2103, 1987.

Kinney WK, Alvarez RD, Reid GC et al. The value of adjuvant whole pelvis radiation after Wertheim hysterectomy for early stage squamous cell carcinoma of the cervix with pelvic nodal metastasis: A matched control study. *Gynecol Oncol* 34:258, 1989.

Kinney WK, Egorshin EV, Ballard DJ et al. Long-term survival and sequeli after surgical management of invasive cervical carcinoma diagnosed at the time of simple hysterectomy. *Gynecol Oncol* 44:24, 1992.

Komacki R, Cox JD, Hanson RM et al. Malignant lymphoma of the uterine cervix. *Cancer* 54:1699, 1984.

Lewandowski GS, Copeland LJ. A potential role for intensive chemotherapy in the treatment of small cell neuroendocrine tumors of the cervix. *Gynecol Oncol* 48:127, 1993.

Lotocki RJ, Krepart GV, Paraskeves M et al. Glassy cell carcinoma of the cervix: A bimodal treatment strategy. *Gynecol Oncol* 44:254, 1992.

Lovecchio JL, Averette HE, Donato D et al. Five year survival of patients with paraaortic nodal metastasis in clinical stage IB and IIA cervical carcinoma. *Gynecol Oncol* 34:43, 1989.

Miller B, Morris M, Rutledge F et al. Aborted exenterative procedures in recurrent cervical cancer. *Gynecol Oncol* 50:94, 1993.

Morrow CP. A panel report: Is pelvic radiation beneficial in postoperative management of stage IB squamous cell carcinoma of the cervix with pelvic node metastasis treated by radical hysterectomy and pelvic lymphadenectomy. *Gynecol Oncol* 10:105, 1980.

Park RC, Thigpen T. Chemotherapy in advanced and recurrent cervical cancer. A review. *Cancer* 71:1446, 1993.

Perez CA, Camel HM, Waltz BJ et al. Radiation therapy alone in the treatment of carcinoma of the uterine cervix: A 20 year experience. *Gynecol Oncol* 23:127, 1986.

Piver MS, Barlow JJ, Krishnamsetty R. Five year survival (with no evidence of disease) in patients with biopsy confirmed aortic node metastasis from cervical carcinoma. *Am J Obstet Gynecol* 139:575, 1981.

Piver MS, Barlow JJ, Vongtama V et al. Hydroxyurea: A radiation potentiator in carcinoma of the uterine cervix. *Am J Obstet Gynecol* 147:803, 1983.

Piver MS, Chung WS. Prognostic significance of cervical lesion size and pelvic node metasasis in cervical carcinoma. *Obstet Gynecol* 46:507, 1975.

Piver MS, Marchetti DL, Patton TJ et al. Radical hysterectomy and pelvic lymphadenectomy versus radiation therapy for small (≤ 3 cm) stage IB cervical carcinoma. *Am J Clin Oncol* 11:21, 1988.

Piver MS, Rose PG, Friedman MF. Change in International Federation of Gynecologists and Obstetricians staging. *Am J Obstet Gynecol* 158:678, 1988.

Piver MS, Rutledge FN, Smith JP. Five classes of extended hysterectomy for women with cervical cancer. *Obstet Gynecol* 44:265, 1974.

Potish RA, Downey GO, Adcock LL et al. The role of surgical debulking in cancer of the uterine cervix. *Int J Radiat Oncol Biol Phys* 17:979, 1989.

Roman LD, Morris M, Mitchell MF et al. Prognostic factors for patients undergoing simple hysterectomy in the presence of invasive cancer of the cervix. *Gynecol Oncol* 50:179, 1993.

Rose P, Baker S, Fournier L et al. Serum squamous cell carcinoma antigen levels in invasive cervical cancer. Prediction of response and recurrence. *Am J Obstet Gynecol* 168:942, 1993.

Rose PG. Locally advanced cervical carcinoma: The role of chemoradiation. *Semin Oncol* 21:47, 1994.

Rose PG, Piver MS, Malfetano JH. A phase II study of weekly cisplatin followed by cisplatin and ifosfamide in advanced and recurrent cervical carcinoma. *Cancer* 71:2245, 1993.

Sagae S, Kuzumaki N, Hisada T et al. Ras oncogene expression and prognosis of invasive squamous cell carcinomas of the uterine cervix. *Cancer* 63:1577, 1989.

Soper JT, Berchuck A, Creasman WT et al. Pelvic exenteration: Factors associated with major surgical morbidity. *Gynecol Oncol* 35:93, 1989.

Stehman FB, Bundy BN, Keyes H et al. Randomized trial of hydroxyurea versus misonidazole adjunct to radiation therapy in carcinoma of the cervix. *Am J Obstet Gynecol* 159:87, 1988.

Stitt JA. High dose rate intracavitary brachytherapy for gynecologic malignancies. *Oncology* 6:59, 1992.

Sutton GP, Blessing JA, McGuire WP et al. Phase II trial of ifosfamide and mesna in patients with advanced or recurrent squamous carcinoma of the cervix who had never received chemotherapy: A Gynecologic Oncology Group study. *Am J Obstet Gynecol* 168:805, 1993.

Sutton GP, Bundy BN, Delgado G et al. Ovarian metastasis in stage IB carcinoma of the cervix. A Gynecologic Oncology Group study. *Am J Obstet Gynecol* 166:50, 1992.

Thoms WT, Eifel PJ, Smith TL et al. Bulky endocervical carcinoma: A 23 year experience. *Int J Radiat Oncol Biol Phys* 23:491, 1992.

van Nagell JR Jr, Donaldson ES, Gay EC et al. Carcinoembryonic antigen in carcinoma of the uterine cervix. Part II. Localization and correlation with plasma antigen concentration. *Cancer* 44:944, 1979.

Vokes EE and Weichselbaum RR. Concomitant chemoradiotherapy; rationale and clinical experience in patients with solid tumors. *J Clin Oncol* 8:911, 1990.

Wimbush PR, Fletcher GH. Radiation therapy of carcinoma of the cervical stump. *Radiology* 93:655, 1969.

III Uterine Cancer

8

Premalignant Conditions of the Endometrium (Endometrial Hyperplasia and Adenocarcinoma in Situ)

Trudy R. Baker

Endometrial Hyperplasia

Endometrial hyperplasias can be described as proliferative lesions of the endometrial glands and, to a lesser extent, the endometrial stroma. The etiologic factor in most cases is thought to be unopposed estrogen stimulation of the endometrial lining. This could result from either chronic anovulation, such as is associated with polycystic ovarian disease, estrogen-producing ovarian neoplasms, obesity, or exogenous unopposed estrogen administration. Any age group can be affected.

CLASSIFICATION

The International Society of Gynecological Pathologists classification of endometrial hyperplasia is seen in Table 8-1. This classification system is based on architectural as well as cytologic features.

Simple Hyperplasia

Simple hyperplasia is characterized by an increased glandular to stroma ratio with glands that are round or irregular in shape. Glands can be dilated or cystic (cystic hyperplasia) and are lined by proliferative-type endometrial cells (Fig. 8-1). The stroma is more densely packed than that of normal proliferative endometrium. Nuclear atypia is absent.

Complex Hyperplasia

Glands in complex hyperplasia exhibit increased crowding with less intervening stroma between glandular elements. Glandular architecture is more complex, with budding and papillary infoldings noted. Cellular stratification can be present within glands, but the nuclei preserve normal polarity.

Adenomatous hyperplasia is an acceptable but a less preferred term for complex hyperplasia in the present classification system.

Atypical Hyperplasia

Atypical hyperplasia, which is classified as either simple or complex, is characterized by cytologic atypia (see Fig. 8-1E). Usually focal, the atypia is characterized by loss of polarity, increased nuclear to cytoplasmic ratio, large nuclei of various sizes and shapes, irregularly clumped chromatin, thickened nuclear membrane, and prominent nucleoli. Mitotic activity is not a reliable diagnostic criterion, and stromal findings are also variable. Grading the degree of atypia does not add to information concerning the chance of progression to carcinoma. Point mutations in the k-*ras* oncogene, which have been

Table 8-1. International Society of Gynccological Pathologists classification of endometrial hyperplasia

Parameter	*Simple hyperplasia*	*Complex hyperplasia*	*Atypical hyperplasia*
Synonyms	Cystic hyperplasia	Adenomatous hyperplasia	Severe adenomatous hyperplasia or adenomatous hyperplasia with atypia
Major characteristics	Increased glandular to stroma ratio but no glandular crowding; no cellular atypia; no stromal invasion.	Glands more numerous with moderate crowding; glandular budding and papillary infoldings; no cellular atypia or stromal invasion	Cytologic atypia; no stromal invasion
Malignant potential	1% over 15 years	3% over 13 years	23% over 11 years (simple hyperplasia with atypia: 8%) (complex hyperplasia with atypia: 29%)

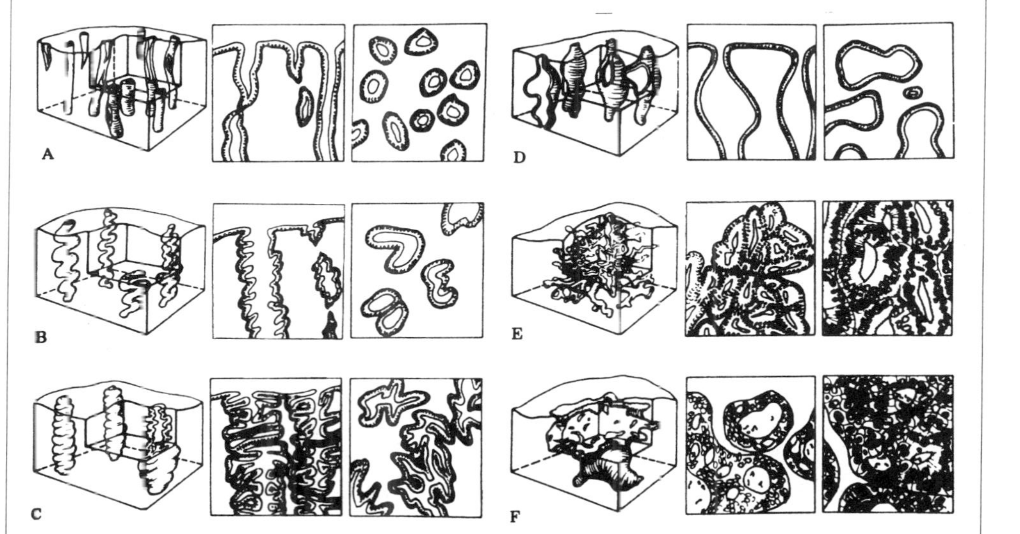

Fig. 8-1. Commonly encountered glandular architectural configurations. A. Early proliferative. B. Midproliferative. C. Late proliferative. D. Mild (cystic) hyperplastic. E. Atypical hyperplastic. F. Carcinomatous. The two-dimensional frames of A–D show a longitudinal section (left) and a section parallel to the surface of the endometrium (right); those of E and F, which are low-power (left) and high-power (right) views, are sections through the glands. Note the minimally stratified epithelium of the closely approximated glands of atypical hyperplasia (E) and the epithelial stratification and cribriform pattern of carcinoma (F).

reported in some endometrial adenocarcinomas and which have been suggested to play a role in tumorigenesis, have also been identified in some atypical hyperplasias. One study noted k-*ras* mutations in seven of 19 endometrial adenocarcinomas and in two of 16 atypical hyperplasias. No k-*ras* mutations were found in 18 hyperplasias without atypia, however. Whether demonstration of these genetic changes will allow identification of lesions that will ultimately progress to carcinoma awaits further study.

Adenocarcinoma In Situ

The term *adenocarcinoma in situ* has been proposed by some as a separate diagnostic category that would exist between atypical hyperplasia and a grade 1 endometrial adenocarcinoma. However, definitions of this lesion have not been agreed on in the literature, and, indeed, it is not certain whether this lesion even exists. Use of the term is not currently recommended, and it is not included in the current classification system accepted by the International Society of Gynecological Pathologists.

DIFFERENTIAL DIAGNOSIS

Not only can one endometrial hyperplasia be difficult to distinguish from another type, but other benign conditions, such as a normal proliferative or secretory endometrium or endometrial polyps, can cause diagnostic difficulties. Cystic (senile) atrophy can also be mistaken for endometrial hyperplasia, but the dilated glands of cystic atrophy are lined by flattened single-layer epithelium, and the associated stroma is also atrophic. In a study of 100 consecutive patients referred with a diagnosis of endometrial hyperplasia, 69 cases were downgraded (17 cases changed to proliferative or secretory endometrium, 27 cases changed to endometrial polyps, nine cases changed to endometrial metaplasia, and 16 cases were downgraded to a lesser severity of hyperplasia). In only three cases was the diagnosis changed to a well-differentiated endometrial adenocarcinoma.

A greater diagnostic problem arises in distinguishing complex hyperplasia with atypia from a grade 1 endometrial adenocarcinoma. The primary criterion for the presence of adenocarcinoma is stromal invasion. This parameter is identified by the finding of at least one of the following: (1) presence of a desmoplastic stromal response in association with the glandular structures; (2) a confluent glandular or cribriform pattern; (3) a papillary pattern; or (4) the replacement of stroma by masses of squamous epithelium. To qualify as invasion, numbers 2, 3, and 4 must occupy at least one-half (2.1 mm) of a low-power field 4.2 mm in diameter. In one study of Kurman that compared the findings in hysterectomy specimens obtained after a diagnosis of atypical hyperplasia or low-grade adenocarcinoma had been made in curettage specimens, carcinoma was found in the uterus in only 17% of cases if no stromal invasion was present in the curettings and all were grade 1 and either confined to the endometrium or superficially invasive. If stromal invasion was identified in the curettings, however, residual carcinoma was present in the uterus in one-half of the cases, one-third of which were grade 2 or grade 3 and one-fourth of which were deeply invasive.

BEHAVIOR OF HYPERPLASIA

The histopathologic features and clinical behavior of hyperplastic endometrial lesions have been correlated. In a study of 170 patients diagnosed with all types of endometrial hyperplasia by endometrial curettings, the patients were followed for at least 1 year before undergoing hysterectomy. Of the 122 patients with hyperplasia (simple and complex), 80% had regression of their disease, 19% had persistence, and only 2% progressed to carcinoma. Of the 48 patients with atypical hyperplasia (both simple and complex), 58% regressed, 19% persisted, and 23% progressed to carcinoma (p = .001). When the groups were analyzed further, progression to carcinoma occurred in 1% of patients with simple hyperplasia, in 3% with complex hyperplasia, in 8% with simple hyperplasia with atypia, and in 29% with complex hyperplasia with atypia. It would appear that increasing degrees of architectural complexity may be a factor in the progression to carcinoma, but cytologic atypia plays the larger role.

The carcinomas that develop in association with hyperplasia, in general, tend to be early, well-differentiated lesions. It is estimated that the time from progression of hyperplasia to carcinoma is approximately 10 years and that the time from progression of atypical hyperplasia to carcinoma is approximately 4 years. It has been noted that 17–25% of patients with atypical hyperplasia diagnosed by dilatation and curettage (D & C) will have a grade 1 carcinoma of the uterus if hysterectomy is performed within 1 month of the D & C.

TREATMENT

Simple and Complex Hyperplasia

In general, these lesions can be treated conservatively, as they are associated with a low risk of progression to carcinoma. Anovulation is usually responsible for the development of these hyperplasias in the reproductive age group. If pregnancy is being considered, induction of ovulation with clomiphene citrate (Clomid) is an option. If pregnancy is not contemplated, medroxyprogesterone acetate (Provera), 10 mg daily for 10 days each month for 3–6 months or 10–20 mg per day for 3–6 months, should reverse these changes. Another option would be expectant management with intermittent endometrial sampling.

For peri- or postmenopausal women who develop simple or complex hyperplasia on estrogen therapy, stopping the hormonal therapy will usually reverse the changes. Alternatively, Provera can be added to the regimen at a dose of 10 mg for 10 days of each month. For women who develop hyperplasias without atypia not related to estrogen replacement therapy, a progestin should be administered for 3–6 months followed by endometrial sampling. Gal treated 38 patients who had complex hyperplasia with daily megestrol acetate (Megace). Endometrial biopsies were performed every 6 months. Ninety-two percent (35 patients) reversed to nonhyperplastic endometrium, two patients progressed to atypical hyperplasia, one continued as complex hyperplasia, and none progressed to endometrial carcinoma.

Atypical Hyperplasia

Patients diagnosed with atypical hyperplasia by office endometrial biopsy require fractional D & C because of the 17–25% incidence of harboring a concomitant endometrial cancer within the uterus. In reproductive-age women who desire pregnancy, ovulation can be induced. In those who do not desire pregnancy, progestin suppression is indicated (Provera, up to 60–70 mg per day; Megace 20–40 mg bid; or Depo-Provera, 150 mg q3months). Close follow-up and periodic endometrial biopsies are required.

In peri- or postmenopausal women, progestin suppression can be attempted with careful follow-up and periodic endometrial sampling. If this is not successful or for patients in whom progestin therapy is contraindicated, hysterectomy is the treatment of choice. For patients who are significant surgical risks, prolonged progestin therapy is a treatment option. Gal used daily Megace to treat 32 patients with atypical hyperplasia who were at significant risk for major surgery; 94% (30 patients) reverted to nonhyperplastic endometrium, two patients remained atypical, but none progressed to endometrial carcinoma. Table 8-2 shows a treatment summary.

Endometrial Adenocarcinoma

Endometrial adenocarcinoma is characterized by a complex architectural pattern, with back-to-back crowding of the glands and cellular atypia. It is distinguished from atypical endometrial hyperplasia by the invasion of tumor cells into the endometrial stroma (see Fig. 8-1F).

Endometrial Polyps

Endometrial polyps are the result of focal overgrowth of endometrial glands and stroma. Histologically, they are composed of weakly proliferative glands but rarely show active proliferative or secretory changes. They are most likely secondary to unopposed estrogen stimulation. They commonly present during the fifth decade and may result in abnormal uterine or postmenopausal bleeding. Benign endometrial polyps are rarely associated with endometrial adenocarcinoma. It has been reported that 0.5% of polyps were associated with endometrial adenocarcinoma. Their malignant potential is zero, but they are important because they can be confused with carcinoma in endometrial curettings.

Endometrial Metaplasia

Endometrial metaplasia is the replacement of normal endometrial glandular epithelium by epithelium not normally found in other müllerian-derived organs such as the fallopian tube. A range of non-neoplastic metaplasias has been described (Table 8-3). Metaplasia tends to occur in relatively young women and has been associated with abnormal uterine bleeding, anovulation, exogenous estrogen use, obesity, and intrauterine contraceptive devices. None of the metaplasias is of clinical significance unless it is confused with endometrial hyperplasia or endometrial adenocarcinoma. It has been reported that metaplasia was associated with endometrial carcinoma in 32% of curettage specimens and 37.5% of hysterectomy specimens. The association of metaplasia with endometrial carcinoma, however, has no obvious clinical significance.

Table 8-2. Treatment of endometrial hyperplasia

Age	*Simple hyperplasia*	*Complex hyperplasia*	*Atypical hyperplasia*
Reproductive years	None or progestins[a] or ovulation induction	None or progestins[b] or ovulation induction	D & C Progestins[b] or ovulation induction
Pre- or postmenopausal years	Progestins[a]	Progestins[b] Hysterectomy if no response to progestins	D & C Hysterectomy If poor surgical risk, progestins[b]

D & C = dilatation and curettage.
[a]Provera 10 mg daily for 10 days out of each month for 3–6 months.
[b]Provera 10–20 mg/day for 3–6 months (for atypical hyperplasia use up to 60–80 days); Megace 20–40 mg/day for 3–6 months; clomiphene citrate 50 mg/day, days 5–9 of menstrual cycle (can increase by 50 mg/day increments to 200 mg/day, days 5–9).

Table 8-3. Types of endometrial metaplasia

Squamous metaplasia
Papillary syncytial metaplasia
Ciliated cell metaplasia
Eosinophilic metaplasia
Mucinous metaplasia
Hobnail cell metaplasia
Clear-cell metaplasia

Source: Adapted from MR Hendrickson, RL Kempson (eds). *Surgical Pathology of the Uterine Corpus*. Philadelphia: Saunders, 1980. Pp. 158–214.

Atypical Secretory Hyperplasia

Little is known about the significance of atypical secretory hyperplasia of the endometrium. It is found most often in young women and is characterized by architectural and cytologic changes similar to those seen in atypical nonsecretory endometrium, except for the additional presence of subnuclear glycogen ridge vacuoles in the glandular epithelium. Its malignant potential is considered to be zero.

Selected Readings

Anderson WA et al. Endometrial metaplasia associated with endometrial adenocarcinoma. *Am J Obstet Gynecol* 157:579, 1987.

Deligdisch L, Cohen CJ. Histologic correlates and virulence implications of endometrial carcinoma associated with adenomatous hyperplasia. *Cancer* 56:1452, 1985.

Enomoto T, Inoue M, Peratoni AO et al. K-ras activation in premalignant and malignant epithelial lesions of the human uterus. *Cancer Res* 51:5308, 1991.

Gal D. Hormonal therapy for lesions of the endometrium. *Semin Oncol* 13:33, 1986.

Hendrickson MR, Kempson RL (eds). *Surgical Pathology of the Uterine Corpus*. Philadelphia: Saunders, 1980. Pp. 158–214.

King A, Seraj IM, Wagner RJ. Stromal invasion in endometrial carcinoma. *Am J Obstet Gynecol* 149:10, 1984.

Kurman RJ, Kaminski PF, Norris HJ. The behavior of endometrial hyperplasia. A long-term study of "untreated" hyperplasia in 170 patients. *Cancer* 56:403, 1985.

Kurman RJ, Norris HJ. Evaluation of criteria for distinguishing atypical endometrial hyperplasia from well differentiated carcinoma. *Cancer* 49:2547, 1982.

Salm R. The incidence and significance of early carcinoma of endometrial polyps. *J Pathol* 108:47, 1972.

Tavassoli FA, Kraus FT. Endometrial lesions in uteri resected for atypical endometrial hyperplasia. *Am J Clin Pathol* 70:770, 1978.

Winkler B, Alvarez S, Richart RM et al. Pitfalls in the diagnosis of endometrial neoplasia. *Obstet Gynecol* 64:185, 1984.

Endometrial Carcinoma

Trudy R. Baker

Incidence

Endometrial adenocarcinoma, although the most common gynecologic malignancy, is one of the least common causes of cancer mortality in women. It accounted for only 4% of all female cancer deaths in 1994. An estimated 31,000 cases occurred in the United States in 1994, with 5,900 of these women succumbing to their disease. The relatively low mortality rate is partly related to the fact that approximately 80% of endometrial adenocarcinomas are clinically confined to the uterus at the time of initial diagnosis.

The incidence of endometrial adenocarcinoma rose in the United States in the early 1970s, which was attributed to the increase in estrogen replacement therapy for menopausal symptoms. Rates have declined since that time, most likely secondary to a decrease in exogenous estrogen administration after a 1976 Federal Drug Administration cancer-related warning and the now routine use of progestins with estrogen replacement therapy in women who have a uterus. However, certain European countries in which estrogens are rarely utilized for menopausal symptoms have also experienced a significant increase in the rate of endometrial carcinoma.

The median age for endometrial cancer is approximately 60 years. Seventy-five percent of endometrial adenocarcinomas occur during the postmenopausal period, primarily during the sixth and seventh decades. Of the one-fourth of women who are premenopausal, 5% are under the age of 40 at the time of initial diagnosis.

Etiology

Most cases of endometrial carcinoma appear related to chronic unopposed estrogen stimulation of the endometrium from either endogenous or exogenous sources. Many of the risk factors identified for the development of this disease are associated with states in which that particular hormonal milieu predominates. These estrogen-related carcinomas tend to develop in a background of hyperplasia and to be better differentiated, and, in general, are associated with a favorable prognosis. An "estrogen independen[illegible] type of endometrial carcinoma has also been described. T[illegible] lesions, which are not associated with the usual risk factor[illegible] in a nonhyperplastic endometrium, are more poorly differ[illegible] and exhibit a more aggressive clinical course.

Risk Factors

Risk factors for the development of endome[illegible] re listed in Table 9-1.

Table 9-1. Risk factors for endometrial cancer

Factor	*Risk*	*Relative risk*
Obesity		
Overweight 10–21 lb	↑	2 ×
Overweight 21–50 lb	↑	3 ×
Overweight >50 lb	↑	10 ×
Menopausal estrogen use	↑	4.5–13.9
Oral contraceptives	↓	0.5
Sequential oral contraceptives	↑	Unknown
Diabetes mellitus	↑	2.0
Nulliparity	↑	2 × with 1 child 3 × with 5 children
Tamoxifen use	↑	7.5
Late menopause	↑	2.4
Early menarche (<12 yrs)	↑	1.6–2.4
Polycystic ovarian syndrome	↑	Unknown
Smoking	↓	0.7–0.9

OBESITY

The primary source of the dominant postmenopausal estrogen, estrone, is the adrenal gland. Androstenedione produced by the adrenal is converted to estrone via aromatization in adipose tissue. The conversion rate of androstenedione to estrone has been noted to correlate strongly with age and obesity. Thus, the obese postmenopausal female has the propensity to chronic unopposed estrogen stimulation that can result in endometrial hyperplasia and carcinoma. It has been suggested that endometrial carcinoma risk may depend not only on the amount of body fat present but also on its distribution pattern. Obesity in premenopausal females frequently results in ovulatory failure, infertility, and abnormal menstruation or amenorrhea, which also results in chronic unopposed estrogen exposure. These women are at increased risk for the development of endometrial cancer even before age 40.

ESTROGEN REPLACEMENT THERAPY

The increased use of estrogen for menopausal symptoms during the 1970s parallelled the rise in the incidence of endometrial cancer. As early as 1975, a 7.6-fold increased risk was observed in women using conjugated estrogens compared to controls. The estimated increase with duration of exposure was 5.6 times for 1–5 years of exposure [illegible] 13.9 times for 7 years or more. The increased risk associated [illegible] estrogen use persists for at least 5 years after discontinuation [illegible]rogen. The addition of a progestin to estrogen replacement [illegible] been shown to reduce the incidence of endometrial can-

SEQU[illegible] COMBINATION ORAL CONT[illegible]

Sequentia[illegible]ves, which consisted of unopposed estrogen during [illegible] resulted in an increased incidence of endometrial [illegible] under age 40. These agents were subsequently [illegible] market. However, the use of combination oral [illegible] resulted in an approximate 50%

reduction in the risk of developing endometrial cancer. The protective effect has been reported to last 20 or more years after the cessation of oral contraceptive use. Some investigators have noted that oral contraceptive use is not protective in women who subsequently used menopausal estrogens for 3 or more years, although others have not noted an alteration of oral contraceptive effect with menopausal estrogen use.

DIABETES

Diabetes has classically been considered a risk factor for the development of endometrial carcinoma, although studies have conflicted. A case control study reported a relative risk of 2.0 (95% CI; 1.1–3.6) for a history of diabetes, an effect that persisted even after adjustment for weight and other factors.

NULLIPARITY

The increased risk in nulliparous married women is probably secondary to anovulation with the resultant unopposed estrogen and not to nulliparity itself.

MENARCHE AND MENOPAUSE

Studies indicate that menarche before age 12 is associated with relative risks of 1.6–2.4 for the development of endometrial carcinoma. Menopause after age 52 is associated with a reportedly 2.4 times greater risk for the development of endometrial cancer, although other studies have not confirmed this finding.

POLYCYSTIC OVARIAN DISEASE

Polycystic ovarian disease is a syndrome of obesity, anovulation, abnormal bleeding or amenorrhea, hirsutism, and polycystic ovaries that predisposes young girls to an increased risk of endometrial carcinoma through the mechanism of anovulation.

SMOKING

The incidence rate of endometrial cancer is significantly decreased for smokers compared to nonsmokers. Although the mechanism of action is thought to result from an increased estrogen metabolism, lower serum estrogen levels among postmenopausal women who smoke compared to nonsmokers has not been reported by most investigators. Studies have, however, consistently reported increased levels of androgens among postmenopausal smokers compared to postmenopausal nonsmokers; therefore, smoking's effect on endometrial cancer risk may be related to its effect on androgens rather than estrogens.

TAMOXIFEN

Tamoxifen, a nonsteroidal antiestrogen, is widely used in the treatment of breast cancer. Since the 1985 report that observed the development of three endometrial cancer cases in breast cancer patients on tamoxifen, approximately 100 cases of endometrial cancer have been reported in this population. This includes those endometrial cancer cases noted in four randomized trials that compared breast cancer patients on tamoxifen with a control arm. Two of those trials, however, showed no increase in endometrial cancer for women on tamoxifen. In a study of the National Surgical Adjuvant Breast and Bowel Project that analyzed node-negative, estrogen receptor–positive breast cancer patients treated either with tamoxifen or placebo, the relative risk of endometrial cancer for the tamoxifen-treated group was 7.5 compared with the placebo group. Notwithstanding the increased risk of endometrial cancer, when the tamoxifen and placebo groups were compared, it was estimated that there was a 38% reduction in the 5-year cumulative hazard rate for breast cancer in those patients treated with tamoxifen.

HYPERTENSION

Rather than being a specific risk factor for endometrial carcinoma, hypertension more likely correlates with age and obesity. A significant risk relationship, in general, has not been noted after adjustment for factors such as weight, age, and socioeconomic status.

DIETARY FACTORS

Case control studies have suggested that the risk of endometrial cancer is increased with greater fat intake while more frequent intake of vegetables, fruit, and whole grain foods offers some protection against the disease. Conflicting results have been reported for frequent consumption of meat and eggs. In general, the use of alcohol has not been associated with a significant increase in risk for endometrial cancer.

Diagnosis

For the evaluation of abnormal uterine bleeding, office endometrial biopsy is accurate in over 90% of cases of endometrial carcinoma. For patients not diagnosed by endometrial biopsy or in whom endometrial biopsy cannot be performed because of cervical stenosis or patient discomfort, fractional dilatation and curettage (D & C) under anesthesia is required. D & C is also required for those women who have persistent symptoms despite a normal biopsy and for those who exhibit adenomatous hyperplasia with atypia to rule out the concomitant presence of an invasive adenocarcinoma. Techniques using cytologic evaluation of endometrial cells are not as accurate as those that obtain endometrial tissue. Cervical and vaginal Papanicolaou (Pap) smears are 80% negative in cases of endometrial carcinoma and cannot be used for evaluating abnormal bleeding.

Histologic Classification

Table 9-2 depicts the most recent histologic classification for endometrial carcinoma.

ENDOMETRIOID

The endometrioid type is the most common and is composed of four variants: (1) papillary or villoglandular, (2) secretory adenocarcinoma, (3) ciliated adenocarcinoma, and (4) adenocarcinoma with squamous differentiation including adenoacanthoma, in which the squamous element is histologically benign, and adenosquamous, characterized by a malignant squamous component. For both types it is the grade of the adenocarcinoma component that determines prognosis. Five-year survivals, grade for grade, are similar for adenocarcinoma, adenoacanthoma, and adenosquamous carcinoma.

Table 9-2. Proposed histologic classification of endometrial carcinoma by the International Society of Gynecologic Pathologists

I. Endometrioid
  A. Ciliated adenocarcinoma
  B. Secretory adenocarcinoma
  C. Papillary or villoglandular
  D. Adenocarcinoma with squamous differentiation
    i. Adenoacanthoma
    ii. Adenosquamous
II. Serous
III. Mucinous
IV. Clear cell
V. Squamous cell
VI. Mixed
VII. Undifferentiated

SEROUS CARCINOMA

Uterine papillary serous carcinoma, a variant of endometrial adenocarcinoma, is histologically similar to ovarian serous papillary adenocarcinoma. Of the 26 surgical stage I patients originally reported, 50% relapsed, and most of the relapses were intra-abdominal (similar to ovarian cancer). Subsequent reports have shown that this lesion is frequently understaged when clinical and surgical staging are compared, is often associated with upper abdominal spread, and carries a poor prognosis. The treatment for this histologic type remains unknown.

MUCINOUS CARCINOMA

Mucinous carcinoma comprises less than 1% of all endometrial carcinomas and is generally associated with good prognosis, as most cases are stage I, are well-differentiated, and invade the myometrium only minimally.

CLEAR-CELL CARCINOMA

Clear-cell carcinomas comprise approximately 4% of all endometrial carcinomas. Most authors have reported that these lesions are associated with a poorer prognosis when compared with endometrioid adenocarcinomas.

SQUAMOUS CELL CARCINOMA OF THE ENDOMETRIUM

A diagnosis of squamous cell carcinoma of the endometrium is based on the following: (1) no coexisting adenocarcinoma; (2) no connection between the tumor and the squamous epithelium of the cervix; and (3) noninvolvement of the cervix. To date there are only 35 reported cases of primary squamous cell carcinoma of the endometrium. Treatment for this tumor is the same, stage for stage, as that for adenocarcinoma.

MIXED CARCINOMA

Mixed carcinoma comprises more than one of the variants described above, and the second type must make up at least 10% of the total volume of the tumor.

Table 9-3. FIGO surgical staging of carcinoma of the corpus uteri, 1988

Stage IA G123	Tumor limited to endometrium
Stage IB G123	Invasion to less than one-half of the myometrium
Stage IC G123	Invasion to more than one-half of the myometrium
Stage IIA G123	Endocervical glandular involvement only
Stage IIB G123	Cervical stromal invasion
Stage IIIA G123	Tumor invades serosa and/or adnexa, and/or positive peritoneal cytology
Stage IIIB G123	Vaginal metastasis
Stage IIIC G123	Metastasis of pelvic and/or para-aortic lymph nodes
Stage IVA G123	Tumor invasion of bladder and/or bowel mucosa
Stage IVB	Distant metastases including intra-abdominal and/or inguinal lymph nodes

UNDIFFERENTIATED CARCINOMA

Undifferentiated carcinoma is an uncommon type that can exhibit different patterns such as small-cell type, in which markers of neuroendocrine differentiation are present, giant-cell type, or spindle cell type.

Staging

In 1988, a surgical staging system for endometrial adenocarcinoma was adopted by the International Federation of Gynecologists and Obstetricians (FIGO) that replaced the previous clinical staging system (Table 9-3). Two prognostic factors—grade and depth of myometrial invasion—have been incorporated into this new system. Surgical staging allows the physician to determine the full extent of the patient's disease so that optimal postoperative therapy can then be planned.

Prognostic Factors

The results of two prospective surgical staging studies conducted by the Gynecologic Oncology Group (GOG) provide much of our knowledge about prognostic factors in endometrial carcinoma. In general, the importance of these prognostic factors is related to their association with pelvic and para-aortic lymph node involvement.

GRADE

Survival for patients with clinical stage I endometrial adenocarcinoma has been correlated with tumor grade, with 80% of grade 1 tumors, 73% of grade 2, and 58% of grade 3 lesions associated with 5-year survival. As the tumor becomes less differentiated, the incidence of deep myometrial invasion increases; however, as many as 10% of grade 1 lesions have been associated with deep myometrial invasion, and 7% of grade 3 lesions have been confined to the endometrium. Of importance, the incidence of pelvic and para-aortic nodal metastases increases as the grade worsens. In the 1984 GOG study of surgical stage I patients (defined as those in which

Table 9-4. Pelvic lymph node metastasis with surgical stage I endometrial cancer

Parameter	*No. of patients*	*Metastasis (%)*
Grade		
1	85	1.2
2	74	5.4
3	35	25.7
Total	*194*	
Myometrial invasion		
Endometrial	87	0.0
Superficial	73	5.5
Intermediate	13	23.1
Deep	21	33.3
Total	*194*	

Source: Adapted from RC Boronow et al. Surgical staging in endometrial cancer: Clinical-pathologic findings of a prospective study. *Obstet Gynecol* 63:825, 1984.

Table 9-5. Para-aortic lymph node metastasis with surgical stage I disease

Parameter	*No. of patients*	*Metastasis (%)*
Grade		
1	64	0.0
2	44	4.5
3	27	25.9
Total	*135*	
Myometrial invasion		
Endometrial	63	0.0
Superficial	48	8.3
Intermediate	8	12.5
Deep	16	25.0
Total	*135*	

Source: Adapted from RC Boronow et al. Surgical staging in endometrial cancer: Clinical-pathologic findings of a prospective study. *Obstet Gynecol* 63:825, 1984.

pathologic study of the surgical specimen did not reveal unanticipated spread to the cervix, adnexa, or intraperitoneal involvement), it was documented that the incidence of pelvic lymph node metastasis in grade 1 or 2 tumors was markedly low but increased significantly for grade 3 lesions (Table 9-4). Similar findings were noted for the para-aortic nodes (Table 9-5).

A third prospective study conducted by the GOG related surgical and pathologic factors and postoperative treatment to recurrence-free interval and recurrence sites in 895 evaluable patients with clinical stage I or II endometrial cancer. Of the patients in that study who demonstrated no evidence of extrauterine risk factors (defined as no nodal, adnexal, isthmic-cervical, or gross extrauterine involvement and negative cytology and capillary space involvement), a recurrence rate of 16.1% was noted for patients with grade 3 lesions versus recurrence rates of 3% and 4% for grade 1 and 2 lesions, respectively.

MYOMETRIAL INVASION

Depth of myometrial invasion has been shown to be an excellent predictor of lymph node metastases. Studies have demonstrated that pelvic lymph node involvement was low for tumor confined to the endometrium or superficially invading the myometrium (see Table 9-4). However, one-third of patients with deeply invading lesions had pelvic lymph node involvement. A similar trend was noted for para-aortic nodal involvement (Table 9-5). Recurrence rates have also been found to positively correlate with depth of myometrial invasion.

CERVICAL INVOLVEMENT

Pelvic and para-aortic lymph node involvement is increased with tumor extension to the isthmic-cervical region. Incidence rates of 16% and 14% for pelvic and para-aortic node metastases, respectively, have been reported compared with 8% pelvic and 4% para-aortic involvement rates when tumor is confined to the uterine fundus. Earlier reports noted pelvic lymph node involvement in 23–40% of patients with cervical involvement.

PELVIC AND PARA-AORTIC NODAL METASTASES

In the 1987 GOG surgical staging study of 621 patients with clinical stage I endometrial adenocarcinoma, 9% of all patients had pelvic lymph node metastases and 6% had para-aortic lymph node involvement. The incidence of para-aortic node involvement without pelvic node involvement was 2%; however, if pelvic node metastases were present, para-aortic involvement was noted approximately one-third of the time.

Nodal metastases are also noted to be increased in the presence of cell types other than endometrioid adenocarcinoma, grade 3 lesions, deep myometrial invasion, positive peritoneal cytology, involvement of the isthmus-cervix, adnexal or other extrauterine involvement, and capillary-like space involvement. One study has shown that the 5-year recurrence-free interval for patients with positive pelvic nodes was 57.8% and for patients with positive para-aortic nodes, 41.2%. These results contrast with a 5-year recurrence-free survival of 92.7% for patients who had no surgical pathologic risk factors other than grade or myometrial invasion.

PERITONEAL CYTOLOGY

The significance of positive cytology in stage I endometrial carcinoma remains controversial. Several studies that have reported positive peritoneal cytology as an adverse factor for survival have included patients with extrauterine disease in their analyses. However, even in those studies of surgically staged patients, including lymph node evaluation, with disease limited to the uterus, there are conflicting results of the significance of peritoneal cytology.

A recently reported prospective trial describes the treatment of surgically staged, stage I endometrial cancer patients with positive peritoneal cytology treated with 1 year of progesterone therapy. Forty-five consecutive patients with surgical stage I endometrial cancer and malignant peritoneal cytology were treated with progesterone therapy and adjuvant radiation therapy depending on the grade and amount of myometrial invasion. Of the 36 patients who underwent second-look laparoscopy after 1 year of treatment, 34 (94.5%) were without evidence of disease and had repeat negative peritoneal cytology; two (5.5%) patients had persistent malignant peritoneal cytology but had no evidence of disease and negative cytology at third-look laparoscopy, 1 year after an additional year of progesterone therapy. Of the 45 women, no patient has developed recurrence, and the estimated 5-year disease-free survival was 88.6%. Progesterone use appears to be safe, but its true effectiveness in patients with positive cytology needs to be determined by a randomized trial.

RECEPTOR STATUS

It has been suggested that progesterone receptor levels are significant prognostic indicators of disease-free survival in clinical stage I endometrial cancer patients. A 3-year disease-free survival rate of 93% was noted in patients demonstrating progesterone receptor levels of greater than 100 fmol/mg of protein compared to 36% 3-year disease-free survival rate for patients with progesterone receptor levels of less than 100 fmol/mg of protein.

Estrogen receptor status has been identified as a significant prognostic factor in endometrial cancer patients by some authors, although it has not been confirmed by others.

OTHER RISK FACTORS

Histologic cell types other than endometrioid adenocarcinoma have been associated with poorer overall survival rates. An 18% incidence of para-aortic node involvement has been reported for histologic types other than endometrioid adenocarcinoma (aortic node involvement <10%). The importance of adnexal involvement and intraperitoneal spread is related to the frequency of associated pelvic and para-aortic lymph node metastases. Pelvic and para-aortic node involvement was reported in 32% and 20%, respectively, of clinical stage I patients with adnexal metastases compared with 8% pelvic lymph node involvement and 5% para-aortic lymph node involvement in patients without adnexal metastases. Similarly, pelvic and para-aortic lymph node involvement was noted in 51% and 23%, respectively, of patients with intraperitoneal spread (absent adnexal involvement), while less than 10% of patients had pelvic or para-aortic node metastasis if no intraperitoneal spread was present.

DNA ploidy and the fraction of cells in the S-phase have also been shown to be prognostic factors in endometrial carcinoma. While most endometrial carcinomas have a diploid DNA content, those exhibiting aneuploidy frequently present in more advanced stages and have been associated with recurrent or persistent disease. An S-phase fraction of 9% or more has correlated with advanced disease, high recurrence rates, and cancer-related deaths.

Lymph-vascular invasion has also been found to be an important prognostic factor in patients with stage I endometrial cancer. A statistically significant increase in tumor recurrence has been reported in the presence of lymph-vascular invasion, with most recurrences occurring in extrapelvic sites. The correlation of recurrence and lymph-vascular invasion was found to be independent of histologic grade or depth of myometrial invasion.

Overexpression of the HER-2/neu oncogene has been shown to occur in 10–15% of endometrial cancers and has been associated with advanced-stage disease. This finding appears to be associated with poor prognosis. In addition, overexpression of the tumor suppressor gene, p53, has been noted in about 20% of endometrial adenocarcinomas and has been associated with advanced stage and poor prognosis.

Treatment

All patients who are medically fit should undergo surgical staging with postoperative therapy planned according to the surgical and pathologic risk factors that are identified.

SURGERY

A vertical midline incision is made that allows adequate access for exploration and for retroperitoneal node dissection, if necessary. Sterile saline, 100 ml, is instilled into the pelvis and right and left paracolic spaces and aspirated for evaluation of peritoneal cytology. Careful evaluation of the entire upper abdomen and pelvis should then be performed. The distal fallopian tubes are ligated to prevent tumor spillage during the course of the surgery. For patients who have no gross evidence of tumor spread outside the uterus, extrafascial hysterectomy and bilateral salpingo-oophorectomy (BSO) are performed and the specimen is sent for frozen-section examination for determination of grade, depth of the myometrial invasion, and presence of cervical involvement. If there is deep (≥ 50%) myometrial invasion or if curettings from a previous D & C or biopsy or the hysterectomy specimen itself demonstrate a grade 3 lesion or if there is cervical involvement, para-aortic lymphadenectomy is performed. Because pelvic lymph node sampling is not complete, especially in elderly obese patients, and because there is a 25–33% chance for pelvic lymph node involvement with a grade 3 or deeply invading lesion, these patients require postoperative pelvic radiation. Therefore, one should perform para-aortic lymphadenectomy to be certain that no disease is present above the pelvis. Pelvic lymph nodes that are grossly involved by tumor or suspicious are excised, however. Because of the low incidence rate of lymph node metastases in patients with grade 1 or 2 tumors and less than 50% myometrial invasion, no para-aortic lymphadenectomy is carried out in that population.

If there is no gross evidence of spread outside the uterus but curettings or evaluation by frozen section reveals the presence of the histologic variant uterine serous papillary adenocarcinoma, surgical staging should include bilateral pelvic and para-aortic lymphadenectomy, omentectomy, and brushings of the diaphragm for cytology based on this tumor's similar spread and relapse pattern to ovarian serous papillary adenocarcinoma. Given the poor prognosis associated with other rare histologic variants (clear-cell, undifferentiated, squamous cell), complete staging evaluation should also be performed for these lesions.

For patients in whom there is obvious extrauterine spread at the time of exploration, extrafascial hysterectomy and BSO are carried out, followed by resection or debulking of gross disease. If the extrauterine disease is confined to the pelvis, any grossly involved pelvic lymph nodes should be excised along with careful upper abdominal evaluation including para-aortic lymphadenectomy, possible omentectomy, and diaphragmatic evaluation. Extrauterine dis-

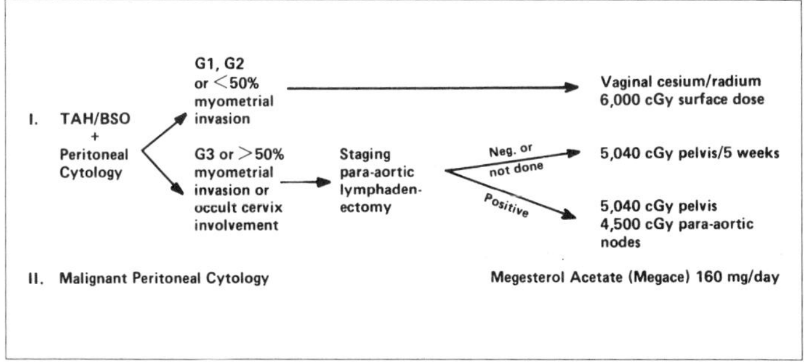

Fig. 9-1. Surgery and irradiation for stage I endometrial carcinoma.

ease that has already spread beyond the pelvis should be resected or debulked with complete upper abdominal evaluation.

Laparoscopically assisted surgical staging of clinical stage I endometrial carcinoma has been reported in which laparoscopically assisted vaginal hysterectomy with pelvic and para-aortic lymphadenectomy (if dictated by the operative findings) was performed. Complications requiring laparotomy occurred in 2 of 59 (3.4%) patients, and both complications were related to the laparoscopically assisted vaginal hysterectomy. Further study will be needed to conclude that this procedure represents a viable alternative to traditional surgical management.

STAGE I

Figure 9-1 shows surgical treatment and irradiation for stage I endometrial carcinoma.

Stage IA or B, Grade 1 or 2

Although patients staged IA or IB are at low risk for pelvic recurrence after surgical therapy, reportedly there is isolated vaginal cuff recurrence in approximately 7–12% of patients. In a randomized study performed at Roswell Park Cancer Institute in which all patients were followed for 10 years or until death, patients randomized to total abdominal hysterectomy (TAH)/BSO and postoperative vaginal radium had a 0% incidence of vaginal recurrence compared to a 4% rate in those who had preoperative intrauterine and vaginal radium followed by TAH/BSO and a 7.5% rate in those who were treated by hysterectomy alone. Because of these results, a prospective trial was begun in 1975 in which all patients who had stage I, grade 1 or 2 disease with less than 50% myometrial invasion and no extrauterine disease were treated by TAH/BSO and postoperative vaginal radium/cesium. A dose of 6,000 cGy to the vaginal vault and 3,000 cGy to the depth of 0.5 cm was delivered. Of the 92 patients, there have been no recurrences, and the estimated 5-year disease-free survival rate was 99%.

Stage I, Grade 3 or IC

The incidence of pelvic lymph node involvement in patients with grade 3 tumors or deep myometrial invasion is significant enough to warrant postoperative pelvic radiation therapy. Of 41 patients with no evidence of para-aortic lymph node metastasis at para-aortic lymphadenectomy so treated, a 5-year estimated disease-free survival rate of 88% has been reported. Four recurrences were noted (9.7%), but only one (2.4%) within the treated field. Studies indicate that external pelvic radiation affords these patients local and regional control of their disease; however, whether it also increases survival rates awaits the results of randomized trials.

STAGE II

The incidence of stage II endometrial cancer varies from 8% to 20% of all endometrial cancers. Varied treatments have been used for stage II disease, including radical hysterectomy, hysterectomy plus radiation therapy (either preoperative or postoperative), and radiation therapy alone. In general, the most favorable results have been obtained with the combination of surgery plus radiation, with 5-year survival rates ranging from 65% to 88% for the combined therapy and from 26% to 74.5% for patients treated with radiation alone. No large studies of surgical stage II patients treated prospectively have been performed; however, given the significant incidence of pelvic lymph node involvement in these patients, postoperative external pelvic radiation therapy should improve local and regional control over that of hysterectomy alone.

MEDICALLY INOPERABLE PATIENTS WITH ENDOMETRIAL CARCINOMA, STAGE I AND II

The 5-year survival rate for patients medically unable to undergo surgery for clinical stage I or II endometrial carcinoma and treated by radiation therapy alone has generally been shown to be decreased by 20–30% compared with patients treated with surgery and radiation. However, a case control study comparing primary radiation to primary surgical therapy with or without radiation therapy in endometrial carcinoma patients and controlled for both clinical stage and tumor grade showed no statistical difference in survival. Because the amount of myometrial invasion or spread to the cervix or adnexa is not known in these patients, all such patients, regardless of grade, should be treated with pelvic radiation (5,040 cGy) plus intracavitary cesium or radium.

STAGE III

Treatment planning for stage III patients is somewhat difficult because of (1) the small number of patients on which to base therapy (<10% of all patients with endometrial cancer are diagnosed in this stage) and (2) treatment has been based on studies that generally have consisted of clinical stage III patients—that is, patients who have not been surgically staged. Several factors that can be gleaned from these studies, however, and that influence treatment decision-making include the following:

1. Improved survival rates have been shown for patients with isolated tubal or ovarian involvement (5-year survival: 60–82%) versus patients with gross adnexal disease (5-year survival: 8–36%).
2. Patients with para-aortic nodal involvement may be salvaged with postoperative radiation therapy to the pelvis and extended para-aortic field radiation. In a 1993 report from Roswell Park Cancer Institute, a 27% 5-year disease-free survival rate was achieved for women with stage I or II endometrial cancer and

positive para-aortic nodes who received pelvic and para-aortic radiation therapy. Others have noted a 5-year disease-free survival rate of 28.6–60.0% for similarly treated patients. However, salvageability appears confined to those with microscopic para-aortic involvement only, as no survivors have been noted in patients with macroscopic para-aortic nodal metastases.

3. Patients with more than one extrauterine site of involvement appear to be at high risk for abdominal and/or distant recurrence.

Stage IIIA

If adnexal or serosal involvement only is documented after complete surgical staging, and complete surgical resection has been performed, postoperative pelvic radiation therapy should be instituted for sterilization of pelvic nodes, which can be involved in up to one-third of these patients.

Patients found to have positive peritoneal cytology after surgical staging should receive 1 year of progestin therapy in addition to treatment as outlined for stage I patients, depending on grade and depth of invasion, or for stage II patients. As previously noted, patients exhibiting more than one site of extrauterine disease appear to be at increased risk for abdominal as well as distant recurrence. For stage IIIA patients with both adnexal involvement and positive peritoneal cytology, pelvic radiation therapy plus a progestin is logical. Whether whole abdominal radiation therapy or adjuvant chemotherapy would result in higher disease-free survival rates in these patients awaits the results of future studies. As well, patients with gross adnexal pelvic disease remaining after surgery would theoretically benefit from systemic chemotherapy, as pelvic radiation therapy is not likely to be curative in this situation.

Stage IIIB

Patients with isolated vaginal involvement should undergo postoperative pelvic radiation therapy with a vaginal boost.

Stage IIIC

Patients who have isolated pelvic nodal metastases should undergo surgical debulking of grossly positive nodes followed by external pelvic radiation therapy. The results of the 1991 GOG staging study noted a 72% 5-year disease-free survival in patients having pelvic nodal metastases as their only evidence of extrauterine disease. If pelvic nodal disease exists along with other extrauterine pelvic sites, external pelvic radiation therapy does not appear adequate, as these patients have a higher risk for abdominal as well as distant recurrences. Systemic chemotherapy should reduce recurrence rates in these patients, but whether or not survival and disease-free survival can be improved by this treatment modality awaits further study.

Almost all cases of para-aortic nodal metastases will be found in patients with positive pelvic nodes, adnexal or intraperitoneal spread, or deep myometrial invasion. In patients who demonstrate microscopic para-aortic nodal metastases as their only evidence of extrapelvic disease, postoperative extended-field radiation to the para-aortic region along with pelvic radiation therapy has resulted in cure for some patients, as discussed above. Systemic chemotherapy may improve disease-free survival in the subgroup of patients as failures appear to occur extra-abdominally, but further study is needed.

At present, there is no effective treatment for patients with macroscopically involved para-aortic disease. Extended-field radiation therapy to the para-aortic region in such patients results in 0% disease-free survival. Effective protocols that incorporate chemohormonal therapy need to be identified for this population.

STAGE IV

While the role of cytoreduction in ovarian cancer seems clear, its role in endometrial cancer is not as well defined. In a study of surgical stage IV patients, however, median survival was significantly improved in those patients who underwent cytoreduction followed by systemic chemotherapy compared to those patients who did not undergo cytoreduction before chemotherapy (18 months versus 8 months, $p = .0001$). Others have also reported improved survival when either radiation or chemotherapy is preceded by cytoreductive surgery. For patients with intra-abdominal disease of less than 2 cm, investigators have reported good results with the use of whole abdominal and pelvic radiation therapy. Prospective studies comparing the use of whole abdominal radiation therapy versus systemic chemotherapy in patients with stage III or IV disease and less than 2 cm of residual disease are currently ongoing. It would appear, however, that aggressive cytoreduction should be carried out if possible, followed by systemic chemotherapy with or without progestins until the results of further studies are complete.

HORMONAL THERAPY FOR METASTATIC OR RECURRENT ADENOCARCINOMA

Early reports of progestin use in patients with metastatic or recurrent endometrial cancer were encouraging. Early studies reported a response rate of approximately 30% in patients with metastatic endometrial carcinoma treated with progestins. In a review of over 1,000 endometrial cancer patients treated with these agents, an overall response rate of 34% was observed. More recent data, however, demonstrate lower response rates in the 10–20% range.

Response to progestins appears to be related to several prognostic factors. In general, higher response rates are noted in well-differentiated tumors, in those recurring after a long disease-free interval, in those with minimal tumor burden, and in those with pulmonary metastases as opposed to nonpulmonary metastatic sites. As well, patients with progesterone-positive and estrogen-positive receptors demonstrate higher responses to hormonal therapy than those with negative receptor status. An overall response rate of 51% is noted for receptor-positive patients, while only 11% of those patients with negative receptors respond.

Tamoxifen therapy has been used for metastatic or recurrent disease with variable responses noted. Given tamoxifen's ability to increase production of progesterone receptors and progesterone's ability to downregulate progesterone receptor production, combination hormonal therapy has been investigated. In general, these combinations do not appear superior to progestin treatment alone.

CHEMOTHERAPY

Active agents consist mainly of doxorubicin (Adriamycin), cisplatin, and carboplatin (Table 9-6). Response to cisplatin varies from a low of 4% in heavily pretreated patients to a high of 42% in patients who had received no prior chemotherapy. The earlier reports of activity

Table 9-6. Single-agent chemotherapy for endometrial cancer

Drug	*Response rate (%)*
Cisplatin	20–35
Carboplatin	30
Adriamycin	20–35
Epirubicin	25
Cyclophosphamide	0–25
Hexamethylmelamine	10–30

Table 9-7. Combination chemotherapy for endometrial cancer

Regimen	*Response rate (%)*
Cyclophosphamide + Adriamycin	31–50
Cyclophosphamide + Adriamycin + cisplatin	31–56
Adriamycin + cisplatin	33–81
Adriamycin + cisplatin + vinblastine	31
Vincristine + VM-26 + cisplatin	52
Cisplatin + Adriamycin + cyclophosphamide + Megace	33–60
Cyclophosphamide + Adriamycin + 5-fluorouracil + Megace	45
Melphalan + 5-fluorouracil + medroxyprogesterone	48
Cyclophosphamide + Adriamycin + Megace *versus*	27
Cyclophosphamide + Adriamycin + 5-fluorouracil + Megace	16
Melphalan + 5-fluorouracil + Megace *versus*	38
Cyclophosphamide + Adriamycin + 5-fluorouracil + Megace	36
Cyclophosphamide + Adriamycin + 5-fluorouracil *versus*	15
Cyclophosphamide + Adriamycin + 5-fluorouracil + alternating methotrexate/tamoxifen	44
Adriamycin *versus*	24
Adriamycin + cyclophosphamide	32
Adriamycin *versus*	35
Adriamycin + cisplatin	66

with the use of either cyclophosphamide or hexamethylmelamine have not been confirmed by other investigators.

Combination regimens are presented in Table 9-7. While many of these regimens have produced high response rates, duration of response is short and median survival less than 1 year.

Regimens that have incorporated progestins do not appear to offer any advantage over combination therapy alone.

Two randomized trials have evaluated Adriamycin alone versus either Adriamycin and cyclophosphamide or Adriamycin and cisplatin. In the first study no significant difference was noted for response rate, median survival, or median progression-free response interval. However, in the second study a significantly higher response rate (66% versus 35%) and progression-free interval (6.2 months versus 3.9 months) were noted for the cisplatin arm. Median survival, however, was not different for the two arms (approximately 9 months).

Endometrial Cancer in the Young

Endometrial carcinoma in women under 40 occurs in less than 5% of cases. Moreover, fewer than 25 cases have been reported in women under the age of 25. Endometrial cancer in the young is primarily associated with (1) polycystic ovarian syndrome (20–25% of cases), (2) significant obesity, (3) use of diethylstilbestrol for the development of secondary sexual characteristics in patients with gonadal dysgenesis, and (4) use of sequential oral contraceptives. Almost all cases are stage I—well-differentiated with no or minimal myometrial invasion. Treatment is the same as for the patients with endometrial carcinoma, although there are reports of treatment by progestational agents alone for the preservation of future fertility.

Selected Readings

Aalders J, Abeler V, Kolstad P et al. Postoperative external irradiation and prognostic parameters in stage I endometrial carcinoma. Clinical and histopathologic study of 540 patients. *Obstet Gynecol* 56:419, 1980.

Austin H, Austin JM, Partridge EE et al. Endometrial cancer, obesity, and body fat distribution. *Cancer Res* 51:568, 1991.

Austin H, Drews C, Partridge EE. A case-control study of endometrial cancer in relation to cigarette smoking, serum estrogen levels and alcohol use. *Am J Obstet Gynecol* 169:1086, 1993.

Boronow RC, Morrow CP, Creasman WT et al. Surgical staging in endometrial cancer: Clinical-pathologic findings of a prospective study. *Obstet Gynecol* 63:825, 1984.

Brinton LA, Berman ML, Mortel R et al. Reproductive, menstrual and medical risk factors for endometrial cancer: Results from a case-control study. *Am J Obstet Gynecol* 167:1317, 1992.

The Cancer and Steroid Hormone Study of the Centers for Disease Control and the National Institute of Child Health and Human Development. Combination oral contraceptive use and the risk of endometrial cancer. *JAMA* 257:796, 1987.

Carcangiu ML, Chambers JT. Uterine papillary serous carcinoma: A study of 108 cases with emphasis on the prognostic significance of associated endometrioid carcinoma, absence of invasion, and concomitant ovarian carcinoma. *Gynecol Oncol* 47:298, 1992.

Childers JM, Brzechffa PR, Hatch KD et al. Laparoscopically assisted surgical staging (LASS) of endometrial cancer. *Gynecol Oncol* 51:33, 1993.

Creasman WT. Prognostic significance of hormone receptors in endometrial cancer. *Cancer* 71:1467, 1993.

Creasman WT, Morrow CP, Bundy BN et al. Surgical pathologic spread patterns of endometrial cancer. A Gynecologic Oncology Group study. *Cancer* 60:2035, 1987.

Dalrymple JC, Russell P. Primary endometrial squamous cell carcinoma with long-term survival. *Aust N Z J Obstet Gynaecol* 33:330, 1993.

Dunton CJ, Pfeifer SM, Braitman LE et al. Treatment of advanced and recurrent endometrial cancer with cisplatin, doxorubicin, and cyclophosphamide. *Gynecol Oncol* 41:113, 1991.

Farhi DC, Nosanchuk J, Silverberg SG. Endometrial adenocarcinoma in women under 25 years of age. *Obstet Gynecol* 68:741, 1986.

FIGO. Corpus cancer staging. *Int J Gynecol Obstet* 28:190, 1989.

Fisher B, Costantino JP, Redmond CK et al. Endometrial cancer in tamoxifen-treated breast cancer patients: Findings from the National Surgical Adjuvant Breast and Bowel Project (NSABP) B-14. *J Natl Cancer Inst* 86:527, 1994.

Goff BA, Goodman A, Muntz HG et al. Surgical stage IV endometrial carcinoma: A study of 47 cases. *Gynecol Oncol* 52:237, 1994.

Greer BE, Hamberger AD. Treatment of intraperitoneal metastatic adenocarcinoma of the endometrium by the whole abdomen moving strip technique and pelvic boost irradiation. *Gynecol Oncol* 16:365, 1983.

Greven KM, Lanciano RM, Corn B et al. Pathologic stage III endometrial carcinoma. *Cancer* 71:3697, 1993.

Grigsby PW, Perez CA, Kuske RR et al. Results of therapy, analysis of failures, and prognostic factors for clinical and pathologic stage III adenocarcinoma of the endometrium. *Gynecol Oncol* 27:44, 1987.

Hammond CB, Soules MR. Endocrine aspects of adenocarcinoma of the endometrium. In J Sciarra (ed), *Gynecology and Obstetrics*. Philadelphia: Lippincott, 1988. Pp. 1–20.

Hanson MB, Van Nagell JR, Powell DE et al. The prognostic significance of lymph-vascular space invasion in stage I endometrial cancer. *Cancer* 55:1753, 1985.

Hendrickson M et al. Uterine papillary serous carcinoma: A highly malignant form of endometrial adenocarcinoma. *Am J Surg Pathol* 6:93, 1982.

Hetzel DJ, Wilson TO, Keeney GL et al. HER-2/neu expression: A major prognostic factor in endometrial cancer. *Gynecol Oncol* 47:179, 1992.

Hicks ML, Piver MS, Puretz JL et al. Survival in patients with paraaortic lymph node metastasis from endometrial adenocarcinoma clinically limited to the uterus. *Int J Radiat Oncol Biol Phys* 26:607, 1993.

Ingram SS, Rosenman J, Heath R et al. The predictive value of progesterone receptor levels in endometrial cancer. *Int J Radiat Oncol Biol Phys* 17:21, 1989.

Kadar N, Homesley HD, Malfetano JH. Positive peritoneal cytology is an adverse factor in endometrial carcinoma only if there is other evidence of extrauterine disease. *Gynecol Oncol* 46:145, 1992.

Kauppila A. Progestin therapy of endometrial, breast and ovarian carcinoma. A review of clinical observations. *Acta Obstet Gynecol Scand* 63:441, 1984.

Killackey MA, Hakes TB, Pierce VK. Endometrial adenocarcinoma in breast cancer patients receiving antiestrogens. *Cancer Treat Rev* 69:237, 1985.

Kohler MF, Berchuck A, Davidoff AM et al. Overexpression and mutation of p53 in endometrial carcinoma. *Cancer Res* 52:1622, 1992.

Levenback C, Burke TW, Silva E et al. Uterine papillary serous carcinoma (UPSC) treated with cisplatin, doxorubicin, and cyclophosphamide (PAC). *Gynecol Oncol* 46:317, 1992.

Morrow CP, Bundy BN, Kurman RJ et al. Relationship between surgical-pathological risk factors and outcome in clinical stage I and II carcinoma of the endometrium: A Gynecologic Oncology Group Study. *Gynecol Oncol* 40:55, 1991.

Muss HB. Chemotherapy of Metastatic Endometrial Cancer. *Semin Oncol* 21:107, 1994.

Park RC, Grigsby PW, Norris HJ. Corpus: Epithelial Tumors. In WJ Hoskins, CA Perez, RC Young (eds), *Principles and Practice of Gynecologic Oncology*. Philadelphia: Lippincott, 1992. Pp. 663–693.

Piver MS, Hempling RE. A prospective trial of postoperative vaginal radium/cesium for grade 1–2 less than 50% myometrial invasion and pelvic radiation therapy for grade 3 or deep myometrial invasion in surgical stage I endometrial adenocarcinoma. *Cancer* 66:1133, 1990.

Piver MS, Recio FO, Baker TR et al. A prospective trial of progesterone therapy for malignant peritoneal cytology in patients with endometrial carcinoma. *Gynecol Oncol* 47:373, 1992.

Piver MS, Yazigi R, Blumenson L et al. A prospective trial comparing hysterectomy, hysterectomy plus vaginal radium, and uterine radium plus hysterectomy in stage I endometrial carcinoma. *Obstet Gynecol* 54:85, 1979.

Podratz KC, Wilson TO, Gaffey TA et al. Deoxyribonucleic acid analysis facilitates the pretreatment identification of high-risk endometrial cancer patients. *Am J Obstet Gynecol* 168:1206, 1993.

Rose PG, Baker S, Kern M et al. Primary radiation therapy for endometrial carcinoma: A case controlled study. *Int J Radiat Oncol Biol Phys* 27:585, 1993.

Rubin SC, Hoskins WJ, Saigo PE et al. Management of endometrial adenocarcinoma with cervical involvement. *Gynecol Oncol* 45:294, 1992.

Salazar OM et al. Adenosquamous carcinoma of the endometrium. *Cancer* 40:119, 1977.

Silverberg SC, DeGeorgi LS. Clear cell carcinoma of the endometrium. *Cancer* 31:1127, 1973.

Smith M, McCartney AJ. Occult, high-risk endometrial cancer. *Gynecol Oncol* 22:154, 1985.

Thigpen JT et al. A randomized comparison of adriamycin with or without cyclophosphamide in the treatment of advanced or recurrent endometrial cancer [abstract]. *Proc Am Soc Clin Oncol* 4:115, 1985.

Thigpen JT et al. Phase III trial of doxorubicin +/– cisplatin in advanced or recurrent endometrial carcinoma. A Gynecologic Oncology Group (GOG) study [abstract]. *Proc Am Soc Clin Oncol* 12:261, 1993.

Ziel H, Finkle W. Increased risk of endometrial carcinoma among users of conjugated estrogens. *N Engl J Med* 293:1167, 1975.

10

Uterine Sarcoma

Peter G. Rose

Incidence and Etiology

INCIDENCE

Uterine sarcoma is rare, accounting for only 1–3% of uterine cancers. However, its virulent course in advanced disease and high recurrence rate, even when initially limited to the uterus, makes it among the most lethal of gynecologic malignancies. Despite its rarity, uterine sarcoma accounts for 15% of uterine malignancy deaths.

Little is known about the global incidence of uterine sarcomas, as most tumor registries do not specify histologic type when reporting uterine malignancy. The National Cancer Institute has collected incidence data on uterine sarcoma since the 1970s, and the age-adjusted incidence has remained unchanged up to 1985.

Patient age at diagnosis is varied, ranging from the second to the eighth decade, with a mean age of 55.7 years. Leiomyosarcoma occurs at a younger age than other uterine sarcomas.

Despite the threefold increased frequency of leiomyoma in black women, the incidence of leiomyosarcoma does not occur more frequently in one race than another. Uterine sarcomas account for a higher percentage (10%) of uterine malignancies in black women. This figure may be explained by the fact that endometrial carcinoma is twice as frequent in the white population as in blacks.

ETIOLOGY

As with endometrial carcinoma, obesity, hypertension, and diabetes are frequently associated diseases, occurring in 18%, 11%, and 8%, respectively, of patients with uterine sarcoma. Their etiologic role is not defined. Marital status has also been reported to be a risk factor, with women who have never been married at a 50% increased risk. Press and Scully reported six endometrial sarcomas following unopposed estrogenic stimulation and suggested that it is an etiologic factor for uterine sarcoma. Subsequent cases of endometrial sarcomas following unopposed estrogenic stimulation and association with tamoxifen have been reported.

Radiation Therapy

Numerous authors have reported uterine sarcoma following radiation therapy for carcinoma of the cervix. Czesnin and Wronkowski reported three uterine sarcomas developing among 8,043 cervical cancer patients treated by radiation therapy. The relative risk was 5.48%.

Malignant Potential

Malignant transformation of leiomyoma is rare. A review at Johns Hopkins University of 13,000 leiomyomas revealed only 38 cases with malignant change (0.29%). This figure represented surgically treated patients.

Signs and Symptoms

Irregular vaginal bleeding is the most common presenting symptom (80%) for all uterine sarcomas. Vaginal bleeding is more frequent with endometrial sarcomas (94%) than with leiomyosarcomas (58%). Other symptoms include pelvic or abdominal pain (16%), an enlarged uterus (12%), a pelvic or abdominal mass (9.5%), and vaginal discharge (9.5%).

Preoperative Evaluation

Because most patients present with uterine bleeding, routine evaluation, including Papanicolaou (Pap) smear and fractional endocervical and endometrial sampling, is often performed. Pap smears are more frequently positive with endometrial sarcoma (46%) than with leiomyosarcoma (22%). Leiomyosarcomas and endometrial stromal sarcomas are also less frequently diagnosed by preoperative uterine curettage (4%) than are mixed mesodermal tumors (91%). A radiograph of the chest is routinely obtained preoperatively and is a useful screen for pulmonary metastasis. However, in patients who are diagnosed as having uterine sarcoma, whole-lung tomograms or computed tomography (CT) of the chest is necessary to exclude early metastatic disease. There have been isolated reports of the use of magnetic resonance imaging (MRI) for preoperative evaluation of leiomyosarcoma. Its impact will require more extensive evaluation. Other radiographic studies and endoscopic procedures are performed as indicated by the patient's symptoms and the results of preliminary laboratory studies.

Pathology

Accurate pathology is important for proper diagnosis and for determining the prognosis of the patient with uterine sarcoma. Ober classified these tumors as pure or mixed with either homologous or heterologous components. Pure sarcomas contain a single recognizable element, whereas mixed sarcomas contain two or more elements. Sarcomatous elements are further classified as homologous, containing tissue native to the uterus (e.g., smooth muscle, endometrial stroma, and blood or lymph vessels), or heterologous, with tissue foreign to the uterus (e.g., bone, cartilage, skeletal muscle, or fat). Because of the rarity of many histologic types, the Gynecologic Oncology Group (GOG) has adopted a simplified version (Table 10-1).

LEIOMYOSARCOMA

Frequency

Although leiomyosarcoma was formerly the most frequently reported uterine sarcoma, studies now report it to be second in frequency after mixed mesodermal tumors. Leiomyosarcoma is a pure tumor arising in the myometrium. Approximately 70% are intramural, 20% are submucosal, and 10% are subserosal. The percentage that involve the cervix is higher than that of leiomyomas. Leiomyosarcomas are classically thought to present as a rapidly enlarging pelvic mass. However, one review found leiomyosarcoma to occur in only 0.23% of such patients. Furthermore, intraoperative frozen-section

Table 10-1. Classification of uterine sarcomas endorsed by the Gynecologic Oncology Group

Leiomyosarcomas
Endometrial stromal sarcomas
Mixed homologous müllerian sarcomas (carcinosarcoma)
Mixed heterologous müllerian sarcomas (mixed mesodermal sarcoma)
Other uterine sarcomas

evaluation for leiomyosarcoma is poor, with only 3 of 16 cases (18%) correctly identified. Gonadotropin-releasing hormone analogues have been used in patients with presumed leiomyosarcoma who are subsequently found to have leiomyosarcoma. The failure of the involute or the presence of increased vaginal bleeding has been suggested as a means of identifying the leiomyosarcoma.

Malignant Potential

The pathologic diagnosis depends on both the number of mitoses per 10 high-powered fields (HPFs) and cellular atypia. Using these criteria, 90% of tumors had 10 or more mitoses per 10 HPFs. However, for tumors with fewer than 10 mitoses per 10 HPFs, mitotic count alone is undependable. Among 27 uterine smooth-muscle neoplasms with 5–9 mitoses per 10 HPFs, 11 (40%) recurred. Even among 42 uterine smooth-muscle tumors with 1–4 mitoses per 10 HPFs, five (12%) recurred. More recently, there have been a number of favorable reports of patients with up to 15 mitoses per 10 HPFs as having a benign course.

Myxoid leiomyosarcomas, which contain smooth-muscle cells separated by myxoid ground substance, are clinically malignant despite their low mitotic count—0–2 per 10 HPFs. In summary, although mitotic count is important and is higher than 10 per 10 HPFs in most patients who subsequently develop recurrent disease, atypical cellular architecture and coagulative tumor necrosis are also important for identification of tumors at high risk for a malignant course.

ENDOMETRIAL STROMAL SARCOMA

Endometrial stromal tumors are classified as high-grade endometrial stromal sarcoma (ESS), low-grade endometrial stromal sarcoma, and endometrial stromal nodule on the basis of mitotic count and tumor border. Both high-grade ESS and low-grade ESS, the latter also known as endolymphatic stromal myosis (ESM), demonstrate infiltrating tumor borders.

High-Grade Endometrial Stromal Sarcoma

High-grade ESS has more than 10 mitoses per 10 HPFs, and its clinical course is highly aggressive, with 5-year survival rates reported from 0% to 55%.

Low-Grade Endometrial Stromal Sarcoma

Low-grade ESS, previously known as endolymphatic stromal myosis, has fewer than 10 mitoses per 10 HPFs, with a more indolent course and a high (100%) 5-year survival rate. With prolonged follow-up, seven of 19 patients reported by Norris and Taylor developed recurrent disease, although there was only one patient death. It has been demonstrated that low-grade ESSs are significantly more positive for estrogen- and progesterone-receptors.

Endometrial Stromal Nodule

Endometrial stromal nodule is a noninfiltrating, well-circumcised stromal tumor with fewer than 10 mitoses per 10 HPFs and a benign clinical course. However, neither mitotic index nor cytologic atypia are completely reliable prognostic factors. Chang et al. reported a 45% recurrence even in stage I patients with rare mitotic counts and minimal atypia. Flow cytometric analyses of the percentage of tumor cells in the S-phase have also been shown to correlate with tumor behavior in a small number of patients.

MALIGNANT MIXED MESODERMAL TUMOR

Malignant mixed mesodermal tumors (MMTs) contain both a sarcomatous element and a carcinomatous element. Sarcomatous elements are again classified as homologous or heterologous. *Carcinosarcoma* specifies a tumor with a malignant epithelial element and a malignant homologous sarcomatous element.

Prognosis

Norris and Taylor reported that homologous MMTs had a better prognosis than heterologous MMTs. The recently reported multivariate analysis of the GOG has confirmed the improved prognosis for homologous MMTs. In this study, among 301 MMTs, the recurrence rate for homologous tumors was 44% and for heterologous tumors was 63%. Certain heterologous elements such as cartilage or skeletal muscle have been reported to affect survival. The tumor marker CA-125 has been reported to correlate with disease status.

Malignant Potential

Only one of the elements may be malignant, as for adenosarcoma. This tumor is believed to have an improved prognosis. Clement and Scully reported 100 patients, with long-term follow-up in 88. Only 15 of the 100 patients had myometrial invasion, with only four having deep myometrial invasion. Twenty-six percent of the patients developed recurrent tumor, which was usually limited to the vagina, pelvis, and abdomen. Myometrial invasion was the only feature associated with recurrence.

Staging and Pattern of Spread

STAGING

There is no accepted staging system for uterine sarcomas. The International Federation of Gynecologists and Obstetricians (FIGO) staging for endometrial cancer is most commonly applied (see Chap. 9). Survival depends on stage, with significantly improved survival in stage I patients. Most patients (55–65%) present with clinical stage I disease, although surgical exploration demonstrates what appears to be more advanced disease than is normally seen in clinical stage I patients in as many as 25–55% of patients.

PATTERNS OF SPREAD

The treatment of uterine sarcoma has been hampered by the inability to accurately stage the disease. The biological behavior and mode of metastasis of these tumors remain poorly understood.

Uterine Sarcomas Metastasize Frequently to Extrapelvic Sites

Salazar et al. collected data from 235 patients with recurrent disease from the literature and noted that 85% of recurrences included extrapelvic sites. Among 45 patients with distant recurrence who were studied, metastatic sites included the lung (69%), upper abdomen (60%), bone (24%), and brain (4%). However, both distant and local recurrences are common.

High Recurrence Rate

The high recurrence rate of stage I disease (50–80%) despite hysterectomy implies that subclinical metastases are present. In a study by the GOG that included 453 patients, lymph node involvement correlated with histologic type, depth of invasion, the presence of vascular or lymphatic involvement, and isthmic or cervical location of the tumor. Positive peritoneal cytology is frequently found in advanced-stage disease. The significance of positive peritoneal cytology in stage I MMT has been reported. Among 18 pathologic stage I patients, 10 of 10 with positive cytology died of disease in contrast to six of 23 dying with negative cytology. Positive cytology appears to be predictive of subclinical extrauterine intraperitoneal metastasis. Whether lymphatic and peritoneal spread is the only mode for distant metastases is not known. In an autopsy study, a high percentage of patients had pulmonary metastasis in the absence of retroperitoneal nodal or intraperitoneal involvement. This finding supports a hematogenous route for metastasis.

Primary Therapy

SURGERY

The traditional surgical therapy for uterine sarcoma has been total abdominal hysterectomy and bilateral salpingo-oophorectomy (TAH/BSO). Of the cumulative reports of stage I patients treated in this manner, the 2-year survival rate is approximately 45%.

Surgical Staging

The presence of extrauterine disease significantly affects prognosis. A number of studies have examined the role of surgical staging in uterine sarcoma. The GOG studied 453 patients with clinical stage I and II uterine sarcoma who underwent comprehensive surgical staging; 301 cases had MMTs. Among 287 eligible patients the frequency of pelvic or para-aortic node metastasis was 17.8%. Pelvic nodes were involved twice as frequently as para-aortic nodes. Factors associated with nodal involvement include adnexal metastasis, positive peritoneal cytology, outer 50% myometrial invasion, and cervical or isthmic tumor location. Other sites of known intra-abdominal recurrence including the omentum, peritoneum, bowel, and liver should be evaluated. In contrast, nodal involvement was seen in only two of 57 patients (3.5%) with leiomyosarcoma.

Cytoreduction

For patients with disease extending outside the uterus, a TAH/BSO is recommended if it will effect significant tumor reduction. The role of radical debulking surgery is not well-documented, but isolated responses have been reported.

Table 10-2. Results of adjuvant radiation therapy

	Stage I (no. of patients)		*Stage II (no. of patients)*	
Author	*Surgery*	*Surgery + irradiation*	*Surgery*	*Surgery + irradiation*
DiSaia et al.	5 (3)	24 (10)	5 (5)	11 (8)
Gilbert et al.	12 (12)	4 (1)	—	—
Vongtama et al.	54 (30)	28 (7)	7 (7)	3 (0)
Salazar et al.	24 (10)	14 (7)	—	—
Perez et al.	6 (3)	17 (6)	3 (3)	8 (5)
Omura et al.	44 (21)	23 (14)	9 (6)	5 (2)
Rose et al.	32 (24)	16 (9)	—	—
Total	177 (103)	126 (54)	24 (21)	27 (15)
Recurrence rate	58.2%	42.9%	87.5%	55.6%

Myomectomy

Van Dinh and Woodruff reported nine patients who were discovered to have leiomyosarcoma after myomectomy for infertility. Only one patient developed a recurrence during follow-up ranging from 1 to 13 years. Three patients subsequently became pregnant. Although these authors had good outcome with conservative therapy, a standard recommendation for such therapy cannot be made.

RADIATION THERAPY

For medically inoperable patients, a small percentage can be effectively treated with primary irradiation. Among 37 patients reported by Badib et al., five (14%) achieved 5-year survival. When evaluated by stage, four of nine (44%) stage I patients survived 5 years compared to one of nine stage II patients and no stage III (n = 10) or stage IV (n = 9) patients.

CHEMOTHERAPY

There are no reports of primary chemotherapy achieving a cure.

Adjuvant Therapy for Stage I and II Disease

ADJUVANT RADIATION THERAPY

As demonstrated above, surgery alone resulted in only a 45% 2-year survival rate. To decrease recurrence, many centers have used adjuvant radiation therapy after primary hysterectomy. The cumulative results are presented in Table 10-2. Improved survival following adjuvant radiation therapy has been noted with MMTs but not leiomyosarcoma. In summary, most studies demonstrate that adjuvant radiation therapy increases pelvic disease control, with only occasional improved survival. The lesions generally recur outside the radiation field, implying that subclinical metastasis existed.

ADJUVANT CHEMOTHERAPY

In view of frequent distant recurrence and the proved, although limited, effectiveness of chemotherapy for advanced disease, there is great interest in prophylactic chemotherapy for early-stage disease. The cumulative results of adjuvant chemotherapy are presented in Table 10-3. The GOG performed a randomized study with 156 patients comparing Adriamycin for 6 monthly cycles to no further therapy. The recurrence rate was 41% for those treated with chemotherapy compared to 53% for those not receiving chemotherapy. The progression-free interval was 73.7 months for the chemotherapy arm versus 55 months for the untreated arm. These differences were not statistically different. The distant spread of uterine sarcoma implies the need for adjuvant systemic therapy. Whether current agents or combinations are effective enough to result in long-term cure is under study and requires longer follow-up.

ADJUVANT HORMONAL THERAPY

Because of the high (50%) recurrence rate for stage I uterine endolymphatic stromal myosis and objective response to progestational agents, a number of authors have advocated adjuvant progesterone therapy. In view of the high frequency of estrogen- and progesterone-receptors in uterine sarcomas, castration should be part of primary therapy.

Advanced Disease (Stage III and IV)

The survival rate for patients with stage III and IV disease is poor, ranging from 0% to 10%. In patients with disease limited to the pelvis on laparotomy (stage III), radiation therapy has occasionally resulted in prolonged survival. However, these patients are at risk of having subclinical extrapelvic disease, and treatment should include systemic therapy. With the advent of more effective chemotherapy, such an approach may be justified. In studies of patients with advanced or recurrent disease, the ability to excise all gross tumor confers prognostic benefit. Pulmonary metastases frequently respond to chemotherapy, and their presence is not a contraindication to surgical abdominal debulking.

Recurrent Disease

Most recurrences are at distant sites and require systemic therapy. Isolated late pulmonary recurrences have responded to local excision and have been associated with up to a 35% 10-year survival. Isolated pulmonary recurrences are rare and seen in only one of 25 patients with stage I leiomyosarcoma. Rarely, isolated pelvic recurrences have been treated with exenterative surgery. The success of these local therapies may in part be due to the indolent nature of some low-grade sarcomas. Occasionally, recurrences in the pelvis have responded to radiation therapy alone. Smith et al. treated 38 patients with recurrent or advanced disease with pelvic radiotherapy and concomitant vincristine followed by vincristine, actinomycin-D, and cyclophosphamide (VAC) chemotherapy for 2 years. Fourteen patients were alive 10–79 months without disease, although the complications of therapy were severe.

Table 10-3. Results of adjuvant chemotherapy

		Stage I (no. of patients)		*Stage II (no. of patients)*	
Author	*Regimen*	*Surgery*	*Surgery/chemotherapy*	*Surgery*	*Surgery/chemotherapy*
Buchsbaum et al.	VAC		12 (7), 58%		
Kolstad	Adriamycin		29 (3), 10%		
Omura et al.	Adriamycin	44 (21), 48%	41 (16), 39%	9 (6), 67%	3 (3), 100%
Van Nagell et al.	VAC		7 (2), 29%		
Piver et al.	Adriamycin	11 (7), 64%	8 (2), 25%		
	CYVADIC		11 (2), 18%		
Total recurrence		55 (28), 50.9%	108 (32), 29.6%	9 (6), 67%	3 (3), 100%

VAC = vincristine, dactinomycin-D, cyclophosphamide; CYVADIC = cyclophosphamide, vincristine, Adriamycin, dacarbazine.

Table 10-4. Effective single agents for uterine sarcoma

Adriamycin
Cisplatin
Dactinomycin
Diaziquone (AZQ)
Etoposide
5-Fluorouracil
Ifosfamide
Lomustine (CCNU)
Methotrexate
Methyl-CCNU
Mitoxantrone
Piperazinedione

Table 10-5. Effective combination chemotherapy regimens used for uterine sarcoma

Adriamycin, cisplatin
Adriamycin, cyclophosphamide
Adriamycin, dacarbazine
Adriamycin, ifosfamide
Cisplatin, dacarbazine
Cisplatin, Adriamycin, and dacarbazine
Cisplatin, vincristine, Adriamycin, dacarbazine
Cisplatin, ifosfamide
Hexamethylmelamine, cyclophosphamide, Adriamycin, cisplatin
Vincristine, Adriamycin, dacarbazine
Vincristine, dactinomycin, cyclophosphamide

Chemotherapy

The chemotherapy of uterine sarcoma has been integrally based on the results of other soft-tissue sarcoma regimens. Effective single agents used for uterine sarcoma are listed in Table 10-4. Only through cooperative studies has the chemosensitivity of this heterogenous group of tumors been subdivided and studied. In MMTs, ifosfamide and cisplatin are the most active agents, with response rates of approximately 30% and 20%, respectively. Doxorubicin (Adriamycin) is much less active, with a 10% response rate. In contrast, in leiomyosarcoma, doxorubicin is the most active agent, with a 25% response rate. Ifosfamide also demonstrates activity with an approximate 14% response rate. However, cisplatin has no significant activity (3–5%). Combination chemotherapy regimens used for uterine sarcoma are listed in Table 10-5. Doxorubicin with or without dacarbazine and doxorubicin with or without cyclophosphamide demonstrated no difference in activity. The combination of ifosfamide and cisplatin is currently being studied against ifosfamide in a phase III trial. Similarly, the combination of doxorubicin and ifosfamide resulted in a 37% response rate in leiomyosarcoma.

HORMONAL THERAPY

Despite the high frequency of estrogen- and progesterone-receptors in uterine sarcoma tissue, response to hormonal therapy is rare

(3%). Consistent response to hormonal therapy has been limited to low-grade endolymphatic stromal sarcoma. Hormonal therapy is the treatment of choice for these tumors.

Other Sarcomas

LYMPHOMAS

Primary lymphomas of the cervix and uterus are rare. Involvement as part of a generalized process is well-recognized and in reported series varies from 16% to 40% of patients. When disease is limited to the vagina, cervix, or uterus, a 5-year survival rate of 73% is reported compared to 40% when the disease involves the ovaries. If discovered at laparotomy, assessment of splenic and lymph node disease status, as well as liver biopsy, is advocated. Granulocytic sarcoma, also known as chloroma because of its green color, has been reported in the female genital tract and may precede the diagnosis of acute myelogenous leukemia.

HEMANGIOPERICYTOMAS

Hemangiopericytomas are a rare uterine sarcoma best treated surgically. They respond poorly to chemotherapy or radiation therapy. Gelfoam embolization preoperatively has aided in surgical excision.

Entities Mimicking Sarcoma

LEIOMYOBLASTOMA

Leiomyoblastoma is a smooth-muscle tumor with borderline malignant activity. Grossly it is softer than a leiomyoma and contains areas of hemorrhage and necrosis. Approximately 20% develop recurrent disease.

INTRAVENOUS LEIOMYOMATOSIS

Intravenous leiomyomatosis is a smooth-muscle tumor characterized by its direct growth into venous channels. It is believed to arise from the muscular wall of veins or from a leiomyoma with vascular invasion and subsequent extension beyond the leiomyoma from which it originated. Because of suspected estrogen dependence, oophorectomy is advocated. Therapy includes local excision and resection of involved veins. In some cases excision of lung metastasis and removal of tumor from the vena cava and right atrium have resulted in long-term survival.

BENIGN METASTASIZING LEIOMYOMA

Benign metastasizing leiomyoma is a smooth-muscle tumor with multiple intrapulmonary nodules. It is thought to arise from a cellular leiomyoma or intravenous leiomyomatosis that gains access to the vascular system and is transplanted to the lungs, where it is implanted and grows. Some authors have suggested that it results after incomplete primary surgery such as curettage, myomectomy, or supracervical hysterectomy.

DISSEMINATED PERITONEAL LEIOMYOMATOSIS

Disseminated peritoneal leiomyomatosis is important in that it must be differentiated from metastatic leiomyosarcoma. It is characterized by multiple peritoneal implants generally measuring less than 1 cm in diameter that involve the pelvic and abdominal peritoneal cavity. Leiomyosarcoma, in contrast, is characterized by fewer but larger metastatic lesions. On histologic examination, the lesion appears benign, with few mitotic figures and minimal nuclear atypia. The lesion is generally associated with an excess of estrogen and is found in conjunction with pregnancy, granulosa cell tumor, and oral contraceptive use. Radical excision is unnecessary, as the lesion regresses following estrogen normalization. However, sarcomatous degeneration has been reported.

Selected Readings

Akkersdijk GJM, Flu PK, Giard RWM et al. Malignant leiomyomatosis peritonealis disseminata. *Am J Obstet Gynecol* 163:591, 1990.

Altaras MM, Aviram R, Cohen I et al. Role of prolonged stimulation of tamoxifen therapy in the etiology of endometrial sarcomas. *Gynecol Oncol* 49:255, 1993.

Badib AO, Vongtama V, Kurohara SS et al. Radiotherapy in the treatment of sarcomas of the corpus uteri. *Cancer* 24:724, 1969.

Baker TR, Piver MS, Caglar H et al. Prospective trial of cisplatin, Adriamycin, and dacarbazine in metastatic mixed mesodermal sarcomas of the uterus and ovary. *Am J Clin Oncol* 14:246, 1991.

Buchsbaum HJ, Lifshitz S, Blythe JG. Prophylactic chemotherapy in stages I and II uterine sarcoma. *Gynecol Oncol* 8:346, 1979.

Chang KL, Crabtree GS, Lim-Tan SK et al. Primary uterine endometrial stromal neoplasms. *Am J Surg Pathol* 14:415, 1990.

Chen SS. Propensity of retroperitoneal lymph node metastasis in patients with stage I sarcoma of the uterus. *Gynecol Oncol* 32:215, 1989.

Clement PB, Scully RE. Mullerian adenosarcoma of the uterus: A clinicopathologic analysis of 100 cases with a review of the literature. *Hum Pathol* 21:363, 1990.

Czesnin K, Wronkowski Z. Second malignancies of the irradiated area in patients treated for uterine cervix cancer. *Gynecol Oncol* 6:309, 1978.

DiSaia PJ, Castro JR, Rutledge FN. Mixed mesodermal sarcoma of the uterus. *Am J Roentgenol* 117:632, 1973.

Gilbert HA, Kagan AR, Lagasse L et al. The value of radiation therapy in uterine sarcoma. *Obstet Gynecol* 45:84, 1975.

Goff BA, Rice LW, Fleischhacker D et al. Uterine leiomyosarcoma and endometrial stromal sarcoma: Lymph node metastases and sites of recurrence. *Gynecol Oncol* 50:105, 1993.

Hannigan EV, Gomez LG. Uterine leiomyosarcoma: A review of prognostic clinical and pathologic features. *Am J Obstet Gynecol* 134:557, 1979.

Harris NL, Scully RE. Malignant lymphoma and granulocytic sarcoma of the uterus and vagina. *Cancer* 53:2530, 1984.

Kanbour AI, Buchsbaum HJ, Hall A et al. Peritoneal cytology in malignant mixed mullerian tumors of the uterus. *Gynecol Oncol* 33:91, 1989.

Kolstad P. Adjuvant chemotherapy in sarcoma of the uterus: A preliminary report. In CP Morrow et al. (eds), *Recent Clinical Developments in Gynecologic Oncology*. New York: Raven, 1983. Pp. 123–129.

Major FJ, Blessing, JA, Silverberg SG et al. Prognostic factors in early-stage uterine sarcoma. *Cancer* 71:1702, 1993.

Montague ACW, Swartz DP, Woodruff JD. Sarcoma arising in a leiomyoma of the uterus. *Am J Obstet Gynecol* 92:421, 1965.

Norris HJ, Taylor HB. Mesenchymal tumors of the uterus: A clinical and pathological study of 53 endometrial stromal tumors. *Cancer* 19:755, 1966.

Norris HJ, Taylor HB. Mesenchymal tumors of the uterus: A clinical and pathologic study of 31 carcinosarcomas. *Cancer* 19:1459, 1966.

Ober WB. Uterine sarcomas: Histogenesis and taxonomy. *Ann NY Acad Sci* 75:568, 1959.

Omura GA, Blessing JA, Major F et al. A randomized clinical trial of adjuvant Adriamycin in uterine sarcomas: A Gynecologic Oncology Group study. *J Clin Oncol* 9:1240, 1985.

Parker WH, Fu Yao S, Berek JS. Uterine sarcoma in patients operated on for presumed leiomyoma and rapidly growing leiomyoma. *Obstet Gynecol* 83:414, 1994.

Peters WA, Howard DR, Andersen WA et al. Uterine smooth-muscle tumors of uncertain malignant potential. *Obstet Gynecol* 83:1015, 1994.

Piver MS, Lele SB, Marchetti DL et al. The effect of adjuvant chemotherapy on time to recurrence and survival of stage I uterine sarcomas. *J Surg Oncol* 38:233, 1988.

Piver MS, Rutledge FN, Copeland L et al. Uterine endolymphatic stromal myosis: A collaborative study. *Obstet Gynecol* 64:173, 1984.

Prayson RA, Hart WR. Mitotically active leiomyomas of the uterus. *Am J Clin Pathol* 97:14, 1992.

Press MF, Scully RE. Endometrial sarcomas complicating ovarian thecoma, polycystic ovarian disease and estrogen therapy. *Gynecol Oncol* 21:135, 1985.

Rose PG, Boutselis JG, Sachs L. Adjuvant therapy for stage I uterine sarcoma. *Am J Obstet Gynecol* 156:660, 1987.

Rose PG, Piver MS, Tsukada Y et al. Patterns of metastasis in uterine sarcoma: An autopsy study. *Cancer* 63:935, 1989.

Salazar OM, Bonfiglio TA, Patten SF et al. Uterine sarcomas: Analysis of failures with special emphasis on the use of adjuvant radiation therapy. *Cancer* 42:1161, 1978.

Schwartz LB, Diamond MP, Schwartz PE. Leiomyosarcomas: Clinical presentation. *Am J Obstet Gynecol* 168:180, 1993.

Smith JP, Rutledge F, Delclos L et al. Combined irradiation and chemotherapy for sarcomas of the pelvis in females. *Am J Roentgenol* 123:571, 1975.

Sutton GP, Blessing JA, Malfetano JH. A phase II trial of doxorubicin, ifosfamide and mesna in patients with advanced or recurrent uterine leiomyosarcoma. *Proc Am Soc Clin Oncol* 12:271, 1993.

Thigpen JT, Blessing JA, Beecham J et al. Phase II trial of cisplatin as first-line chemotherapy in patients with advanced or recurrent uterine sarcomas: A Gynecologic Oncology Group study. *J Clin Oncol* 9:1962, 1991.

Van Dinh T, Woodruff JD. Leiomyosarcoma of the uterus. *Am J Obstet Gynecol* 144:817, 1982.

van Nagell JR, Hanson MB, Donaldson ES et al. Adjuvant vincristine, dactinomycin, and cyclophosphamide therapy in stage I uterine sarcomas. *Cancer* 57:1451, 1986.

Vongtama V, Karlen JR, Piver MS et al. Treatment, results and prognostic factors in stage I and II sarcomas of the corpus uteri. *Am J Roentgenol Radium Ther Nucl Med* 126:139, 1976.

11

Hydatidiform Mole and Gestational Trophoblastic Tumors

John R. Lurain

Gestational trophoblastic disease encompasses four clinicopathologic forms of growth disturbance of the human trophoblast: (1) hydatidiform mole, (2) invasive mole, (3) choriocarcinoma, and (4) placental site trophoblastic tumor. The term *gestational trophoblastic tumor* has been applied to the latter three conditions because the diagnosis and decision to institute treatment are often undertaken without knowledge of the histology. These diseases are unique because of (1) the elaboration of the tumor marker human chorionic gonadotropin (hCG), (2) the inherent sensitivity of trophoblastic tumors to chemotherapy, and (3) the immunobiological relationship between the disease and its host.

Incidence

The incidence of hydatidiform mole in the United States and Europe is approximately 1 in 1,500 pregnancies. In other areas, especially the Far East, the incidence has been reported to be more than 1 in 100 normal pregnancies. Much of this geographic variation may in fact be due to reporting differences rather than true incidence differences. Repeat hydatidiform moles occur in 0.5–2.6% of patients, and these patients have a subsequent greater risk of developing invasive mole or choriocarcinoma than after an initial molar pregnancy. There is an increased risk of molar pregnancy for women over the age of 40 and at the lower end of the reproductive range, although there does not appear to be any significant association with gravidity. The overall incidence of invasive mole has been estimated to be 1 per 15,000 pregnancies. Approximately 10–17% of hydatidiform moles will result in invasive mole. Choriocarcinoma is reported to occur in 1 in 40,000 pregnancies. Approximately 2–3% of hydatidiform moles progress to choriocarcinoma, which accounts for almost 50% of cases; 25% of cases follow abortion or tubal pregnancy, and 25% are associated with term gestation.

Etiology

The etiology of hydatidiform mole remains unclear, but it appears to be due to abnormal gametogenesis and fertilization. Two main theories have been proposed to explain the sequence of events that produces hydatidiform mole. Hertig and Edmonds considered that the lesion was due to retention of a blighted ovum, with cessation of development of the villus stromal circulation and continued secretory activity of the trophoblast nourished by the material blood, resulting in varying degrees of fluid accumulation within the villus stroma and trophoblastic proliferation. Inconsistent with this theory is the fact that fetal death does not necessarily lead to hydatidiform molar change. Park believed that the primary abnormality lay in the trophoblast. Dysplasia and resultant proliferation of the trophoblast cause an oversecretion of fluid into the villus stroma. Neither theory can completely explain (1) the absence of a fetus or fetal tissues in complete moles; (2) the reasons for varying degrees of hydropic change and trophoblastic proliferation seen in complete moles, partial moles, and abortuses; or (3) the cytogenetic differences between complete and partial moles. No environmental exposure, infectious agents, or nutritional factors have definitely been implicated in the etiology of trophoblastic diseases, although a possible link between dietary carotene and vitamin A deficiency and hydatidiform mole has been suggested.

Pathology

HYDATIDIFORM MOLE

Hydatidiform mole is a pregnancy characterized by vesicular swelling of placental villi and usually the absence of an intact fetus. Microscopically, there is proliferation of the trophoblast (both cytotrophoblast and syncytiotrophoblast) with varying degrees of hyperplasia and dysplasia. The chorionic villi are fluid-filled and distended, and blood vessels are scant. Two syndromes of hydatidiform mole have been described based on both cytogenetic and morphologic criteria.

Complete or Classic Hydatidiform Mole

Complete or classic hydatidiform mole undergoes early and total hydatidiform enlargement of villi in the absence of an ascertainable fetus or embryo, and the trophoblast is consistently hyperplastic. It usually has a 46,XX karyotype derived from a paternal haploid set that totally replaces the maternal contribution and reaches the 46,XX status by its own duplication. Occasionally, a 46,XY karyotype occurs as a result of dispermic fertilization of an empty egg. Trophoblastic sequelae (invasive mole or choriocarcinoma) follow complete hydatidiform mole in 15–20% of cases and may be more commonly associated with heterozygote moles.

Partial Hydatidiform Mole

Partial hydatidiform mole is characterized by slowly progressive hydatidiform change in the presence of functioning villus capillaries that affects only some of the villi. It is associated with an identifiable abnormal fetus or embryo (alive or dead), fetal membranes, or fetal red blood cells. Trophoblastic immaturity is constant, and there is only focal hyperplasia. Partial moles have a triploid karyotype, usually 69,XXY. The reported incidence of trophoblastic sequelae following partial mole varies between 4% and 11%, with metastases occurring rarely. A histopathologic diagnosis of choriocarcinoma has not been confirmed following a partial hydatidiform mole.

INVASIVE MOLE

Invasive mole, a benign tumor arising from a hydatidiform mole, invades the myometrium by direct extension or by venous channels. It metastasizes to distant sites in about 15% of cases, most commonly to the lungs and vagina. The tumor is characterized by swollen placental villi and accompanying trophoblast with hyperplasia and usually dysplasia located in sites outside the uterine cavity. Invasive mole tends to undergo spontaneous regression.

CHORIOCARCINOMA

Choriocarcinoma, a malignant disease, is characterized by abnormal trophoblastic hyperplasia and anaplasia, absence of chorionic villi, hemorrhage and necrosis, direct uterine invasion, and vascular spread to the myometrium and distant sites, the most common of which are the lungs, brain, liver, pelvis/vagina, spleen, intestines, and kidney.

PLACENTAL-SITE TROPHOBLASTIC TUMOR

Placental-site trophoblastic tumor is an extremely rare tumor that arises from the placental implantation site and resembles syncytial endomyometritis. Pathologically, tumor cells infiltrate the myometrium and grow between smooth-muscle cells, but unlike syncytial endomyometritis there is vascular invasion. Placental site trophoblastic tumor differs from choriocarcinoma primarily in the absence of an alternating pattern of cytotrophoblast and syncytiotrophoblast, in that the cells are of one type (intermediate trophoblast), and in that hemorrhage and necrosis are less evident. There are no placental villi. Human placental lactogen is present in tumor cells, whereas immunoperoxidase staining for hCG is positive only in scattered cells. Serum hCG levels are relatively low compared to those seen with choriocarcinoma. There appears to be a direct correlation between the mitotic activity and the clinical behavior of the tumor. Although several reports have noted a benign course for some of these tumors, they are relatively chemotherapy-resistant, and deaths from metastatic disease have occurred. Surgery has been the mainstay of treatment.

Diagnosis

HYDATIDIFORM MOLE

The outstanding clinical feature of hydatidiform mole is uterine bleeding, which occurs during the sixth to sixteenth week of gestation in over 95% of patients. Toxemia of pregnancy during the first or second trimester or hyperemesis occurs in about one-fourth of patients. Clinical hyperthyroidism and trophoblastic emboli with signs and symptoms of pulmonary edema occur in a small number of patients. Occasionally, the diagnosis is based on the spontaneous passage of typical molar tissue.

On physical examination, about 50% of patients will have uterine enlargement greater than expected for the gestational date. Bilateral theca lutein enlargement of the ovaries occurs in about 15% of cases. Fetal heart tones are usually absent.

Diagnostic procedures that may confirm the diagnosis of hydatidiform mole are (1) a radiograph that fails to visualize a fetal skeleton after 16 weeks' gestation, (2) amniography, and (3) ultrasonography that demonstrates multiple echoes and holes within the placental mass and usually no fetus. Ultrasound has virtually replaced all other means of preoperative diagnosis of hydatidiform mole. hCG levels are usually, but not always, elevated above levels seen with normal pregnancy.

Differential diagnosis of hydatidiform mole includes (1) normal intrauterine pregnancy; (2) a threatened or missed abortion; (3) an intrauterine pregnancy complicated by multiple gestation or diseases associated with an enlarged placenta and elevated hCG levels (e.g., erythroblastosis fetalis and intrauterine infections); and (4) an enlarged uterus secondary to uterine leiomyomas with a small normal intrauterine pregnancy.

GESTATIONAL TROPHOBLASTIC TUMORS (INVASIVE MOLE AND CHORIOCARCINOMA)

The symptom most suggestive of invasive mole or choriocarcinoma is continued uterine bleeding after evacuation of a molar pregnancy or following any pregnancy event. Bleeding from uterine perforation or metastatic lesions may be expressed as abdominal pain, hemoptysis, melena, or evidence of increased intracranial pressure from intracerebral hemorrhage leading to headache, seizures, or hemiplegia. Patients may also present with pulmonary symptoms such as dyspnea, cough, or chest pain secondary to extensive lung metastases.

After evacuation of a hydatidiform mole, signs suggestive of postmolar trophoblastic tumor are an enlarged, irregular uterus and persistent bilateral ovarian enlargement. Occasionally, a metastatic lesion is noted on examination, most commonly in the vagina. Choriocarcinoma associated with a nonmolar gestation has no characteristic physical signs but may produce findings as a result of metastatic disease.

Most often the diagnosis of trophoblastic tumor is made clinically by the finding of a persistently elevated or rising hCG level after any pregnancy event. Metastatic lesions may be identified by radiologic studies and scans of various organs. Angiography or color flow Doppler ultrasonography may be used to identify intramyometrial lesions.

Pathologic diagnosis can sometimes be made by curettage or biopsy of metastatic lesions, or occasionally by examination of hysterectomy specimens or placentas. Biopsy of a vaginal lesion is infrequently performed because of the massive, uncontrolled bleeding that may occur.

Differential diagnosis of trophoblastic tumors includes (1) retained products of conception or endometritis as causes of postpartum uterine bleeding and subinvolution, (2) primary or metastatic tumors of other organ systems, and (3) another pregnancy occurring shortly after the first.

Management of Molar Pregnancy

When the diagnosis of hydatidiform mole is established, the molar pregnancy should be evacuated. The preferred method of evacuation, independent of uterine size, is suction curettage followed by sharp curettage. An oxytocic agent should be infused intravenously after the start of evacuation and continued for several hours to enhance uterine contractility. Hysterectomy is an alternative to suction curettage if fertility is no longer desired. There is no place for hysterotomy or medical induction of labor in the management of molar evacuation. Before evacuation, the hCG level should be determined, a radiologic examination of the lungs performed, and blood typed and cross-matched.

Follow-up of patients after evacuation of a hydatidiform mole indicates that this therapy is curative in over 80% of patients. At postoperative examination, the clinical findings of prompt uterine involution, ovarian cyst regression, and cessation of bleeding are optimistic signs. Definitive follow-up, however, requires serial hCG testing using an assay of sufficient sensitivity. Quantitative serum hCG levels should be obtained every 1–2 weeks until negative for three consecutive determinations, followed by every 3 months for 1 year. Contraception should be practiced during this follow-up period.

Patients at highest risk for postmolar trophoblastic tumors are those with (1) pre-evacuation uterine size larger than expected for gestational duration or more than 20 weeks' size; (2) bilateral ovarian enlargement (theca lutein cysts); (3) age greater than 40 years; (4) very high hCG levels; (5) medical complications of molar pregnancy such as toxemia, hyperthyroidism, and trophoblastic embolization; and (6) repeat hydatidiform mole. Prophylactic chemotherapy at the time of or immediately following molar evacuation may be considered for these high-risk patients.

Indications for treatment of postmolar trophoblastic tumor include the following:

1. Plateauing hCG levels for three consecutive determinations.
2. Rising hCG levels for two consecutive determinations.
3. High hCG levels (>20,000 mIU/ml) more than 4 weeks after evacuation.
4. Persistently elevated hCG levels 6 months after evacuation.
5. Detection of metastases.
6. Histopathologic diagnosis of choriocarcinoma.

Classification and Staging of Gestational Trophoblastic Tumors

DIAGNOSIS

Gestational trophoblastic tumor is diagnosed by rising or plateauing hCG levels following evacuation of a molar pregnancy, a histopathologic diagnosis of choriocarcinoma or placental site trophoblastic tumor, or persistent elevation of hCG or demonstration of metastases in conjunction with an elevated hCG following any pregnancy event.

EVALUATION

Once the diagnosis of a trophoblastic tumor has been made, it is necessary to determine the extent of disease. After a thorough history and physical examination, the following studies should be obtained: chest radiograph with computed tomography (CT) scan of lungs if negative, CT scan of the abdomen and pelvis, CT scan or magnetic resonance imaging (MRI) of the brain, complete blood and platelet counts, serum chemistries including liver and renal function studies, and a quantitative serum hCG assay.

STAGING

After these initial studies, patients are categorized based on anatomic extent of disease and likelihood of response to various chemotherapeutic protocols. Treatment is based on this classification.

Table 11-1. FIGO staging for gestational trophoblastic tumors

Stage I	Disease confined to uterus.
Stage IA	Disease confined to uterus with no risk factors.
Stage IB	Disease confined to uterus with one risk factor.
Stage IC	Disease confined to uterus with two risk factors.
Stage II	Gestational trophoblastic tumor extending outside uterus but limited to genital structures (adnexa, vagina, broad ligament).
Stage IIA	Gestational trophoblastic tumor extending outside uterus but limited to genital structures with no risk factors.
Stage IIB	Gestational trophoblastic tumor extending outside uterus but limited to genital structures with one risk factor.
Stage IIC	Gestational trophoblastic tumor extending outside uterus but limited to genital structures with two risk factors.
Stage III	Gestational trophoblastic tumor extending to lungs with or without known genital tract involvement.
Stage IIIA	Gestational trophoblastic tumor extending to lungs with or without genital tract involvement and with no risk factors.
Stage IIIB	Gestational trophoblastic tumor extending to lungs with or without genital tract involvement and with one risk factor.
Stage IIIC	Gestational trophoblastic tumor extending to lungs with or without genital tract involvement and with two risk factors.
Stage IV	All other metastatic sites.
Stage IVA	All other metastatic sites without risk factors.
Stage IVB	All other metastatic sites with one risk factor.
Stage IVC	All other metastatic sites with two risk factors.

Notes on staging: Risk factors affecting staging include the following: (1) serum human chorionic gonadotropin >100,000 mIU/ml, and (2) duration of disease >6 months from termination of antecedent pregnancy.
The following factors should be considered and noted in reporting: (1) Prior chemotherapy has been given for known gestational trophoblastic tumor; (2) placental site tumors should be reported separately; and (3) histologic verification of disease is not required.

FIGO Staging

A system based on anatomic criteria and conforming to the staging systems used for all other gynecologic cancers was adopted by the International Federation of Gynecologists and Obstetricians (FIGO) Cancer Committee in 1982 and was modified in 1992 (Table 11-1). Most treatment centers in the United States and Europe determine therapy and report results of gestational trophoblastic tumors using prognostic factor systems rather than an anatomic system alone.

Prognostic Group Clinical Classification

The prognostic group clinical classification system is used by most major U.S. trophoblastic disease centers to determine treatment and report results (Table 11-2). Patients with gestational trophoblastic tumors are divided into three disease groups: nonmetastatic, low-

Table 11-2. Prognostic group clinical classification for gestational trophoblastic tumors

I. Nonmetastatic gestational trophoblastic tumor
II. Metastatic gestational trophoblastic tumor
   A. Low risk
      1. hCG <100,000 IU/24-hour urine or <40,000 mIU/ml serum
      2. Symptoms present <4 months
      3. No brain or liver metastases
      4. No prior chemotherapy
      5. Pregnancy event is not term delivery (i.e., mole, ectopic, or spontaneous abortion)
   B. High risk
      1. hCG >100,000 IU/24-hour urine or >40,000 mIU/ml serum
      2. Symptoms present >4 months
      3. Brain or liver metastases
      4. Prior chemotherapeutic failure
      5. Antecedent term pregnancy

risk metastatic, and high-risk metastatic. "High-risk" refers to patients who are not likely to be cured by single-agent chemotherapy and who are at the highest risk for treatment failure. Patients are classified as being at high-risk based on the presence of one or more of the following: (1) immediate pretreatment hCG level in excess of 100,000 IU/24-hour urine or 40,000 mIU/ml serum beta-subunit; (2) greater than 4 months from antecedent pregnancy event or onset of symptoms to treatment; (3) metastases to sites other than the lungs or vagina; (4) antecedent term gestation; or (5) prior unsuccessful chemotherapy.

World Health Organization Prognostic Scoring System

In 1983, the World Health Organization (WHO) adopted a modified prognostic scoring system proposed by Bagshawe based on patient's age, parity and type of antecedent pregnancy, time interval between antecedent pregnancy and trophoblastic tumor event, hCG level, paternal and maternal blood type, number and site of metastases, largest tumor mass, and previous chemotherapy (Table 11-3). A weighted score was applied to each factor, each was assumed to act as an independent variable, and their effects were assumed to be additive. Patients with a score of 4 or less were considered to be low risk, those with a score of 5–7 were middle risk, and those with scores of 8 or greater were high risk.

Treatment of Nonmetastatic Gestational Trophoblastic Tumors

Hysterectomy is advisable as initial treatment in patients with nonmetastatic trophoblastic tumors who no longer wish to preserve fertility, and it is the treatment of choice for those with placental-site trophoblastic tumors. The use of hysterectomy to treat nonmetastatic disease results in a reduced number of courses and shorter duration of chemotherapy. Adjuvant single-agent chemotherapy at the time of operation is indicated to eradicate any occult metastases and reduce the likelihood of tumor dissemination. Hysterectomy is gen-

Table 11-3. WHO scoring system based on prognostic factors for gestational trophoblastic tumors*

	Score			
Risk factors	*0*	*1*	*2*	*4*
Age (years)	≤ 39	>39		
Antecedent pregnancy	H. mole	Abortion	Term	
Pregnancy event to treatment interval (months)	<4	4–6	7–12	>12
hCG (IU/L)	$<10^3$	10^3–10^4	10^4–10^5	$>10^5$
ABO blood groups (female x male)		0 x A A x 0	B AB	
No. of metastases		1–4	4–8	>8
Site of metastases		Spleen Kidney	GI tract Liver	Brain
Largest tumor mass, including uterine (cm)		3–5	>5	
Prior chemotherapy			Single drug	Two or more drugs

*The total score for a patient is obtained by adding the individual scores for each prognostic factor. Total score: ≤ 4 = low risk; 5–7 = middle risk; ≥ 8 = high risk.

erally performed midway through the chemotherapy protocol; no increase in postoperative morbidity has been reported with this sequence.

Single-agent chemotherapy is the treatment of choice for patients wishing to preserve their fertility. Several chemotherapy protocols have been used, all yielding excellent and comparable remission rates (Table 11-4). Methotrexate, 0.4 mg/kg (maximum 25 mg) IV or IM daily for 5 days per treatment course, has been the traditional treatment of choice. An alternate uses slightly higher doses of methotrexate, 1.0–1.5 mg/kg every other day, for doses with folinic acid, 0.10–0.15 mg/kg given IM 24 hours after each dose of methotrexate. This protocol has the advantage of decreased toxicity, especially stomatitis, but the disadvantages of increased cost, patient inconvenience, and an increased need for a change in chemotherapy to achieve remission. These methotrexate chemotherapy courses are repeated as often as toxicity permits, usually every 2 weeks (9-day window). Methotrexate has also been given in single weekly doses of 30–50 mg/m^2 IM for nonmetastatic postmolar disease, producing results only slightly less satisfactory.

Actinomycin-D, 10–13 mg/kg IV daily for 5 days per course every other week, has alternately been used and is the appropriate therapeutic regimen for patients with liver or renal disease or effusions contraindicating the use of methotrexate. Actinomycin-D may also be given as a single dose of 1.25 mg/m^2 IV every 2 weeks, yielding satisfactory results in nonmetastatic postmolar disease with greater patient convenience and improved cost-effectiveness.

Chemotherapy is changed to the alternate agent if the hCG level plateaus or if toxicity precludes an adequate dose or frequency of

Table 11-4. Chemotherapy for nonmetastatic and low-risk metastatic gestational trophoblastic tumors

Methotrexate 0.4 mg/kg IV or IM qd × 5 d; repeat every 14 days (9-day window)
Methotrexate 1.0–1.5 mg/kg IM days 1, 3, 5, 7; folinic acid 0.10–0.15 mg/kg IM days 2, 4, 6, 8; repeat every 15–18 days (7- to 10-day window)
*Methotrexate 30–50 mg/m² IM weekly
Actinomycin-D 10–13 μg/kg IV qd × 5 days; repeat every 12–14 days (9-day window)
Actinomycin-D 1.25 mg/m² IV; repeat every 14 days

*Recommended only for treatment of persistent, nonmetastatic postmolar gestational trophoblastic tumors

treatment. If there is a significant elevation in hCG level or development of metastases, multiagent chemotherapy should be started.

Treatment is continued until three consecutive normal hCG levels have been obtained and two courses have been given after the first normal hCG level. No course of chemotherapy should be started if the white blood cell count is below 3,000/mm³ or the platelet count is below 100,000/mm³. Actinomycin D should be administered as an injection over 5–10 minutes through a well-running IV infusion, as extravascular extravasation results in extensive tissue necrosis and slough.

The most common toxic reactions to these drugs are oropharyngeal ulcerations (stomatitis), other gastrointestinal ulcerations, conjunctivitis, pleuritic or peritoneal pain, vulvovaginitis, and skin rash. Significant hair loss, leukopenia, and thrombocytopenia are rare.

Cure is anticipated in all patients with nonmetastatic disease. Approximately 85% of patients are cured by the initial chemotherapy regimen. Most of the remaining patients achieve permanent remission with additional chemotherapy. Fewer than 5% of patients require hysterectomy for cure, resulting in preservation of reproductive function in more than 95% of patients.

Treatment of Low-Risk Metastatic Gestational Trophoblastic Tumors

Single-agent chemotherapy with methotrexate or actinomycin-D, as described above and in Table 11-4, is the treatment for patients in this category. When resistance to sequential single-agent chemotherapy develops, combination chemotherapy as for high-risk disease is used. Hysterectomy may be necessary to eradicate persistent, chemotherapy-resistant uterine disease, or it may be performed as adjuvant treatment coincident with chemotherapy to shorten the duration of therapy.

Cure rates should approach 100% in this group of patients if treatment is administered properly. As many as 40–50% of patients in this category will develop resistance to the first chemotherapeutic agent, however, and will require alternate treatment. It is there-

Table 11-5. EMA-CO regimen for high-risk metastatic gestational trophoblastic tumors*

Day 1	Etoposide 100 mg/m^2 IV infusion in 250 ml NS over 30 mins Actinomycin-D 0.5 mg IV push Methotrexate 100 mg/m^2 IV push 200 mg/m^2 IV infusion in 1,000 ml D_5W over 12 hrs
Day 2	Etoposide 100 mg/m^2 IV infusion in 250 ml NS over 30 mins Actinomycin-D 0.5 mg IV push Folinic acid 15 mg IM every 12 hrs for 4 doses beginning 24 hrs after starting methotrexate
Day 8	Vincristine 1.0 mg/m^2 IV push Cyclophosphamide 600 mg/m^2 IV

*Repeat cycle on days 15, 16, and 22 (every 2 weeks).

fore important to carefully monitor patients undergoing treatment for evidence of drug resistance (plateau or rise in hCG level and/or development of new metastases) so that chemotherapy can be changed as early as possible. Approximately 10–15% of patients treated for low-risk metastatic disease with sequential single-agent chemotherapy will require combination chemotherapy with or without surgery to achieve remission.

Treatment of High-Risk Metastatic Gestational Trophoblastic Tumors

CHEMOTHERAPY

Multiagent chemotherapy with or without adjuvant radiotherapy or surgery should be the initial treatment for patients with high-risk metastatic gestational trophoblastic tumors.

The EMA-CO chemotherapy regimen formulated by Newlands and Bagshawe, using etoposide, high-dose methotrexate infusion with folinic acid rescue, actinomycin-D, cyclophosphamide, and vincristine (Table 11-5), or some variation of it, is the treatment of choice for patients with high-risk disease. When brain metastases are detected, the methotrexate infusion dosage is increased to 1 g/m^2, and 30 mg of folinic acid is given every 12 hours for 3 days starting 32 hours after infusion initiation. The MAC triple chemotherapy regimen (methotrexate, actinomycin-D, and cyclophosphamide or chlorambucil) and the modified Bagshawe protocol CHAMOCA (cyclophosphamide, hydroxyurea, actinomycin-D, methotrexate, vincristine, and doxorubicin) are no longer acceptable for treatment of patients with high-risk disease. In 1984, Bagshawe initially reported an 83% survival rate in high-risk patients treated primarily with EMA-CO. A subsequent report from Charing Cross Hospital updating their experience with the regimen demonstrated an 80% complete response rate and an 82% survival rate and minimal toxicity. Schink et al. and Soper et al. have confirmed these excellent results.

The other chemotherapeutic agents with proven activity in trophoblastic tumors are cisplatin, bleomycin, and ifosfamide. These drugs have been used in combination with etoposide or vinblastine to produce cures in some patients who failed initial therapy. When these agents are used as components of primary therapy, however, significant cumulative toxicity often occurs before complete remission is accomplished, and the ability to deliver adequate salvage chemotherapy is severely compromised. Use of high doses of chemotherapy and colony-stimulating factors may also play an important role in the management of these patients.

Toxicity is significantly greater in combination chemotherapy than in single-agent treatment. Toxic reactions are similar to those listed for methotrexate and actinomycin-D, except complete alopecia occurs, nausea and vomiting may be moderately severe, and bone marrow suppression can be significant. Vincristine may cause neurotoxicity and acts as a vesicant agent if extravasation occurs. Bleomycin causes cutaneous changes and fever and may result in cumulative dose-dependent pulmonary toxicity. The dose-limiting toxicity of cisplatin is usually peripheral neuropathy or ototoxicity, although progressive renal insufficiency can result. Ifosfamide may produce progressive somnolence and coma as well as hemorrhagic cystitis.

Chemotherapy is continued until three consecutive normal hCG levels are reached and two to four courses have been given after the first normal hCG level. Only rarely should a course of chemotherapy be started if the white blood cell count is below 3,000/mm^3 or the platelet count is less than 100,000/mm^3.

RADIATION THERAPY

When central nervous system metastases are present, whole-brain irradiation (2,000–3,000 cGy in 200-cGy fractions) is given simultaneously with the initiation of combination chemotherapy using high-dose (1 g/m^2) infusion methotrexate with folinic acid rescue. Approximately 50–60% of patients with brain metastases will achieve sustained remission using this treatment plan.

SURGERY

Adjuvant surgical procedures, especially hysterectomy and thoracotomy, may be of use in removing known foci of chemotherapy-resistant disease, controlling hemorrhage, relieving bowel or urinary obstruction, treating infection, or dealing with other life-threatening complications.

RESULTS

Intensive multimodality therapy with appropriate combination chemotherapy and adjuvant radiotherapy and surgery, when indicated, has resulted in cure rates of 80–90% in patients with high-risk metastatic gestational trophoblastic tumors. The factors most important in determining prognosis in these patients are (1) clinicopathologic diagnosis of choriocarcinoma, (2) metastases to sites other than the lung and vagina, (3) number of metastases, and (4) failure of previous chemotherapy. Treatment failures in these patients are primarily due to (1) presence of extensive choriocarcinoma at the time of diagnosis, (2) lack of appropriately aggressive initial treatment in high-risk patients, and (3) failure of presently used treatment protocols to control advanced disease.

Follow-Up After Successful Treatment of Gestational Trophoblastic Tumors

TROPHOBLASTIC DISEASE SURVEILLANCE

Quantitative serum hCG levels should be obtained monthly for 6 months, every other month for the remainder of the first year, every 3 months during the second year, and at 6-month intervals indefinitely thereafter. Physical examinations are performed at 6- to 12-month intervals and other examinations (e.g., chest radiographs) as indicated.

Contraception should be maintained for 1 year after the completion of chemotherapy. Barrier methods and oral contraceptives are both acceptable forms of contraception, but the latter suppresses pituitary luteinizing hormone, which may interfere with the accurate measurement of hCG.

With a subsequent pregnancy, pelvic ultrasound examination is recommended during the first trimester to confirm a normal gestation, as these patients are at increased risk for another gestational trophoblastic disease event. Also, the products of conception or placentas from future pregnancies should be carefully examined histopathologically and an hCG level obtained 6 weeks after pregnancy termination.

REPRODUCTIVE PERFORMANCE

The successful treatment of gestational trophoblastic tumors with chemotherapy has resulted in a large number of women whose reproductive potential has been retained despite exposure to drugs that have teratogenic potential. A large number of successful pregnancies has been reported in this group of patients. In general, these patients experience no increase in abortions, stillbirths, congenital anomalies, prematurity, or major obstetric complications. There has been no evidence for reactivation of disease due to a subsequent pregnancy. Patients who have had one trophoblastic disease episode are, however, at greater risk for the development of a second episode during a subsequent pregnancy (1%), but this possibility is unrelated to whether or not they have received chemotherapy previously. Patients are advised to delay conception for 1 year from cessation of chemotherapy. This period not only allows uninterrupted hCG follow-up to ensure cure but may permit mature ova, damaged by exposure to cytotoxic drugs, to be eliminated, thereby allowing more immature oocytes to produce gametes for subsequent fertilization.

SUBSEQUENT MALIGNANCIES

Because many anticancer drugs are know carcinogens, there is concern that the chemotherapy used to induce long-term remissions or cures of one cancer may induce second malignancies. There have been no reports, however, of increased susceptibility to the development of other malignancies after successful chemotherapy of trophoblastic tumors. This may be due to the relatively short exposure of these patients to chemotherapeutic drugs and the infrequent use of alkylating agents.

Selected Readings

Bagshawe KD. Treatment of high-risk choriocarcinoma. *J Reprod Med* 29:813, 1984.

Berkowitz RS, Goldstein DP, Bernstein MR. Ten years' experience with methotrexate and folinic acid as primary therapy for gestational trophoblastic disease. *Gynecol Oncol* 23:111, 1986.

Berkowitz RS, Goldstein DP, Bernstein MR et al. Subsequent pregnancy outcome in patients with molar pregnancy and gestational trophoblastic tumors. *J Reprod Med* 32:680, 1987.

Gordon AN, Kavanagh JJ, Gershenson DM et al. Cisplatin, vinblastine and bleomycin combination therapy in resistant gestational trophoblastic disease. *Cancer* 58:1407, 1986.

Hertig AT, Edmonds HW. Genesis of hydatidiform mole. *Arch Pathol* 30:260, 1940.

Homesley HD, Blessing JA, Schlaerth J et al. Rapid escalation of weekly intramuscular methotrexate for nonmetastatic gestational trophoblastic disease. *Gynecol Oncol* 39:305, 1990.

Lurain JR. Chemotherapy of Gestational Trophoblastic Disease. In G Deppe (ed), *Chemotherapy of Gynecologic Cancer*. New York: Alan R Liss, 1990. Pp 273–301.

Lurain JR. The Natural History of Gestational Trophoblastic Diseases. In AE Szulman, HJ Buchsbaum (eds), *Gestational Trophoblastic Disease*. New York: Springer-Verlag, 1987. Pp 69–76.

Lurain JR, Brewer JI. Invasive mole. *Semin Oncol* 9:174, 1982.

Lurain JR, Brewer JI, Torok EE et al. Gestational trophoblastic disease. Treatment results at the Brewer Trophoblastic Disease Center. *Obstet Gynecol* 60:354, 1982.

Lurain JR, Brewer JI, Torok EE et al. Natural history of hydatidiform mole after primary evacuation. *Am J Obstet Gynecol* 145:591, 1983

Lurain JR, Casanova LA, Miller DS et al. Prognostic factors in gestational trophoblastic tumors. A proposed new scoring system based on multivariate analysis. *Am J Obstet Gynecol* 164:611, 1991.

Miller DS, Lurain JR. Classification and staging of gestational trophoblastic tumors. *Obstet Gynecol Clin North Am* 15:477, 1988.

Newlands ES, Bagshawe KD, Begent RHJ et al. Results with the EMA-CO (etoposide, methotrexate, actinomycin-D, cyclophosphamide, vincristine) regimen in high-risk gestational trophoblastic tumours. *Br J Obstet Gynecol* 98:550, 1991.

Park WW. *Choriocarcinoma: A Study of Its Pathology*. London: Heinemann, 1971.

Rustin GJS, Rustin F, Dent J et al. No increase in second tumors after cytotoxic chemotherapy for gestational trophoblastic tumors. *N Engl J Med* 308:473, 1983.

Schink JC, Singh DK, Rademaker AW et al. Etoposide, methotrexate, actinomycin-D, cyclophosphamide, and vincristine for the treatment of metastatic, high-risk gestational trophoblastic disease. *Obstet Gynecol* 80:817, 1992.

Soper JT, Evans AC, Clarke-Pearson DL et al. Alternating weekly chemotherapy with etoposide-methotrexate-dactinomycin/cyclophosphamide-vincristine for high-risk gestational trophoblastic disease. *Obstet Gynecol* 83:113, 1994.

Sutton GP, Soper JT, Blessing JA et al. Ifosfamide alone and in combination in the treatment of refractory malignant gestational trophoblastic disease. *Am J Obstet Gynecol* 167:489, 1992.

Szulman AE, Surti U. The syndromes of hydatidiform mole. I. Cytogenetic and morphologic correlations. *Am J Obstet Gynecol* 131:665, 1978.

Theodore C, Azab M, Droz JP, et al. Treatment of high-risk gestational trophoblastic disease with chemotherapy combinations containing cisplatin and etoposide. *Cancer* 64:1824, 1989.

Weed JC Jr, Woodward KT, Hammond CB. Choriocarcinoma metastatic to the brain: Therapy and prognosis. *Semin Oncol* 9:208, 1982.

IV

Vulvar and Vaginal Cancer

12

Vulvar Intraepithelial Neoplasias and Vulvar Non-Neoplastic Disorders

John H. Malfetano

Terminology for Vulvar Intraepithelial Neoplasia

During the past two decades, there have been major terminology changes for vulvar non-neoplastic disorders (vulvar dystrophies), intraepithelial neoplasias, and superficially invasive carcinomas. The International Society for the Study of Vulvar Disease (ISSVD) has been the major contributor in clarifying the existing confusing terms in vulvovaginal disorders. Historically, the literature is saturated with names and terms for intraepithelial vulvar diseases, including Bowen's disease, carcinoma in situ, erythroplasia of Queyrat, carcinoma simplex, hyperplastic dystrophy with atypia, Bowenoid papulosis, and Bowenoid dysplasia. Since the clinical descriptions, histologic appearance, and clinical behavior are similar for these entities, the term *vulvar intraepithelial neoplasia* (VIN) was accepted in 1986 to replace these terms.

The diagnosis of VIN is solely histopathologic and is characterized by the loss of epithelial architecture associated with nuclear hyperchromasia and pleomorphism, the presence of atypia, abnormal mitosis, dyskeratosis, parakeratosis, and hyperkeratosis (Fig. 12-1). These squamous intraepithelial lesions are then subgrouped according to the extent of atypia throughout the thickness of the epithelium:

1. Squamous vulvar VIN
2. VIN I mild dysplasia
3. VIN II moderate dysplasia
4. VIN III severe dysplasia, carcinoma in situ
5. Nonsquamous vulvar intraepithelial neoplasia
6. Paget's disease
7. Tumors of melanocytes

Similar terminology has been used for squamous intraepithelial lesions of the cervix (SIL or CIN) and the vagina (VAIN).

The anogenital epithelium is of cloacal origin and extends from the cervix to the vagina, vulva, anus, and lower 3 cm of rectal mucosa (up to the dentate line). There are similar etiologic factors and clinical presentations for pathologic entities of the lower genital tract, including the potential for preinvasive diseases (CIN, VAIN, and VIN).

Age and Incidence

There is no racial predisposition to VIN, with blacks and whites having the same prevalence. The frequency of carcinoma in situ of the

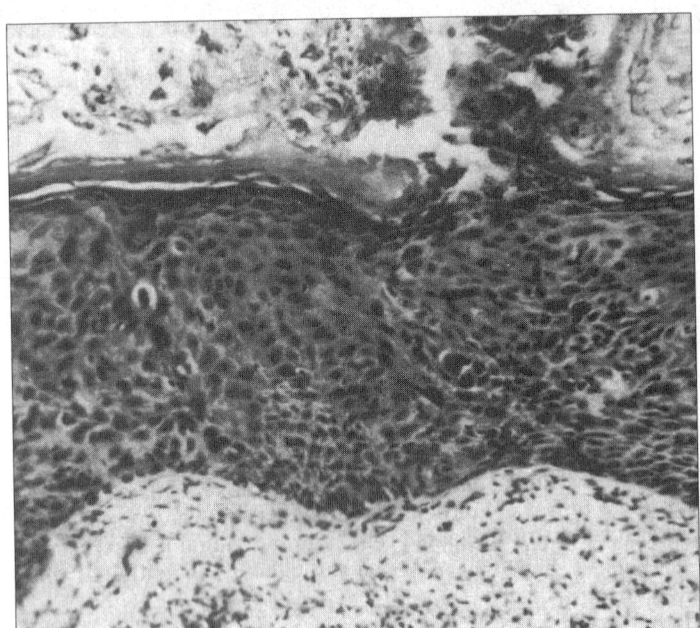

Fig. 12-1. In situ carcinoma of the vulva. Atypical cells involve the full epithelial thickness.

vulva appears to be increasing, and the average age is shifting toward young women, particularly those of reproductive age. Approximately 75% of lesions occur during the premenopausal period. The median age for women with intraepithelial vulvar carcinoma is approximately 40, with a significant number of women developing it between the ages of 20 and 39. In the study by Caglar et al. of 50 patients with VIN, the ages ranged from 14 to 83 years (median 46). Nineteen (38%) of the patients were under the age of 40. By contrast, invasive carcinoma of the vulva is primarily a disease of women between the ages of 60 and 80, suggesting a possible latent period of approximately 30 years. With much of the increase in intraepithelial vulvar carcinoma of recent origin, it may be more than two decades before we witness a rise in the incidence of invasive vulvar carcinoma similar to that seen with the progression of in situ cervical cancer to invasive cervical cancer.

Epidemiology of Vulvar Intraepithelial Neoplasia

There is still uncertainty about the etiologic factors and natural history of VIN. A strong association exists between certain sexually transmitted diseases (STDs) and VIN, including human papillomavirus (HPV), gonorrhea, syphilis, trichomonas, gardnerella vaginalis, and human immunodeficiency virus (HIV). Other investigators have suggested an association with immunosuppressed states, including renal transplants, systemic lupus erythromatosus, lymphoproliferative disorders, Fanconi's anemia, long-term corticosteroid use, and chemotherapy. Other risk factors include smoking and other genital precancers or cancers. In the study of 50 patients with VIN III by Caglar et al., 12% of the patients had preinvasive disease of the lower genital tract other than the vulva, and 12% had genital tract or extragenital invasive carcinomas.

Vulvar Non-Neoplastic Epithelial Disorders

As with the terminology for vulvar intraepithelial lesions, there has been considerable confusion with the terminology for white lesions of the vulva, which have been described as leukoplakia, senile vulvitis, kraurosis vulvae, lichen simplex chronicus, and hyperplastic dystrophy. The ISSVD discarded these terms and replaced them with the following classification:

Lichen sclerosis
Squamous cell hyperplasia (formerly hyperplastic dystrophy)
Other dermatoses

Clinically, lichen sclerosis is a thin, white or pinkish epithelial lesion that has been likened to crinkled cigarette or parchment paper. Associated vulvar changes may include atrophy with almost complete disappearance of the labia minora, Fisher's introital stenosis, and telangiectasias. The squamous cell hyperplasias of the vulva are frequently localized, elevated, and well-delineated and have a white or dusky red appearance depending on the degree of hyperkeratosis. Histopathologically, both conditions have inflammatory infiltrates. With lichen sclerosis the epithelium is thin, rete ridges are lost, and the dermis underneath the squamous epithelium has an acellular homogenous appearance. Lichen sclerosis rarely, if ever, progresses to carcinoma. Squamous cell hyperplasia histologically has hyperkeratosis (increase in the thickness of the horny layer); acanthosis (irregular thickening of the malpighian layer), which causes distortion of the rete pegs; and frequently parakeratosis. The malignant potential of this lesion is very controversial, with reports of a 1–5% likelihood of developing vulvar carcinoma. Squamous cell hyperplasia is also seen in about one-third of the patients with lichen sclerosis.

Treatment of Non-Neoplastic Vulvar Disorders

LICHEN SCLEROSIS

Multiple biopsies must be performed on several areas of the vulva prior to institution of therapy. Any other associated factors such as candidiasis, trichomoniasis, or uncontrolled diabetes should be treated concomitantly. Surgery is contraindicated because it can result in delayed healing and unsightly scarring. Topical testosterone proprionate (2%) in white petrolatum jelly twice a day for at least 6 months is the treatment of choice. Lifetime maintenance therapy is required for permanent control of the disease. The response rates to this therapy are quite variable. In patients who demonstrate little or no response or who experience the adverse side effects of increased libido, clitoral enlargement, or other androgenic effects, a topical preparation of 1–2% progesterone in petrolatum may be of benefit. Rarely, the vulvar pruritus is so intense that it is not relieved by these topical measures and interdermal injections of triamcinolone (10 mg/ml diluted 2 to 1 in saline) may be tried; 0.1 ml is injected at 1-cm intervals over the affected area and massaged into the dermis. A last resort for intense pruritus is 0.1 ml of absolute alcohol injected SC at 1-cm intervals and massaged to disperse the alcohol evenly.

Lichen sclerosis may occasionally be seen in children. Topical corticosteroids or progesterone in oil (400 mg in 4 oz of Aquaphore) used twice a day for 4–6 weeks are effective for the relief of pruritus and avoid the side effects of testosterone.

SQUAMOUS CELL HYPERPLASIA

Topical corticosteroids comprise the primary therapy. Any of the fluorinated steroids used 2–3 times a day will relieve the pruritus. For severe pruritus, crotamiton (Eurax) is added to the steroid therapy to enhance the antipruritic effect. Friderich recommended seven parts betamethasone valerite (Valisone) cream mixed with three parts Eurax used twice a day for 4 weeks.

Although surgical removal is not recommended, over a 10-year period Caglar et al. performed skinning vulvectomy with split-thickness skin graft reconstruction in three patients, carbon dioxide (CO_2) laser therapy in two patients, and simple vulvectomy in one patient because of resistance to topical therapy and severe disability from progressive vulvar dystrophy. The three patients who underwent skinning vulvectomy and the two patients treated by CO_2 laser developed recurrences in the newly grafted skin or laser site areas. However, recurrences were less severe than the original lesions and were easily controlled with steroid therapy.

MIXED VULVAR NON-NEOPLASTIC DISORDERS

Lichen sclerosis and squamous cell hyperplasia may occur together. The use of corticosteroid therapy for 6 weeks until the hyperplasia recedes followed by testosterone therapy, and then the steroid and testosterone preparations on alternate days, has been recommended.

HUMAN PAPILLOMAVIRUS INFECTION

The papilloma viruses are widespread in nature, causing characteristic proliferations on epidermal and mucosal surfaces. These lesions are benign, presenting as flat, cutaneous warts or condylomas. Since the late 1970s the incidence of genital condyloma acuminata has increased at an alarming rate. Certain subtypes of HPV are potentially oncogenic, and there is substantial evidence that they may cause cervical, vaginal, and vulvar neoplasias. Most of the condylomas of the vulva contain the more benign HPV subtypes 6 and 11, and the higher grade VINs most often contain the oncogenic HPV subtypes 16, 18, and 31.

Vigorous and effective treatment of condyloma acuminata is important. A variety of treatment regimens have been tried with limited success, including topical agents such as podophyllin resin, trichloroacetic acid, bleomycin, 5-fluorouracil, and dinitrochlorobenzene. Other therapeutic methods include surgical excision, cryosurgery, cautery, CO_2 laser, loop electrosurgical excision procedure (LEEP), and immunotherapy. Interferon is now commercially available for lesions that fail more standard therapies. The CO_2 laser has an 82% cure rate as primary therapy and a 90–96% cure rate with repeat therapy for recurrences. Any or all of these modalities should be used to remove and then control the disease while producing minimal scarring or disfiguring of the vulva.

GRANULOMATOUS LESIONS OF THE VULVA AND OTHER VENEREAL INFECTIONS

Thirteen percent of patients with VIN III have a history of previously diagnosed syphilis. A series by Sengupta of 119 Jamaican women with vulvar carcinoma noted 51% of the patients had a history of chronic granulomatous disease and syphilis. There is also an association with herpes simplex virus 2 (HSV-2) in a small number of patients with carcinoma in situ of the vulva. Frequently, patients also have concomitant trichomonal infection, gardnerella vaginalis, a history of gonorrhea, or HIV. HIV-positive status may be associated with vulvar in situ cancer or vulvar dysplasia. Korn et al. reported on 52 HIV-infected patients undergoing screening colposcopy as part of routine gynecologic care and noted cervical dysplasia in 50% and vulvar dysplasia in an additional 15%.

Clinical Presentation of Vulvar Intraepithelial Neoplasia

The clinical appearance of VIN is quite variable, with lesions being predominantly white, but gray, pink, brown, or pigmented ones may be seen. The distribution of intraepithelial neoplasia appears to have two distinct related forms that may be age-dependent: One is seen predominantly premenopausally where there are multifocal lesions, and the other form is seen in the postmenopausal woman and is more unifocal in nature. White lesions representing intraepithelial disease are the most common and are seen in about 65% of patients. The lesion previously was called leukoplakia because of its thickened white appearance. It presents as a thickened layer of keratin over the epidermis that develops in response to nonspecific irritation. The underlying subcutaneous blood vessels become obscured by the thickened hyperkeratotic layer.

The most common presenting symptom is pruritus and is present in 60% of the patients. This symptom is generally long-standing, having been present for many months to years. This frequently produces a chronic "itch-scratch" cycle until medical attention is sought. Many women are totally asymptomatic and the disease is discovered on routine inspection of the vulva during an annual examination or during colposcopy of the cervix or vagina because of an abnormal Pap smear. The minority of patients may present with perineal pain or discharge; generally this is after chronic itching and scratching of the vulva.

Diagnosis of Vulvar Intraepithelial Neoplasia

EXAMINATION AND INSPECTION OF THE VULVA

The initial part of any gynecologic examination begins with visual inspection of the vulva. Any lesion on the vulva that appears white, red, or pigmented is considered abnormal and warrants biopsy. Diagnostic measures to enhance a suspicion of an abnormality include staining the vulva with toluidine blue, colposcopy including acetic acid staining, cytologic evaluation, and biopsy.

CYTOLOGY

Although cytology has its primary role in screening for cervical abnormalities, it may aid in the diagnosis of vulvar neoplasia. Unfortunately, with hyperkeratotic skin, abnormal intraepithelial cells are frequently hidden under this layer and not obtainable by the Pap technique. Nauth and Schilke, using a moistened cotton swab and subsequent biopsy, demonstrated a 57% incidence of severely dyskeratotic cells in precancerous lesions and a 77% incidence in malignant lesions using cytology.

TOLUIDINE BLUE

Toluidine blue is a nuclear stain that reflects increased nuclear activity from ulceration, infection, or neoplasia of the vulvar skin. The vulva is painted with 1% toluidine blue, which, after 2 minutes, is washed off with 1% acetic acid. Abnormal areas will retain the pale blue dye, whereas normal skin will be devoid of the dye. The areas of dye retention represent abnormal tissue and should be biopsied. False-negative reactions can be seen with areas that are ulcerated or abraded or in some hyperkeratotic lesions that can only absorb a small amount of dye.

COLPOSCOPY

The colposcope has been an invaluable aid for the diagnosis of cervical and vaginal intraepithelial disease and is quite helpful for the experienced colposcopist when examining the vulva. Three to five percent acetic acid is applied to the vulva and left for a minimum of 3 minutes. Intraepithelial neoplasia will produce a predominant aceto-whitening of the skin with or without punctation; this denotes the area for biopsy. It is also quite valuable in assessing HPV infection of the vulva, especially in patients with known HPV infection of the lower genital tract.

BIOPSY

Biopsy remains the definitive method for the diagnosis of any pigmented vulvar lesion. The Keys dermatologic punch is essential for vulvar biopsies. The specimen obtained from this punch biopsy allows the most accurate orientation for evaluation of the specimen's full thickness. Technique for biopsy is cleansing the skin with an antiseptic solution and infiltrating the skin and subcutaneous tissue with 1% lidocaine using a 25- or 27-gauge needle. A 4-mm Keys dermatologic punch is pressed firmly into the lesion or at its periphery and rotated in a circle and the specimen is removed. If there is any bleeding, Monsel's solution (ferric subsulfate) or silver nitrate can be applied for hemostasis. Intraepithelial disease is frequently multifocal and several biopsies are required. Excisional biopsy of the vulva should be reserved for those lesions that have extensive induration or ulceration and when the punch biopsy has not yielded a satisfactory pathologic specimen.

Treatment for Intraepithelial Neoplasia

Treatment for intraepithelial diseases of the vulva must be individualized. It is based on the patient's symptoms, the amount of disease found on the vulva, and the results of inspection, palpation, colposcopy, and multiple biopsies.

Spontaneous regression of untreated VIN III has been reported, but it is relatively uncommon and has usually been associated with HPV infection. Untreated, VIN III may progress to an invasive carcinoma, although the latent period at present is unknown.

TOPICAL 5-FLUOROURACIL AND DINITROCHLORBENZINE

Five percent topical 5-FU cream (Efudex) may be applied to the vulva for treatment of intraepithelial neoplasia. This cream will cause a chemical desquamation of the lesion, which generally causes a significant amount of burning, pain, inflammation, and edema to the vulva that most patients find unsatisfactory. The overall response rate for VIN III with Efudex cream is 63%, and the cream probably should be reserved for use after traditional methods fail. Topical dinitrochlorbenzine (DNCB) is another treatment regimen that is only indicated when all other measures have failed. A report by Foster and Woodruff indicated a complete response to DNCB in five of six patients that had previous surgery and/or topical 5-FU.

CARBON DIOXIDE LASER

The CO_2 laser was introduced as an alternative to surgical excision. The goal of CO_2 laser vaporization is to treat the entire area of abnormal vulvar epithelium with resultant rapid healing. With the laser, the depth of tissue destruction can be seen colposcopically and be controlled. In nonhairy areas, destruction to a depth of less than 1 mm will ablate the lesion and preserve the desired cosmetic effect. In hairy areas of the vulva, because the hair root sheet may extend to a depth of 2.5 mm, vaporization to a depth of 3 mm is required. This depth of vaporization may cause destruction of skin appendages and result in hypertrophic scar formation, thereby negating the cosmetic advantage of laser therapy. The cure rate for VIN with one laser application is about 70%. One-third of these patients need a second or third laser operation to control the disease.

CRYOTHERAPY

Cryotherapy has little use for intraepithelial diseases of the vulva because of delayed and painful healing and the inability to treat large geographic areas on the vulva.

PHOTODYNAMIC THERAPY

Photochemical destruction of cells sensitized with a light-activated compound such as hematoporphyrin has been applied to intraepithelial diseases of the vulva.

LOOP ELECTROSURGICAL EXCISION PROCEDURE

LEEP uses an electrosurgical generator and a high-frequency alternating current passed through a monopolar electrode (wire loop) to cut or coagulate tissue. This new technology has emerged for evaluation and treatment of premalignant diseases of the vulva, vagina, and cervix. There is considerable experience using this technique for cervical dysplasia (CIN). Less clinical information exists for diagnosis and therapy of VIN. One of the problems in applying this technique to vulvar diseases is that the epithelium of the vulva is much thinner than that of the cervix, and extreme care must be taken to avoid thermal damage to the subepithelial tissues, causing noninterpretable specimens and cosmetic disfigurement.

SURGERY

Surgery remains the hallmark treatment modality for intraepithelial carcinomas of the vulva. The major advantages of surgery are that the lesion is completely removed and a pathologic specimen is available to review to rule out any occult invasive carcinoma. In a series of 50 patients reported by Caglar with carcinoma in situ of the vulva, pretreatment colposcopic evaluation and biopsy failed to reveal an invasive carcinoma in five patients (10%). In three of these patients (6%), invasion was an incidental finding at the time of the therapeutic wide local excision. Other advantages of surgery include a lower recurrence rate than is seen with CO_2 laser, topical 5-FU, photodynamic therapy, or cryotherapy. Disadvantages of surgery include the need for general anesthesia, increased postoperative pain, and possible scar formation.

WIDE LOCAL EXCISION

For unifocal lesions, a wide local excision with a 1-cm margin of noninvolved skin is generally curative. Particularly with patients with HPV-associated intraepithelial disease, the failure rate from a wide excision will be high because of the multifocal nature of the disease and the presence of subclinical viral infections in the normal-appearing adjacent skin. Intraepithelial disease of the vulva involves only the epidermis and not the dermis. Therefore, in performing a wide excision, only the epidermis and not the underlying fibrofatty tissue, muscle, or glands should be excised. These defects can be closed primarily with a fine absorbable suture, and excellent cosmetic results should be obtained.

SKINNING VULVECTOMY

In patients with extensive carcinoma in situ of the vulva, a skinning vulvectomy operation was developed to avoid the more mutilating procedure of vulvectomy. Underneath the epidermis is a relatively avascular plane that allows easy excision of the overlying epidermis and the intraepithelial disease. Frequently, the remaining defect can be closed primarily with fine suture. However, at times the defect is so large that it will require application of a full-thickness skin graft to the remaining superficial fascia, generally taken from the thigh. This operation is generally reserved for extensive multifocal disease that cannot be treated with wide local excision (Fig. 12-2).

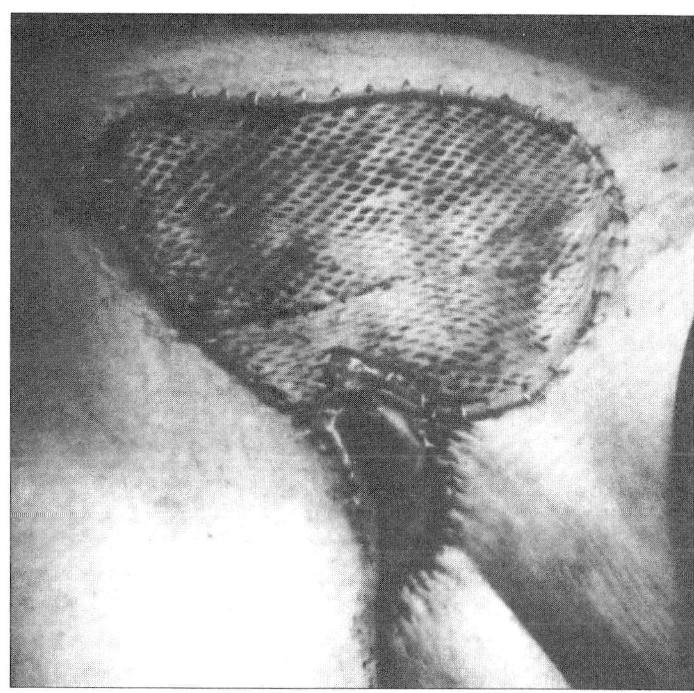

Fig. 12-2. Total skinning vulvectomy including the vulva, perineum, anus, and anal canal. Note the full-thickness skin graft.

Nonsquamous Intraepithelial Vulvar Lesions: Paget's Disease

Paget's disease is an intraepithelial disease that predominately affects postmenopausal white women. Clinically, women present with pruritus and vulvar discomfort. Paget's disease has a characteristic erythematous scaly appearance and histologically shows large, pale, vacuolated cells with vesicular nuclei (Paget's cell) within the epidermis and particularly in the rete ridges (Fig. 12-3). Unlike mammary Paget's disease, in which there is almost always an underlying ductal carcinoma, vulvar Paget's disease is associated with an underlying adenocarcinoma in only 20% of patients.

The mainstay of therapy is surgery. Excision of the involved vulva can be accomplished by wide local excision or simple vulvectomy for more extensive cases. Care must be taken when using wide local excisions since the disease frequently extends beyond the gross lesion. If an underlying adenocarcinoma is diagnosed, then radical vulvectomy and staging lymphadenectomy are required.

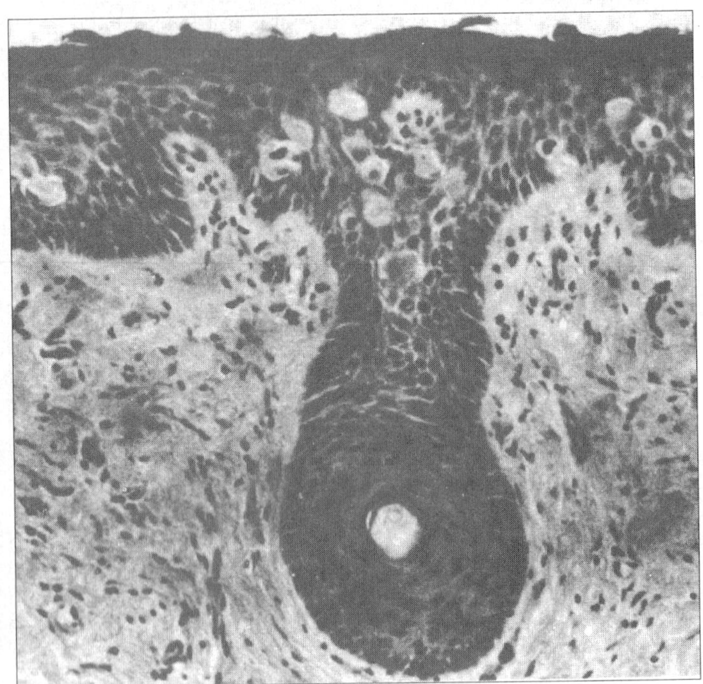

Fig. 12-3. Paget's disease of the vulva. Note the large, pale Paget's cells within the epithelium.

Selected Readings

Ansink AC, Krul MRL, Deweger RA et al. Human papillomavirus, lichen sclerosis and squamous cell carcinoma of the vulva: Detection and prognostic significance. *Gynecol Oncol* 52:180, 1994.

Bloss JD. The use of electrosurgical techniques in the management of premalignant diseases of the vulva, vagina and cervix: An excisional rather than an ablative approach. *Am J Obstet Gynecol* 169:1081, 1993.

Caglar H, Erk M, Hreshchyshyn MM. Carbon dioxide laser surgery of female genital, perineal and anal condyloma acuminata. *NY State J Med* 87:365, 1987.

Caglar H, Tamer S, Hreshchyshyn MM. Vulvar intraepithelial neoplasia. *Obstet Gynecol* 60:346, 1982.

Foster DC, Woodruff JD. The use of Dinitrochlorobenzene in the treatment of vulvar carcinoma in situ. *Gynecol Oncol* 11:330, 1981.

Friedman-Kien AE, Eron LJ, Conant M et al. Natural interferon alfa for treatment of condylomata acuminata. *JAMA* 259:538, 1988.

Hart W, Millman J. Progression of intraepithelial Paget's disease of the vulva to invasive carcinoma. *Cancer* 40:2333, 1977.

Hart W, Norris H, Helwig E. Relation of lichen sclerosis et atrophicus of the vulva to development of carcinoma. *Obstet Gynecol* 45:369, 1975.

Korn AP, Autry M, DeRemer PA et al. Sensitivity of the papanicalaou smear in human immunodeficiency virus-infected women. *Obstet Gynecol* 83:401, 1994.

Nauth HF, Schilke E. Cytology of the exfoliative layer in normal and diseased vulvar skin: Correlation with histology. *Acta Cytol* (Baltimore) 26:269, 1982.

Reid R, Greenberg MD, Lorinez AT et al. Superficial laser vulvectomy. IV. Extended laser vaporization and adjunctive 5-fluorouracil therapy of human papillomavirus-associated vulvar disease. *Obstet Gynecol* 76:439, 1990.

Rettenmaier M, Berman ML, DiSaia PJ et al. Photoradiation therapy of gynecologic malignancies. *Gynecol Oncol* 17:200, 1984.

Rutledge F, Sinclair M. Treatment of intraepithelial carcinoma of the vulva by skin excision and graft. *Am J Obstet Gynecol* 102:806, 1968.

Sengupta BS. Carcinoma of the vulva in Jamaican women. *Acta Obstet Gynecol Scand* 60:537, 1981.

Wilkinson EJ. The 1989 Presidential Address. International Society for the Study of Vulvar Disease. *J Reprod. Med* 35:981, 1990.

Wright VC, Davies E. Laser surgery for vulvar intraepithelial neoplasia. *Am J Obstet Gynecol* 156:374, 1987.

13

Vulvar Cancer

John H. Malfetano

Carcinoma of the vulva should be amenable to early diagnosis. Any physician caring for women must thoroughly examine the vulva prior to evaluation of the vagina or the cervix. The vulva should be inspected for any obvious masses, ulcers, or color changes within the epithelium. White, red, or pigmented lesions are considered abnormal and warrant biopsy. Careful palpation of the inguinal regions and the vulva for subcutaneous lesions is important after the visual examination.

Patient and physician delay is common in making vulvar diagnoses. Earlier detection of vulvar carcinomas coupled with the prognostic factors that have been clearly defined within the last decade will allow more conservative cosmetic surgery and improved survival.

Incidence

Vulvar carcinoma is a disease of the aged, accounting for 4–5% of all gynecologic malignancies. With 2,500 new cases annually in the United States, it remains the fourth most common genital tract malignancy, surpassed only by carcinomas of the endometrium, ovary, and cervix. The disease is seen in the postmenopausal woman, with the highest incidence in the seventh decade of life and a median/average age of 63. Seventy-five percent of the patients are over the age of 50, with nearly one-third being at least 70 years of age. Fifteen percent of the patients will develop the disease under the age of 40, and this incidence may be rising.

Etiology

PRURITUS

Many hypotheses for etiologic factors in carcinoma of the vulva have been proposed; however, no specific causative agent has been identified. The only common variable in all theories is a chronic itch-scratch cycle. The intense pruritus that accompanies vulvar carcinoma causes profuse itching. This perpetual sequence persists until the patient seeks medical attention and a pathologic diagnosis is made. Delays in diagnosis are frequently affected by the patient's social and cultural background as well as physician delay in taking a biopsy.

WETNESS

The vulva and adjacent labial crural folds are inherently moist or wet, so there is excellent absorption of any foreign substances through the vulvar skin. The degree of absorption frequently depends on the hydration state of the stratum corneum in the vulvar epidermis. Obesity and poor hygiene are important predisposing factors for carcinoma of the vulva.

HISTORICAL PERSPECTIVES (INDUSTRIAL WASTE AND ARSENICALS)

In England, Stacey reported on toxic substances that were associated with carcinomas of the vulva. He recognized that women working with bituminous oils in cotton-spinning areas of Lancashire and in several dye works near Halifax had contamination of their undergarments by these substances. He also noted a number of cases of vulvar carcinoma near Sheffield in women working in steel and silver plants who reported using oily cotton wastes instead of toilet paper. Arsenic was a substance frequently found in medications to treat illnesses such as syphilis, leukemia, anemia, and skin diseases. Fowler's solution (liquour arsenicalis) was prescribed by dermatologists for many years for the treatment of pruritus vulvae. Other detergents contained arsenic, which, if not completely rinsed from the underclothing, led to chronic vulvar irritation and the itch-scratch cycle.

HYGIENIC AGENTS

Vaginal deodorants, perfumed soaps, and hygenic sprays may be carcinogenic.

HYGIENE

Vulvar hygiene remains most important in preventing epithelial changes in the vulva that develop from chronic itching and scratching. Dyes and underclothing can be irritants to the skin and therefore white underwear is preferred when the vulva has been irritated. Tight pants and synthetic underwear, such as nylon, produce poor ventilation and can initiate local irritation. Rinsing the vulva with water after voiding, especially in patients with stress urinary incontinence, and the use of powders as drying agents are important to good vulvar hygiene.

VULVAR INTRAEPITHELIAL NEOPLASIA

It is well recognized that untreated cervical intraepithelial neoplasia (CIN) may progress to invasive carcinoma of the cervix. However, this continuum from a precancerous lesion to an invasive lesion is not well documented for intraepithelial lesions of the vulva (VIN). VIN is usually seen in women under the age of 40 and invasive carcinomas of the vulva after the age of 60. With respect to cervical intraepithelial disease, it is widely accepted that there is a 5- to 10-year latent period before the appearance of an invasive carcinoma. However, with invasive diseases of the vulva, the latent period appears to be 25–30 years.

INFECTIONS

Chronic granulomatous venereal diseases and syphilis have been implicated in the etiology of carcinoma of the vulva. Sengupta, in a series of 119 Jamaican women with vulvar carcinoma, noted that 51% of the patients had a history of chronic granulomatous disease and syphilis. These diseases are seen infrequently today in the United States, and their association with carcinoma of the vulva remains less well substantiated.

VULVAR NON-NEOPLASTIC DISORDERS (DYSTROPHIES)

The malignant potential of squamous cell hyperplasia and lichen sclerosis remains controversial. Historically, it was reported that

50% of patients with white lesions (leukoplakia) would develop vulvar carcinoma. Lichen sclerosis rarely, if ever, will progress to an invasive carcinoma of the vulva. However, squamous cell hyperplasia is seen concomitantly in about one-third of the patients with lichen sclerosis, and the malignant potential of the squamous cell hyperplasia is 1–5%.

HUMAN PAPILLOMAVIRUS

There has been much research done on human papillomavirus (HPV) as an etiologic factor in squamous cell carcinomas of the cervix and carcinoma of the vulva. Most of the HPV infections of the vulva are of a benign subtype 6 and 11, producing characteristic condylomas. HPV subtypes 16, 18, and 31 are considered more oncogenic and are frequently associated with higher-grade VIN. However, to date, there is no definite series suggesting that HPV infection is a causative factor of invasive diseases of the vulva, other than having a possible association.

OTHERS

Other potential etiologic factors that have been studied include smoking, presence of other genital intraepithelial lesions or cancers, immunosuppressed states, and the human immunodeficiency virus (HIV).

Presentation and Symptoms

PRESENTATION

There is generally a long period of delay before seeking medical attention in this group of patients and also in making the diagnosis of vulvar carcinoma. Most of these patients are elderly and frequently embarrassed, so they deny the condition and rarely speak to their friends or family about their genital problems until a mass or bleeding occurs. Frequently, the family notices an unusual odor or discharge and inquires about the problem. Nearly 60% of patients have had a mass, lesion, or sore for 10 months prior to seeking therapy. Once medical attention is sought, there usually is another delay of 3 months or longer in making the diagnosis. These lesions are treated with salves, ointments, and creams without a biopsy until the condition worsens or consultation is sought. Twenty-five percent of patients are under medical treatment without a biopsy.

SYMPTOMS

Eighty percent of patients with vulvar carcinoma will present with pruritus. This symptom is usually present for years before the patient seeks medical attention. Less commonly a mass, swelling, ulcer, or bleeding lesion is noted. Pain is a common symptom when a lesion is near the clitoris or urethra because of discomfort with micturition. Superinfection of the malignancy also causes pain and more irritation from the discharge that ensues. Only about 5% of patients present with a groin lump or abscess as the presenting complaint.

DIAGNOSIS

Any lesion on the vulva—red, white, pigmented, ulcerative, raised, exophytic, or new—warrants biopsy. The biopsy can be accomplished in the office with local anesthesia in the majority of patients. The vulva is prepared with an antiseptic solution and infiltrated with a local anesthetic solution. The Keyes dermatologic punch (4 mm) is an excellent instrument for performing the vulvar biopsy. Otherwise, a small excisional biopsy can be performed with little discomfort. Cytology (Papanicolaou smear), colposcopy, and toluidine blue staining of the vulva can be performed to delineate the extent of some lesions. However, definitive diagnosis must be made histopathologically.

Lymphatics of the Vulva

Nearly 60% of carcinomas are present on the labia majora, with 20% on the labia minora or vestibule, 12% near the clitoris, and 6% on the perineal body. Primary epidermoid carcinoma of the vulva spreads contiguously to adjacent structures (i.e., urethra, bladder, vagina, and rectum and via lymphatic embolization to the regional inguinal and femoral lymph nodes). Hematogenous spread to distant organs is rare and usually a late phenomenon. The vulva has a rich lymphatic network covering its entire surface.

There are delicate anastomoses and lymphatic channels from one side of the vulva to those on the opposite side. Understanding the lymphatic network allows individualization and less radical operative procedures in some patients. Contralateral involvement of the inguinal nodes without ipsilateral spread is almost never seen. Malfetano et al. reported a series of 169 patients from Roswell Park Cancer Institute; 58 had inguinal lymph node metastasis, and only one had contralateral metastasis. The primary lymphangitic route of spread to the inguinal nodes is via the superficial femoral nodes, then the deep femoral nodes, and finally the pelvic lymphatics via the external iliac, obturator, common iliac, and paraaortic nodes. The inguinal nodes are found along the inguinal ligament and along the saphenous vein underneath the skin in Camper's fascia and above the cribriform fascia. These nodes remain the primary nodal group for metastatic disease. The secondary nodal group includes the deep femoral nodes, which are located along the femoral artery, vein, and nerve and underneath the fascia lata and cribriform fascia. Cloquet's node, or the node of Rosenmüller, has been thought of as a sentinel node for metastatic disease to the pelvis. This node lies at the entrance of the femoral canal (the lowest of the external iliac nodes below the inguinal ligament) (Fig. 13-1).

The location of the primary tumor frequently dictates the extent and type of surgery indicated secondary to the nodal drainage. Lesions on the labia majora, labia minora, and clitoris drain to the superficial and deep inguinal nodes on the same side (ipsilateral) as the primary lesion. If the metastatic disease is present within the inguinal nodes, then the contralateral nodes and pelvic nodes are at risk for metastases. The clitoris also has alternative lymphatics that drain over the pubic symphysis to the external iliac or obturator nodes via the dorsal vein of the clitoris. Clitoral lesions were once thought to have a higher incidence of pelvic nodal disease without inguinal disease because of the lymphatic network of the clitoris, but this has not been proven clinically. Lesions that primarily involve the vagina may drain directly to the pelvic lymphatics, and lesions encroaching on the anus can metastasize via the hemorrhoidal lymphatic system to aortic nodes.

A thorough understanding of the lymphatic supply of the vulva is important for managing treatment of vulvar carcinomas. Clinically

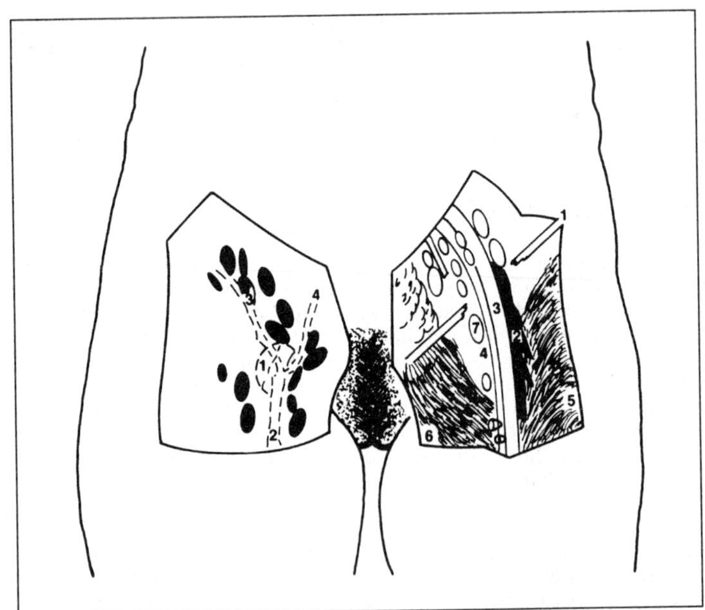

Fig. 13-1. Right (patient's): Superficial inguinal nodes. (1 = cribriform fascia covering fossa ovalis; 2 = saphenous vein; 3 = superficial epigastric vein; 4 = superficial circumflex iliac vein.) Left (patient's): Deep inguinal nodes after the cribriform fascia has been removed. (1 = inguinal ligament; 2 = femoral nerve; 3 = femoral artery; 4 = femoral vein; 5 = sartorius muscle; 6 = adductor longus muscle; 7 = Cloquet's node.)

we cannot rely on our assessment of inguinal nodes when formulating any treatment plan since palpation is frequently unreliable. There is 25–50% error in our clinical estimation by palpation of nodal metastases.

Staging

The staging system for vulvar carcinoma was previously based on clinical examination to include the tumor size, tumor location, and lymph node status. With the poor predictiveness of inguinal node palpation, the significance of lymph node metastases for survival, and the fact that the majority of patients undergo radical vulvectomy and groin node dissection, the staging system was changed to a surgical system. The new surgical staging system incorporates the actual pathologic status of the inguinal nodes (Table 13-1).

Treatment

SURGERY

Standard therapy for invasive squamous cell carcinoma of the vulva remains radical vulvectomy and bilateral inguinal femoral lymphadenectomy. The mortality and morbidity rates from this proce-

Table 13-1. FIGO staging of vulvar carcinoma

		TNM	*Classification of carcinoma of the vulva*
Stage 0			
Tis	Carcinoma in situ, intraepithelial carcinoma	T	Primary tumor
Stage I			
T1 N0 M0	Tumor confined to the vulva and/or perineum—≤ 2 cm in greatest dimension, nodes are not palpable	Tis	Preinvasive carcinoma (carcinoma in situ)
Stage II			
T2 N0 M0	Tumor confined to the vulva and/or perineum—>2 cm in greatest dimension, nodes are not palpable	T1	Tumor confined to the vulva and/or perineum—≤ 2 cm in greatest dimension
Stage III			
T3 N0 M0 T3 N1 M0 T1 N1 M0	Tumor of any size with: (1) Adjacent spread tothe lower urethra and/or the vagina, or the anus, and/or (2) Unilateral regional lymph node metastasis	T2	Tumor confined to the vulva and/or perineum—>2 cm in greatest dimension
Stage IVA			
T1 N2 M0 T2 N2 M0	Tumor invades any of the following: upper urethra, bladder mucosa, rectal mucosa, pelvic bone, and/or bilateral regional node metastasis	T3	Tumor of any size with adjacent spread to the urethra and/or vagina and/or to the anus

Table 13-1. (continued)

		TNM	*Classification of carcinoma of the vulva*
Stage IVB Any T Any N M1	Any distant metastasis including lymph nodes	T4	Tumor of any size infiltrating the bladder mucosa and/or the rectal mucosa, including the upper part of the urethral mucosa and/or fixed to the bone
		N	Regional lymph nodes
		N0	No lymph node metastasis
		N1	Unilateral regional lymph node metastasis
		N2	Bilateral regional lymph node metastasis
		M	Distant metastasis
		M0	No clinical metastasis
		M1	Distant metastasis (including pelvic lymph node metastasis)

Source: Adapted from the International Federation of Gynecology and Obstetrics. Annual report on the results of treatment in gynecologic cancer. *Int J Gynecol Obstet* 28:189, 1989.

dure, which had been great in the past, have been drastically reduced with earlier detection, improvement in surgical techniques, and the ancillary support of blood banking, antibiotics, and improved anesthesia. Unfortunately, problems of body image and sexual dysfunction persist, although they generally affect only a small group of younger women. Within the past decade, there has been a trend toward less radical operations, with the integration of both surgery and radiation therapy in an attempt to decrease the morbidity of the standard operation.

PROGNOSTIC FACTORS

Many attempts have been made to identify a set of clinical pathologic variables to predict survival in patients with carcinoma of the vulva. The single most important variable remains the presence or absence of groin node metastases (Table 13-2). Other variables—for example, tumor size, grade, lymphovascular invasion, tumor confluence, depth of invasion, and age—may contribute to inguinal nodal disease and ultimate survival but cannot be isolated as single prognostic factors.

SURVIVAL

The overall survival rate for patients with carcinoma of the vulva and negative inguinal-femoral nodes is 90% or better. However, the rate drastically drops to 38–40% when the nodes contain metastases.

Minimally Invasive Carcinoma

CONSERVATIVE SURGERY

There has been a recent effort to do less-radical surgery in a select group of patients with early invasive carcinoma of the vulva. It must be stressed that to do less-radical surgery in a select group of patients, one cannot jeopardize the cure rate—which is more than 90% in patients with negative inguinal nodes—to improve cosmetic or sexual well-being. The optimal management of early invasive cancer must be individualized, and one must consider the most appropriate surgical procedure for both the primary tumor and the groins.

DEFINITION OF INVASIVENESS

The definition of microinvasive or minimally invasive carcinoma of the vulva has been controversial. The International Society for the Study of Vulvar Disease (ISSVD) unanimously recommended that superficially invasive carcinoma of the vulva (stage IA) be rigidly defined, as conservative operations may lead to an increased risk of recurrence and death. Stage IA carcinoma of the vulva was defined as a single lesion measuring 2 cm or less in diameter with a depth of invasion of 1 mm or less. Patients with more than one site of invasion are not included in this category. The depth of invasion is measured as the distance from the epithelial stromal junction (basement membrane) of the adjacent, most superficial dermal papillae to the deepest point of tumor invasion. The thickness of the tumor is defined as the distance from the surface of the tumor or granular layer when a keratin layer is present to the deepest point of invasion (Figs. 13-2 and 13-3).

Table 13-2. Incidence of positive groin nodes according to FIGO stage

FIGO stage	*No. of patients*	*% positive*
I	142	10
II	191	31
III	195	55
IV	5	5

Source: Adapted from HD Homesley. Carcinoma of the Vulva. In HF Cann (ed), *Conn's Current Therapy*. Philadelphia: Saunders, 1985. P 98.

Table 13-3. Incidence of lymph node metastasis versus depth of invasion in patients undergoing vulvectomy and inguinal lymphadenectomy (61 patients)

Depth (mm)	*No. of cases*	*Nodal metastasis (%)*
<1	6	0
>1	55	27.3
<2	16	18.8
>2	45	26.7
<3	22	13.6
>3	39	30.8
<4	34	14.7
>4	27	37.0
<5	42	16.7
>5	17	42.1

Source: Adapted from JH Malfetano, MS Piver, Y Tsukada et al. Univariate and multivariate analysis of 5-year survival, recurrence and inguinal node metastasis in stage I and II vulvar carcinoma. *J Surg Oncol* 30:124, 1985.

These definitions were needed when several reports in the literature appeared using the term *microinvasive carcinoma* with no universal definition. The incidence of lymph node metastases was unacceptably high at 11.1% and recurrence rates of 12.6% in a disease that appeared to be cured with a more radical operation. More recently, Malfetano et al. reported on 61 patients undergoing radical vulvectomy and bilateral groin node dissection with lesions clinically confined to the vulva, and no patient with less than 1 mm of invasion had nodal metastasis compared with 18.8% of those with less than 2 mm of invasion (Table 13-3). Hacker et al. confirmed this data with a report of 77 patients who had stromal invasion of 5 mm or less. Thirty-four patients had less than 1 mm of invasion, and no patient had inguinal nodal disease, although there was significant nodal metastasis as the depth of invasion increased beyond 1 mm.

GUIDELINES

Minimally invasive carcinoma of the vulva may be treated in a more conservative fashion. If the tumor is unifocal, a wide radical local excision with surgical margins of at least 1 cm may be performed for stage I lesions (<2 cm in diameter) and with a depth of invasion of 1 mm or less. The risk for groin node metastasis in this particular group is negligible and a groin node dissection is not required. All other patients with unilateral lesions and more than 1 mm of invasion should under-

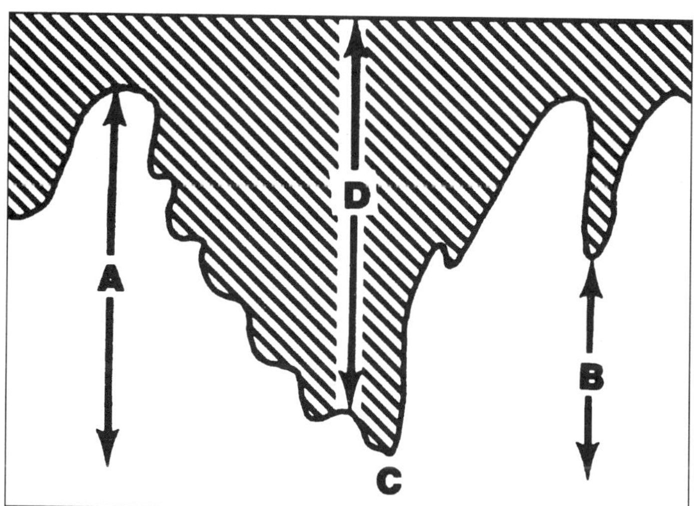

Fig. 13-2. ISSVD definition for measuring the depth of invasion. A. Top of most superficial dermal papilla. B. Deepest ridge. C. Deepest part of tumor invasion. D. Tumor thickness.

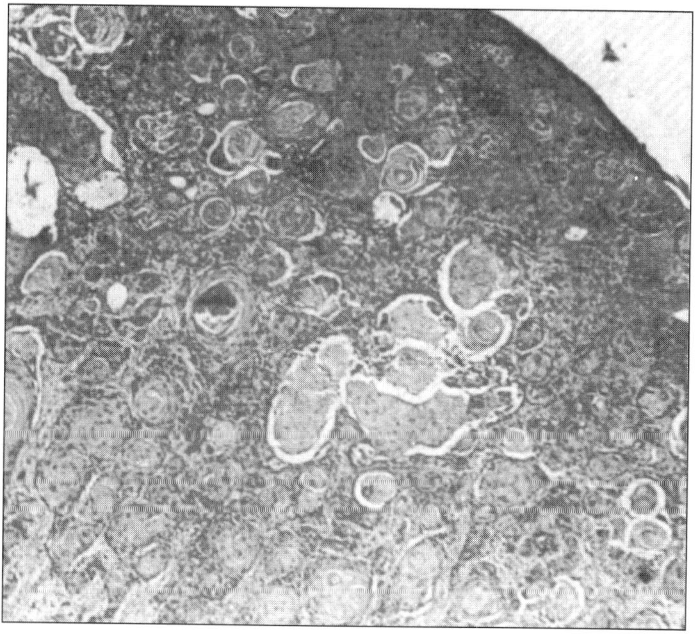

Fig. 13-3. Squamous cell carcinoma with 3 mm depth of invasion.

go ipsilateral groin node dissection to document the presence or absence of nodal disease. Bilateral inguinal femoral lymphadenectomy is still required for those patients with bilateral lesions or lesions crossing the midline.

Ongoing clinical trials are attempting to resolve this issue of less radical surgery. Many centers are advocating a conservative approach for solitary lesions 2 cm or less and a depth of invasion of 5 mm or less. The primary lesion is resected by a wide radical excision, and the ipsilateral inguinal nodes are dissected. This treatment is considered sufficient as long as the primary lesion has no lymphatic or vascular space involvement and the inguinal nodes are negative for metastasis. The operating surgeon must be prepared to perform the standard operation of radical vulvectomy and bilateral groin node dissection if the groin nodes are positive or the primary lesion contains lymphatic and vascular space involvement or is more invasive than 5 mm. Long-term results from this type of conservative surgery are not yet available, so such treatment must remain in centers with research protocols.

Complications of Radical Vulvectomy and Bilateral Inguinal Lymphadenectomy

WOUND INFECTION

Wound breakdown or infection of the vulvar or groin incisions occurs in more than 50% of patients. Careful attention to hemostasis and ligation of efferent and afferent lymphatics as well as not devascularizing the skin flaps of the groin help decrease this occurrence. The use of prophylactic antibiotics and suction drains in the groin also help reduce this complication. Today, many centers advocate doing the radical vulvectomy and dissecting the groin nodes through separate incisions to decrease the morbidity from the operation. However, concern for recurrences within the "skin bridges" between the vulva and the groin must be considered when undertaking the operation in this fashion. The management of wound breakdown includes local care with cleansing and sharp debridement as necessary. Appropriate cultures and antibiotics are needed when the patient has developed an infection clinically. With meticulous wound care the wound heals by secondary intention.

LYMPHEDEMA

Lymphedema is a rather unsightly and unfortunate complication of radical vulvectomy, and bilateral groin node dissection is reported in nearly one-third of patients. The occurrence of chronic lymphedema may lead to lymphangitis or erysipelas. Support stockings, pneumatic calf compression stockings, and antibiotics are helpful for managing this problem.

FEMORAL NERVE PARASTHESIAS

Trauma to the femoral nerve when dissecting the inguinal nodes causes some degree of numbness and pain over the upper anterior surface of the thigh in nearly all patients postoperatively. This common occurrence is rather self-limited and usually resolves within 2 months. In more extreme cases, physical therapy is frequently helpful.

SECONDARY HEMORRHAGE

Hemorrhage from the femoral vein or artery is a potential problem, although it rarely occurs. This condition may appear with infection of the groin leading to disruption of the vessels. Transplantation of the sartorius muscle to cover these great vessels has been advocated as a routine procedure when doing a groin node dissection. Obviously, careful, meticulous hemostasis is important for preventing this complication. The use of suction drains may also be helpful for preventing accumulation of blood and lymph and for decreasing infection rates.

LYMPHOCYSTS

Lymphocysts are more common than previously reported. A lymphocyst is a unilocular lymph-filled space without a distinct epithelial lining. Its presence causes accumulation of lymph within the groin, producing a cystic mass that becomes painful and frequently secondarily infected. Previous irradiation, metastatic disease to the lymph nodes, ultraradical lymphadenectomy, and heparin may contribute to this problem. Careful surgical ligation of efferent and afferent lymphatics as well as suction drains and pneumatic calf compression stockings may encourage the obliteration of this dead space and prevent the problem. Drainage of the lymphocyst under aseptic techniques is necessary if this complication occurs.

THROMBOEMBOLIC DISEASE

Radical surgery involving extensive dissection about great vessels can predispose to phlebitis and pulmonary embolus. Prophylactic heparin or pneumatic calf compression stockings reduces these risks. Appropriate anticoagulation is necessary if these conditions arise.

URINARY TRACT INFECTIONS

Postoperatively, patients undergoing radical vulvectomy and bilateral groin node dissection have an indwelling Foley catheter for several days. Urinary tract infections are frequent with indwelling catheters. Difficulty controlling micturition occurs when the catheter is removed. Spraying of the urinary stream is common with removal of the labia. Another common problem is incontinence if a radical urethrectomy is needed for removal of the primary tumor or anatomically the bladder base has been moved or sutured.

SEXUALITY

There has been increased awareness of problems with body image and sexuality after this operation. There is markedly reduced acceptance by the patient of her body image as well as of coital activity after this procedure. Other concerns include sexual dysfunction with a high frequency of reduced libido, orgasmic dysfunction, and dyspareunia. Appropriate preoperative information and teaching may lessen this problem. Sexual or psychiatric counseling may be necessary.

Other Cell Types

Nearly 90% of all carcinomas of the vulva are of the squamous cell variety. Other histologic cell types that can occur on the vulva (in descending order of frequency) are melanoma, Paget's disease, basal cell carcinoma, adenocarcinoma, and sarcoma.

MELANOMA

Malignant melanoma of the vulva is the second most common vulvar malignancy. Nearly 5% of all melanomas occur on the vulva, which accounts for only 1% of the total body skin surface. The disease is more frequently seen on the labia minora and clitoris than is squamous cell carcinoma. There is frequent extension to the vagina and urethra on presentation. There appears to be a slight predilection for fair-complexioned, blue-eyed women, with increasing incidence with age, and the lesions appear to be familial. Presenting symptoms are similar to those of squamous cell carcinoma. All pigmented lesions on the vulva demand excision, especially the junctional nevus, which may be a precursor lesion to melanoma.

Staging

The initial stage at presentation appears to be the most important prognostic factor along with the microscopic staging. The International Federation of Gynecologists and Obstetricians (FIGO) staging system is not applicable to melanomas because the prognosis is mainly related to the depth of tumor penetration. There are two microscopic staging systems that have been used for vulvar melanoma. Clark's staging system depends on the anatomic level of the skin invaded by the melanoma. Survival correlates with the specific subepidermal layer of penetration. Breslow's classification appears to be more appropriate for vulvar melanoma, as the vulvar skin lacks a well-defined papillary dermis and interpretation is sometimes difficult. Breslow's system includes a numerical value (in millimeters) of the distance from the surface epithelium to the site of deepest tumor penetration (Table 13-4). Survival appears to correlate with depth of invasion.

Treatment

Appropriate therapy must be individualized to the site and extent of the primary lesion as well as the microscopic staging system. The treatment of vulvar melanoma remains controversial; however, the primary lesion should be removed with a margin of at least 2 cm. For those melanomas with a depth of invasion of greater than 0.75 mm, a radical vulvectomy and regional lymphadenectomy should be considered.

ADENOCARCINOMA

Adenocarcinomas are unusually rare and generally arise from Bartholin's gland. Any inflammatory process within this gland may produce pain and swelling and must be evaluated for the possibility of a malignancy. Other presenting symptoms can include dyspareunia, a palpable mass, or an ulcer in the region of Bartholin's gland. Treatment consists of radical vulvectomy and bilateral inguinal femoral lymphadenectomy.

BASAL CELL CARCINOMA

Basal cell carcinomas can occur on all hair-bearing areas of the body and are occasionally seen on the labia majora. They may present as (1) a red or brown macule or superficial plaque or (2) a small nodule with a central ulceration—the so-called rodent ulcer. These lesions almost never metastasize to lymphatics, and wide local excision is the treatment of choice.

Table 13-4. Breslow's classification of melanoma

Level	*Thickness of lesion (mm)*
1	<0.76
2	0.76–1.5
3	1.5–3.0
4	>3.0
5	>4.0

Source: A Breslow. Thickness, cross-sectional areas, and depth of invasion in the prognosis of cutaneous melanoma. *Ann Surg* 172:901, 1970.

PAGET'S DISEASE

Paget's disease is an intraepithelial lesion of the vulva frequently associated with an underlying adenocarcinoma arising from the apocrine glands. There is a 20–25% incidence of an underlying adenocarcinoma in association with this lesion. The origin of the Paget's cell remains controversial, with some authors believing it arises from the apocrine glands underlying the squamous epithelium and others believing that it originates from an undifferentiated basal cell of the squamous epithelium that embryologically gives rise to the skin appendages. The usual presentation is a bright red, pruritic, scaly lesion with raised white patches, giving the appearance of leukoplakia. The treatment is wide local excision with careful sectioning of the underlying apocrine-bearing tissue for histologic study to detect an occult adenocarcinoma. If no carcinoma is identified, wide excision is all that is necessary; however, recurrences at the skin margins are frequent, and re-excision may be necessary. Radical vulvectomy and bilateral inguinal femoral lymphadenectomy is the treatment of choice if an underlying adenocarcinoma is discovered on wide excision of the primary lesion.

VERRUCOUS CARCINOMA

Verrucous carcinoma is a pathologic variant of epidermoid carcinoma of the vulva with its own distinct clinicopathologic features. Patients present with an exophytic cauliflower-like or papillary growth that resembles condyloma acuminatum. This lesion was originally called the giant condylomas of Buschke-Löwenstein. Generally, the lesion is locally aggressive, with contiguous growth and infrequent metastasis. Therefore, histology becomes important for differentiating these lesions from papillomas or a condyloma acuminatum. A superficial biopsy can make this diagnosis more difficult. Histologically, a papillomatous tumor with hyperkeratosis and parakeratosis is seen. There is pronounced acanthosis and deeply penetrating tongues of highly differentiated epithelium, without nuclear pleomorphism and occasional mitoses. The treatment for these lesions is wide local excision. Radiation therapy has been implicated in the transformation of these lesions to anaplastic carcinoma and thus should be avoided.

SARCOMAS

Sarcomas are rare on the vulva, but distant metastases are common. Leiomyosarcoma appears to be the most common variant, although liposarcoma, lymphoma, rhabdomyosarcoma, fibrosarcoma, angiosarcoma, and epithelioid sarcoma have been reported. The treatment must be individualized to the location and extent of the primary lesion, although wide local excision appears to be the most appropriate treatment. The role of adjuvant radiation therapy or chemotherapy is to be considered, although there are no data to substantiate these modalities.

Recurrence

Nearly 80% of recurrent carcinoma of the vulva occurs within the first 24 months. Treatment modalities depend on whether the recurrences are local, inguinal, or distant. Generally, local recurrences can be treated with wide excision. Groin node metastasis can be re-excised, and pelvic and inguinal radiation therapy may be considered. The role of chemotherapy has been slow to evolve with carcinoma of the vulva, and there appear to be no active agents at the present time for this disease.

Radiation Therapy

Radical vulvectomy and bilateral inguinal femoral lymphadenectomy are curative in 90% of patients with no evidence of metastasis to the inguinal nodes. Unfortunately, patients with metastasis to the groin nodes have a significantly less favorable survival. It appears that the number of positive nodes or bilaterality of positive nodes is related to prognosis. Patients with three or fewer positive unilateral nodes continue to have a good prognosis; however, for those with bilateral positive nodes or more than three positive nodes, the prognosis is dismal.

A Gynecologic Oncology Group protocol compared pelvic and groin irradiation to pelvic lymphadenectomy in patients with metastatic disease in the inguinal femoral nodes. A significantly superior progression-free interval of 70% versus 51% and survival rate of 79% versus 54% at 2 years were seen with the radiation therapy regimen. There was also a decrease in groin node recurrence from 42.1% to 11.8% in the group that underwent radiation therapy. Therefore, it is recommended that patients with two or more inguinal metastases or bilateral metastases to the groin nodes undergo inguinal and pelvic irradiation after primary surgery.

There are many ongoing clinical trials and preliminary reports on the role of a combined chemotherapy-radiation treatment approach. Patients with advanced vulvar carcinomas whose disease is not suitable for surgical resection because of rectal or bladder involvement that would necessitate an exenterative procedure or those who have unresectable inguinal nodes would be candidates. The attempt is to cause sufficient regression of the primary or metastatic lesions to allow lesser nonexenterative surgery to be contemplated. The majority of these trials are using cisplatin and 5-fluorouracil infusion with radiation therapy. There appears to be a significant response rate to this aggressive combined treatment modality; however, significant data are still not available to recommend this treatment approach.

Selected Readings

Boronow RC. Combined therapy as an alternative to exenteration for locally advanced vulvo-vaginal cancer: Rationale and results. *Cancer* 49:1085, 1982.

Breslow A. Thickness, cross-sectional areas and depth of invasion in the prognosis of cutaneous melanoma. *Ann Surg* 172:901, 1970.

Clark WH et al. The histogenesis and biologic behavior of primary human malignant melanomas of the skin. *Cancer Res* 29:705, 1979.

Creasman WT, Gallagher HS, Rutledge F. Paget's disease of the vulva. *Gynecol Oncol* 3:133, 1975.

DiSaia PJ, Rutledge F, Smith VP. Sarcoma of the vulva: Report of 12 patients. *Obstet Gynecol* 38:180, 1971.

Hacker NF et al. Individualization of treatment for stage I squamous cell vulvar carcinoma. *Obstet Gynecol* 63:155, 1984.

Hacker NF et al. Management of regional lymph nodes and their prognostic influence in vulvar cancer. *Obstet Gynecol* 61:408, 1983.

Homesley H et al. Radiation therapy versus pelvic node resection for carcinoma of the vulva with positive groin nodes. *Obstet Gynecol* 68:733, 1986.

International Society for the Study of Vulvar Disease. Microinvasive cancer of the vulva: Report of the ISSVD Task Force. *J Reprod Med* 29:454, 1984.

Japaze H, Van Dina T, Woodruff JD. Verrucous carcinoma of the vulva. Study of 24 cases. *Obstet Gynecol* 60:462, 1982.

Keys H. Gynecologic Oncology Group. Randomized trials of combined technique therapy for vulvar cancer. *Cancer* 71:1691, 1993.

Leuchter RS et al. Primary carcinoma of the Bartholin gland: A report of 14 cases and review of the literature. *Obstet Gynecol* 60:361, 1982.

Malfetano JH, Piver MS, Tsukada Y. Stage III and IV squamous cell carcinoma of the vulva. *Gynecol Oncol* 23:192, 1986.

Malfetano JH, Piver MS, Tsukada Y et al. Univariate and multivariate analysis of 5-year survival, recurrence and inguinal node metastases in stage I and II vulvar carcinoma. *J Surg Oncol* 30:124, 1985.

Piver MS, Xynos FP. Pelvic lymphadenectomy in women with carcinoma of the clitoris. *Obstet Gynecol* 49:592, 1977.

Piver MS, Malfetano JH, Lele SB et al. Prophylactic anticoagulation as a possible cause of inguinal lymphocyst after radical vulvectomy and inguinal lymphadenectomy. *Obstet Gynecol* 62:17, 1983.

Rose PG, Piver MS, Tsukada Y et al. Conservative therapy for melanoma of the vulva. *Am J Obstet Gynecol* 159:52, 1988.

Sengupta BS. Carcinoma of the vulva in Jamaican women. *Acta Obstet Gynecol Scan* 60:537, 1981.

Stacey JE. Epithelioma of the vulva. *Proc Royal Soc Med* 32:304, 1939.

14

Vaginal Cancer

Michael L. Hicks

A primary malignancy originating in the vagina is an exceptionally rare condition representing approximately 1–2% of all gynecologic malignancies. The most common malignant cell type originating in the vagina is squamous cell carcinoma. Other primary lesions of the vagina can occur, most notably adenocarcinoma, melanoma, sarcoma, and endodermal sinus tumor. However, secondary or metastatic carcinomas (cervical cancer, gestational trophoblastic disease, endometrial cancer, ovarian cancer, colorectal carcinoma, urogenital carcinoma, and vulvar carcinoma) are identified much more frequently in the vagina than primary lesions.

Squamous Cell Carcinoma

EPIDEMIOLOGY

Squamous cell carcinoma of the vagina has its peak incidence between the ages of 50 and 60. The majority of cases of squamous cell carcinoma of the vagina have been reported to occur in the posterior wall of the upper third of the vagina. However, because of the multicentricity of the disease, several lesions also may occur at any site simultaneously.

Vaginal exposure to the human papillomavirus, early hysterectomy, and previous irradiation have been suggested as possible risk factors for the development of squamous cell carcinoma of the vagina. To date, specific etiologic factors are yet to be validated.

PRESENTATION

Postmenopausal vaginal bleeding and/or vaginal discharge are the most common symptoms in patients presenting with primary vaginal carcinoma. Other symptoms, although less common, are pelvic pain and pressure, dyspareunia, dysuria, and postcoital bleeding. These symptoms are usually associated with more advanced stages of the disease. It should be mentioned that the Papanicolaou (Pap) smear may identify asymptomatic patients with squamous cell carcinoma of the vagina, especially in patients who have undergone a hysterectomy.

DIAGNOSTIC EVALUATION

Asymptomatic Patients with Previous Hysterectomy

In the presence of a Pap smear that is suspicious for squamous cell carcinoma, the patient should undergo colposcopic evaluation and directed biopsies of the vagina. This is imperative to identify and diagnose the presence of an invasive vaginal lesion.

Symptomatic Patients

Symptomatic patients presenting as described above must undergo complete inspection of the vagina during speculum examination. Any gross lesions seen should be biopsied for histologic confirmation of invasive disease. This will also aid in adequately documenting the location of the lesion.

Table 14-1. FIGO clinical staging for primary vaginal cancer

Stage 0	Carcinoma in situ (intraepithelial carcinoma)
Stage I	Carcinoma is limited to the vaginal mucosa
Stage II	Carcinoma has involved the subvaginal tissue but has not extended into the pelvic wall
Stage III	Carcinoma has extended into the pelvic wall
Stage IV	Carcinoma extension with involvement of the mucosa of the bladder or rectum or extension beyond the true pelvis

Staging

All patients should have a thorough history and physical examination. After tissue confirmation, the patient must be evaluated for the extent of local and possible metastatic disease. The following diagnostic studies should be performed: chest x-ray, intravenous pyelogram (IVP), cystoscopy, and proctosigmoidoscopy. Computed tomography may be useful in evaluating areas in the upper abdomen, such as the liver, proximal ureters, and retroperitoneal lymphatic system.

Staging for vaginal carcinoma is clinical, not surgical. Staging is in accordance with the International Federation of Gynecologists and Obstetricians (FIGO) listed in Table 14-1.

PROGNOSTIC FACTORS

The two most significant factors influencing prognosis in patients with squamous cell carcinoma of the vagina are (1) the depth of tumor penetration into the vaginal wall and local structures and (2) the volume of disease. The location of the lesion, age of the patient, and tumor differentiation have not been found to influence prognosis significantly.

TREATMENT

In the past, vaginal cancer has been treated variably with radical surgery, radiation therapy, or a combination of both. By the early 1970s, surgical therapy had become the preferred treatment at several centers. A convincing treatise on this subject in 1970 by Herbst et al. reviewed 68 cases of primary carcinoma of the vagina, 32 of which were treated by radical surgery and 36 by radiation therapy. The 5-year survival rate for surgery was 48.4% versus 21.1% for radiation. The conclusions of this study and others like it, however, did not consider the factors of patient selection (patients with more advanced lesions tended to undergo radiation therapy) and that many of the irradiated patients were treated with equipment and techniques now considered obsolete. In addition, women receiving surgical treatment were usually permanently maimed, losing the vagina and often the bladder or rectum (total pelvic exenteration). Most of these patients have spent the remainder of their lives sexually incapacitated and with surgically created stomata for excretion of urine and feces.

Subsequently, in 1971, the year following the publication by Herbst et al. that advocated surgery for cancer of the vagina, Brown and coworkers published a study in which 76 patients achieved excellent results with a primary radiotherapeutic approach to this disease. In their study, 70% of patients with stage I, II, and III vaginal cancers survived 5 years after treatment. Stage-for-stage, survival was similar to that seen for cancers of the cervix and endometrium, both of which had long been thought to have a significantly better prognosis than cancer of the vagina. In addition, unlike many of the women who underwent radical surgery, patients treated with radiation therapy most often maintained a functional vagina and normal urinary and fecal continence. A high cure rate and low complication rate have now been achieved by many authors using modern radiotherapy techniques. However, even though radiation therapy has become the mainstay of treatment for vaginal cancer, there are still selected cases where surgical extirpation is the preferred method of management.

Radiation Therapy

Treatment of squamous cell carcinoma of the vagina must be tailored to the stage, location, depth, extent of disease, and previous surgery that the patient may have undergone (i.e., hysterectomy). The combination of external beam radiation (teletherapy) and internal or local radiation (brachytherapy) must be used for bulky and deep lesions greater than a depth of 0.5 cm. External beam radiation will usually result in shrinkage of the vaginal neoplasm, which allows for a better anatomic arrangement for successful application of brachytherapy devices. Additionally, external beam radiation decreases tumor burden (volume of disease) in order to improve the effectiveness of brachytherapy.

Stage 0

In situ carcinoma is a noninvasive lesion of the vagina. The entire epithelium of the vaginal mucosa has abnormal cells; however, there is no penetration of the abnormal cells below the basement membrane. The mainstay of treatment of this lesion is either surgical excision or laser vaporization. Colposcopic guidance is recommended to accurately identify the areas of abnormality. Local irradiation with an intracavitary application has been used in the treatment of in situ carcinoma of the vagina. The dose of radiation ranges from 6,500 to 8,000 cGy. It is delivered to the vaginal mucosa only since there is no need for treatment of tissue underlying the basement membrane. Although this treatment is effective, it could result in vaginal stenosis. 5-Fluorouracil (5-FU) topical treatment can also be used for carcinoma in situ of the vagina. The recommended dose is 5 g intravaginally at night for 5 days. This should be repeated every 6–12 weeks after evaluation for response. This treatment can lead to significant vaginal and vulva irritation and therefore compliance is a problem.

Stage I

Treatment of stage I as well as all stages of vaginal carcinoma must be individualized based on location, multifocal sites, size, and depth of invasion of the disease. The patient with an intact uterus who has a lesion in the upper third of the vagina may be treated with brachytherapy alone using a central tandem and ovoids (a Fletcher Suit or similar applicator) similar to the treatment of cervical cancer (Fig. 14-1). Additionally, smaller lesions in other anatomic sites of the upper two-thirds of the vagina may be treated with an intracavitary cylinder overlying the entire vaginal mucosa. The cylinder should deliver 6,000–7,000 cGy to the vagi-

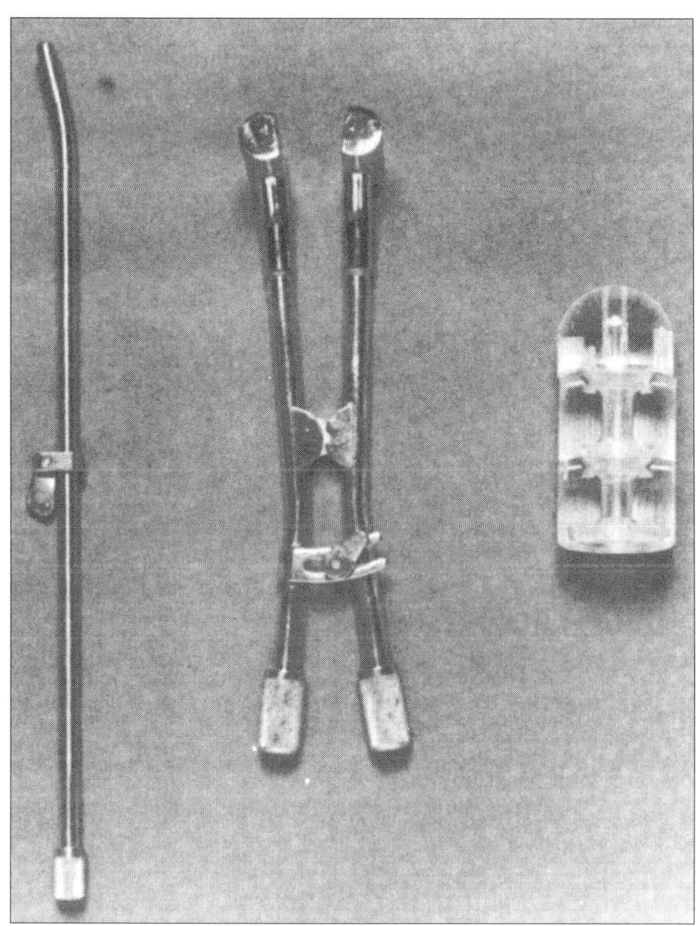

Fig. 14-1. Left to right: Uterine tandem, vaginal ovoids, and vaginal cylinder are used for intravcavitary irradiation in the treatment of vaginal cancer.

nal mucosa and 6,000–7,000 cGy to a depth of 0.5 cm at the site of tumor invasion.

Cases in which there is only one isolated lesion in the upper two-thirds of the vagina are the exception. The majority of patients will present with multifocal or larger lesions. Additionally, because the reported incidence of pelvic recurrence is somewhere between 10% and 20%, local therapy alone will not have a significant impact on decreasing pelvic recurrences.

Therefore, patients with multifocal lesions or a lesion greater than 2 cm should undergo external beam radiation initially. This radiation is given in a fractionated method with a total dose of 4,000–5,040 cGy. Following external beam radiation therapy, if the maximum diameter of the residual disease is less than 0.5 cm, it can be adequately treated with two intracavitary brachytherapy appli-

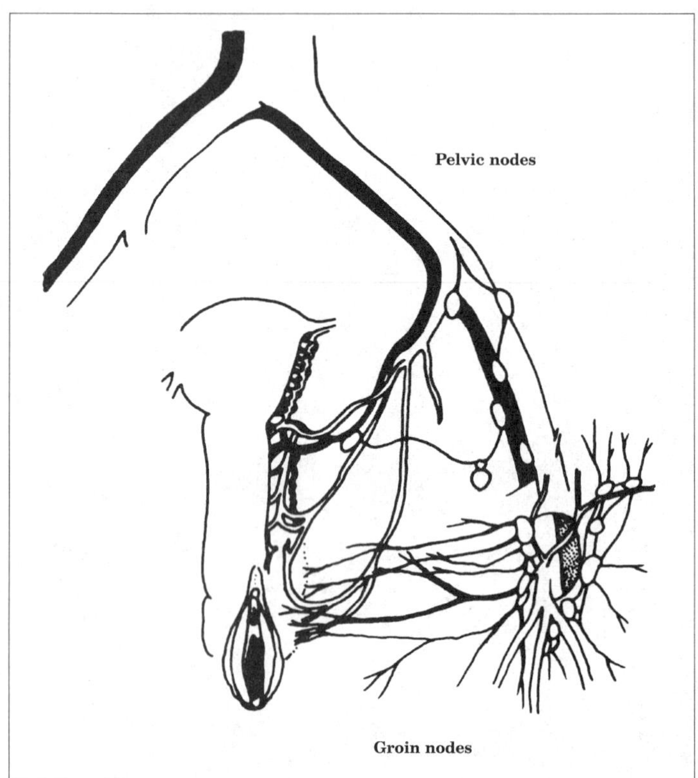

Fig. 14-2. Lymphatic drainage of the upper and lower vagina. The upper two-thirds of the vagina drains directly to the pelvic lymph nodes, and the lower one-third drains to the groin lymph nodes.

cations delivering a total dose (including external beam radiation therapy) of 6,000–8,000 cGy to a depth of 0.5 cm below the vaginal mucosa. Improved survival in stage I squamous cell carcinoma of the vagina has been accomplished with the use of combination radiation therapy (external beam radiation therapy and brachytherapy) compared to external beam radiation therapy or brachytherapy alone.

Stages II–IV

With more advanced stages of disease the tumor volume increases, anatomic deviations occur, regional lymph node metastasis is more likely, and local recurrences are more common, ranging from 25–58%. Therapeutic planning must include the primary lesion and the regional lymphatics (pelvic lymph nodes) at risk for metastasis (Fig. 14-2).

Therapy should begin with whole pelvis radiation (external beam radiation). A dose between 5,000 and 6,000 cGy should be delivered to the pelvis depending on the size, extent, and radiation responsiveness of the lesion. The goals of whole pelvis radiation are (1)

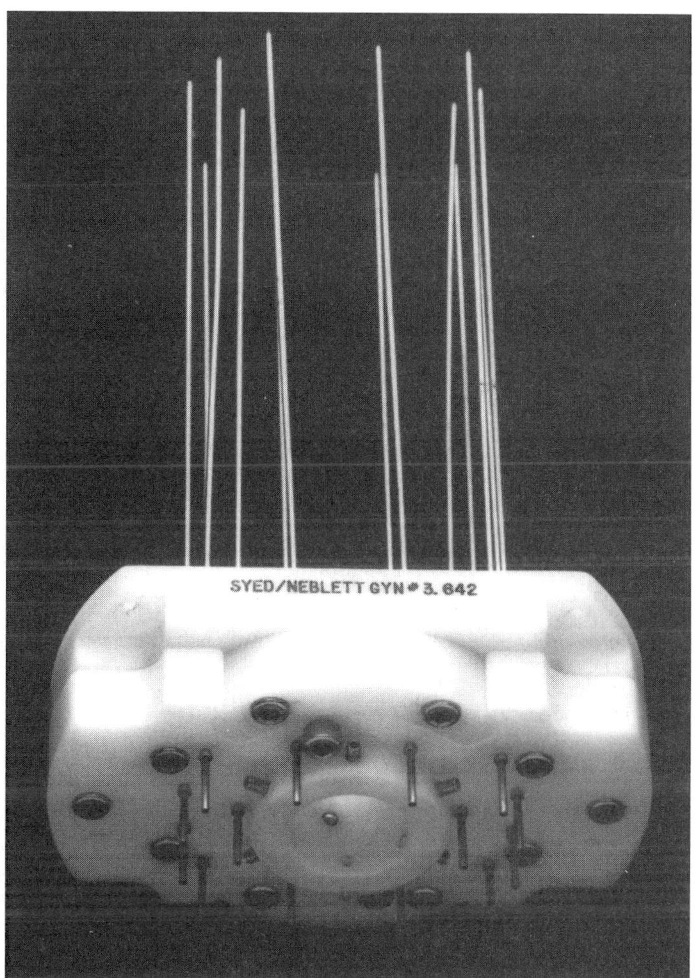

Fig. 14-3. Syed-Neblett interstitial brachytherapy applicator.

shrinkage of the primary tumor, (2) recreation of normal vaginal anatomy, and (3) irradication of metastatic disease that may be in the regional pelvic lymph nodes.

Following external beam radiation, the isodose curve for intracavitary brachytherapy is usually not adequate for further accomplishment of total resolution of deep tumor extension from the primary vaginal lesion. Therefore, interstitial brachytherapy must be used to achieve improved local regional control. This can usually be accomplished with a Syed-Neblett applicator (Fig. 14-3).

In advanced stages of disease, combination therapy incorporating external radiation and interstitial brachytherapy has unequivocally shown improvement in local regional control.

Lesions in the Lower One-Third of the Vagina

Primary squamous cell carcinoma of the lower one-third of the vagina is clinically staged the same as lesions of the upper two-thirds of the vagina. However, because of its embryologic derivation being similar to the vulva, the inguinal and femoral lymph nodes are at risk for metastasis. Prior to starting radiation treatment for this lesion, an inguinal-femoral lymphadenectomy should be performed. If the inguinal or femoral lymph nodes are noted to be involved with metastatic disease, this region should be incorporated into the radiation field during treatment with whole pelvis radiation. Primary vaginal lesions in this region of the vagina should be treated as described above following the same principles.

Patients with a Previous Hysterectomy

The patient that develops primary squamous cell carcinoma of the vagina after a hysterectomy presents a treatment problem that is secondary to the inability to use a central uterine tandem for the brachytherapy application. For a small stage I lesion, vaginal ovoids or transvaginal cones may be effective in delivering the above-described radiation dose. However, in larger lesions or in more advanced stages (stages II–IV) of disease, external beam radiation therapy should be given as described above and an additional 1,000–2,000 cGy of external radiation may be needed for tumor control. This can be given to a reduced cone-downed field that primarily incorporates the residual disease. Additionally, for advanced tumors with large residual volume following external radiation, interstitial brachytherapy may be required. This can be accomplished with a Syed-Neblett applicator. However, instead of using the central uterine tandem, a modification can be accomplished with a perineal template.

Placement of interstitial needles in a patient with an upper vaginal lesion in the absence of a uterus could result in complications, such as injury to the small intestines, rectum, or colon. To prevent these complications, a laparotomy can be performed to remove the small bowel from the pelvis. Also, this will allow the operator to have direct visualization of the placement of the needles to avoid the rectum and colon. Additionally, the omentum can be placed in the pelvis and used as a barrier between the pelvis and the small-bowel viscera.

Surgery

Although radiation therapy is the primary modality of treatment for squamous cell carcinoma of the vagina, surgical management is appropriate for some cases. The patient with preinvasive disease (stage 0) may undergo surgical excision of the vaginal lesion or colposcopic-directed laser vaporization as described above. Additionally, the patient with stage I disease in the upper vagina, which is very close to the cervix, may be effectively treated with a type III radical hysterectomy, upper vaginectomy, and pelvic lymphadenectomy. In the younger patient this method of treatment will not only result in a cure in most cases but also preserve the ovaries.

For patients with stage I disease of the lower one-third of the vagina, if the lesion is in the extreme distal portion of the vagina (close to the vulva), the patient may be effectively treated with a partial radical vaginectomy and bilateral inguinal femoral lymphadenectomy.

Finally, the patient with local recurrence of a vaginal carcinoma following prior treatment with radiation therapy may benefit from a pelvic exenteration. This procedure may provide salvage.

SURVIVAL

Evaluating the outcome of patients with squamous cell carcinoma of the vagina is very complex because the various series reporting survival outcomes are not homogenous. The problems in analyzing survival in the various series are because (1) there are variations in the histologic subtypes; (2) most reported series span several years and there have been major changes in radiation technology that may not be factored into the survival data (i.e., orthovoltage versus megavoltage); (3) patients are treated with different modalities of therapy (external radiation therapy alone, brachytherapy alone, surgery alone, radiation therapy in conjunction with surgery); (4) the prescribed dose of radiation is variable; (5) there are variations in follow-up periods; (6) there are very small numbers in most series; and (7) there are major differences in statistical analysis reporting the survival data. Survival for patients with squamous cell carcinoma of the vagina is directly related to stage and volume of the disease. Stage I has a survival rate ranging from 80% to 100%; stage II, 43–75%, stage III, 0–42%; and stage IV, 0–21% (Table 14-2).

COMPLICATIONS

Complications are directly related to the amount of radiation given. In patients with stage I disease, the amount of radiation needed to completely irradicate a lesion is less in comparison to patients with more advanced stages of disease. Thus, patients with stage I disease usually do not develop major complications. However, minor complications such as vaginal stenosis, temporary vaginal necrosis, transient sigmoiditis, and transient diarrhea may arise, but these complications are usually easily managed. Patients with more advanced disease will require high doses of irradiation (in the range of 80–100 Gy) for tumor control. Therefore, because of the higher radiation exposure these patients are expected to have a higher incidence of major complications. Major complications reported are related to the dose-limiting structure that approximates the vagina (colon, rectum, bladder, ureters, and small bowel). The sequelae are rectovaginal fistulas, vesicovaginal fistulas, small-bowel obstruction, uretero-vaginal fistulas, ureteral stenosis, rectal strictures, severe radiation proctitis, and small- or large-bowel perforations. The rate of major complication ranges from 10% to 15%.

Clear-Cell Adenocarcinoma of the Vagina

Adenocarcinoma of the vagina is an exceptionally rare disorder. Before 1971 this phenomenon was only reported in postmenopausal patients. Herbst and Greenwald in 1971 reported on 8 and 5 cases, respectively, of primary vaginal adenocarcinoma. Significantly, these two reports of 13 cases exceeded the total number of all documented cases in the world literature before 1945. Additionally, they were the first to show an association of vaginal clear-cell adenocarcinoma with intrauterine exposure to diethylstilbestrol (DES). Following these reports, DES was banned by the Food and Drug Administration (FDA) in 1971 and a Registry for Research on Hormonal Transplacental Carcinogenesis was established.

Table 14-2. Survival rates of patients undergoing radiation therapy for vaginal carcinoma

Author	*No. of cases*	*Stage I*	*No. of cases*	*Stage II*	*No. of cases*	*Stage III*	*No. of cases*	*Stage IV*
Marcus et al.	5	80%	10	50%	1	100%	2	30%
Benedet et al.	32	75%	31	68%	16	42%	18	21%
Puthawala et al.	1	100%	16	75%	9	25%	1	0%
Gallup et al.	1	10%	11	54%	3	0%	0	0%
Dixit et al.	6	100%	8	75%	29	29%	2	0%
Perez et al.	50	75%	75	49%	16	32%	8	10%

The summary from the findings of the Registry For Research on Hormonal Transplacental Carcinogenesis is as follows:

1. Currently there are 547 reported cases of clear-cell adenocarcinoma of the vagina and cervix.
2. Of these patients, 60% were exposed to DES or a similar synthetic estrogen in utero.
3. The age range of these patients is 7–34 and the median age is 19.
4. Sixty percent of the primary lesions are vaginal.
5. Ninety percent of the patients were in early stages at the time of diagnosis.
6. The risk of developing adenocarcinoma of the vagina in an exposed female from birth to 34 years of age is approximately 0.1% (or one case per 1,000 women exposed).
7. These tumors are extremely rare among DES-exposed females and DES is not a complete carcinogen.

TREATMENT

In the past, because the majority of cases presented as stage I or II lesions, radical pelvic surgery (radical hysterectomy, pelvic lymphadenectomy, partial or total vaginectomy, and replacement of the vagina with a split-thickness skin graft) was employed. Whole pelvis radiation was used for more advanced and large bulky lesions in the fashion described above for vaginal squamous cell cancers.

Currently treatment is more conservative since the majority of patients with this lesion are in the reproductive age group. The objective of therapy is to irradicate the lesion without compromising fertility. To date there are two reports describing the use of only brachytherapy or brachytherapy in conjunction with limited local surgery resulting in cures and preservation of fertility. In the first report Fletcher and colleagues reported on 19 young women who were treated with brachytherapy alone and two patients who also had brachytherapy in conjunction with limited local surgery. They have followed their patients for approximately 2 years and report only one recurrence and one patient who died from a pulmonary embolism. In the other report Senekjian and associates reported on 43 patients who again had only local excision of the vaginal lesion and/or brachytherapy. The 5-year survival rate was noted to be 92%, which was comparable to the 176 patients who underwent radical excision. In addition, the subgroup of patients who received localized irradiation had a recurrence rate equal to that of the conventional radical therapy group. This outcome was noted to be more favorable than in patients undergoing local excision alone. Both of the authors have demonstrated that with the use of brachytherapy and local limited excision, reproductive capacity can be preserved without compromising survival.

For more advanced stages, combination therapy (whole pelvis radiation and brachytherapy) as described above for treatment of squamous cell carcinoma of the vagina is recommended.

Rhabdomyosarcoma

Of the five types of rhabdomyosarcoma (RMS), the embryonal variant, botryoid sarcoma, represents the most common subtype of RMS presenting as a genital lesion. Vaginal RMS usually occurs early in childhood, before the age of 2. RMS is the seventh leading cause of death in children. On clinical presentation these lesions are usually easily visualized; however, vaginal bleeding may be the only presenting symptom.

TREATMENT

In the past, successful treatment was primarily with multimodality therapy (the combination of radical pelvic surgery, radiation therapy, and adjuvant chemotherapy). Although with multimodality therapy survival was improved, radical pelvic surgery often resulted in the removal of the bladder, rectum, uterus, vagina, ovary, and fallopian tubes. This undoubtedly resulted in significant changes in the quality of life and totally compromised the reproductive capacity and sexual function of these very young patients.

Currently the management of RMS has shifted from radical pelvic surgery to a more conservative approach to preserve fertility. RMS has been shown to be highly chemosensitive, specifically to the combination of vincristine, actinomycin-D, and cyclophosphamide (VAC). Neoadjuvant use of the VAC chemotherapeutic combination has resulted in complete and partial responses. In patients with a partial response, limited local surgery has been successful in rendering the patient completely free of disease.

Following tissue confirmation of RMS in addition to the required radiographic studies (see the discussion under staging for squamous cell carcinoma of the vagina), a bone marrow aspiration should be performed to rule out systemic disease. Primary therapy should begin with VAC chemotherapy, and the response to chemotherapy should be monitored closely. In patients who do not have a complete response, limited local pelvic surgery can be attempted without compromising survival.

Endodermal Sinus Tumor of the Vagina

Endodermal sinus tumor of the vagina is a rare lesion that usually occurs before the age of 2. As with other vaginal malignancies, before the routine use of chemotherapy, radical surgery was the primary method of treatment. Survival rates were poor and fertility and sexual function were compromised. The improved survival rates noted in the treatment of endodermal sinus tumor of the ovaries with combination chemotherapy has been one of the most significant advancements in oncology. The combination of bleomycin, etoposide (VP-16), and cisplatin (BEP) has produced excellent progression-free survival rates. Therefore, complete remission and preservation of fertility can be accomplished.

Melanoma

Primary melanoma of the vagina is very rare, with approximately 150 cases reported. The patient usually presents with vaginal bleeding or discharge. The lesion is most commonly located on the anterior vaginal wall of the lower third of the vagina. Surgery is the only potentially curative treatment. However, there is still controversy about whether radical versus more conservative surgical measures influence survival. With melanoma, the single most prognostic factor is the depth of invasion, as it is in other sites of melanoma. Adjuvant therapy for vaginal melanoma has included local radiation therapy, immunotherapy (bacillus Calmette-Guérin vaccine and interferon-b), and chemotherapy. Fifty percent of patients die of metastatic disease within 2 years, and the 5-year survival rate ranges from 5% to 20%.

Selected Readings

Benedet JL, Murphy KJ, Fairey RN et al. Primary invasive carcinoma of the vagina. *Obstet Gynecol* 62:715, 1983.

Brown GR, Fletcher GH, Rutledge, RN. Irradiation of in situ and invasive squamous cell carcinomas of the vagina. *Cancer* 28:1278, 1971.

Dancuart F, Delclos L, Wharton JT et al. Primary squamous cell carcinoma of the vagina treated by radiotherapy: A failures analysis—The M.D. Anderson Hospital experience 1955–1982. *Int J Radiat Oncol Biol Phys* 14:745, 1988.

Dixit S, Singhal S, Babo HA. Squamous cell carcinoma of the vagina: A review of 70 cases. *Gynecol Oncol* 48:80, 1993.

Fletcher GH. Tumors of the Vagina and Female Urethra. In GH Fletcher (ed), *Textbook of Radiotherapy* (3rd ed). Philadelphia: Lea & Febiger, 1980. Pp. 821–824.

Gallup DG, Talledo OE, Shah KJ et al. Invasive squamous cell carcinoma of the vagina: A 14-year study. *Obstet Gynecol* 69:782, 1987.

Greenwald P, Barlow JJ, Nasca PC et al. Vaginal cancer after maternal treatment with synthetic estrogens. *N Engl J Med* 285:390, 1971.

Herbst AL, Anderson D. Clear cell adenocarcinoma of the vagina and cervix secondary to intrauterine exposure to diethylstilbestrol. *Semin Surg Oncol* 6:343, 1990.

Herbst AL, Green TH Jr, Ulfelder H. Primary carcinoma of the vagina. *Am J Obstet Gynecol* 106:210, 1970.

Herbst AL, Ulfelder H, Poskanzer DC. Adenocarcinoma of the vagina: Association of maternal stilbestrol therapy with tumor appearance in young women. *N Engl J Med* 284:878, 1971.

Levitan A, Gordon AN, Kaplan AL et al. Primary malignant melanoma of the vagina: A report of four cases and a review of the literature. *Gynecol Oncol* 33:85, 1989.

Marcus RB, Million RR, Daly JW. Carcinoma of the vagina. *Cancer* 42:2507, 1978.

Perez CA, Camel HM, Galakatos AE et al. Definitive irradiation in carcinoma of the vagina: Long term evaluation of results. *Int J Radiat Oncol Biol Phys* 15:1283, 1988.

Piver MS, Barlow JJ, Wang JJ et al. Combined radical surgery, radiation therapy and chemotherapy in infants with vulvovaginal embryonal rhabdomyosarcoma. *Obstet Gynecol* 42:522, 1973.

Puthawala A, Syed AM, Nalick R et al. Integrated external and interstitial radiation therapy for primary carcinoma of the vagina. *Obstet Gynecol* 62:367, 1983.

Senekjian EK, Frey KW, Anderson D et al. Local therapy in stage I clear cell adenocarcinoma of the vagina. *Cancer* 60:1319, 1987.

Woodruff JD, Parmley TH, Julian CG. Topical 5-fluorouracil in the treatment of vaginal carcinoma in situ. *Gynecol Oncol* 3:124, 1975.

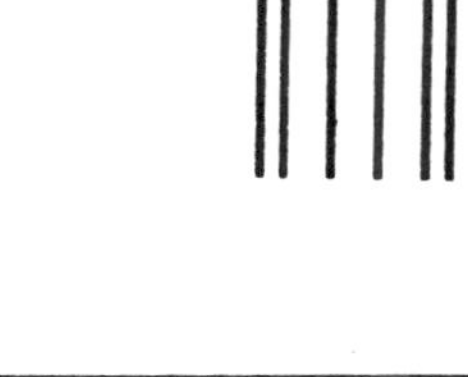

NO POSTAGE
NECESSARY
IF MAILED
IN THE
UNITED STATES

BUSINESS REPLY MAIL

FIRST CLASS MAIL PERMIT NO. 2117 BOSTON, MA

POSTAGE WILL BE PAID BY ADDRESSEE

LITTLE, BROWN AND COMPANY
Attn: George W. Pratt, III
34 Beacon Street
P.O. Box 2158
Boston, MA 02106-9920

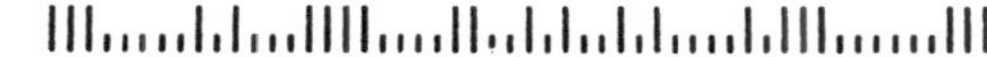

PLEASE HELP US!

Take a moment to complete and return this brief questionnaire.
Return postage is already paid. Thank you very much.

Title Purchased ____________________

Where did you buy this title?

Bookstore ______ Mail ______ Convention ______ Other: ____________

How did you learn about this title?

Colleague ______ Bookstore ______ Brochure ______ Meeting ______ Other: ____________

Please describe yourself:

______ MD ______ DO ______ Nurse ______ Pharmacist ______ Physician Assistant

______ Resident: What year? ______ What specialty? ____________

______ Medical Student: What year? ____________

Sex: ___ Female ___ Male

Age: ___ 21-40 ___ 41-60 ___ 61+

City ____________ State ____________ Zip ____________

What other Manuals/Handbooks do you own/use? ____________

____

Thank you from Little, Brown and Company.

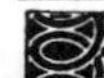

V

Treatment Modalities

15

Principles of Chemotherapy of Gynecologic Cancer

M. Steven Piver

Cell Cycle and Mechanism of Action of Cytotoxic Chemotherapy

Cytotoxic chemotherapy eventually leads to cell death, primarily by preventing cell division and thus further cell proliferation. During normal cell division, actively proliferating cells proceed through the G1, S, G2, and ultimately mitosis (M) phases of the cell cycle to produce two daughter cells. Cells not actively proliferating may be in a resting, or inactive, G0 phase (Fig. 15-1). During the G1 phase of the cell cycle (18–30 hours), enzymes that are essential for the production of RNA and protein, the building blocks of all cells, are produced. In preparation for cell division, during the S phase (16–20 hours), DNA is synthesized by replication of the existing strand to produce a copy. RNA and protein are synthesized during the premitotic G2 phase (2–10 hours). During M phase (0.5–1.0 hours), the four stages of mitosis occur: prophase, metaphase, anaphase, and telophase. Cell division during mitosis results in two daughter cells, each of which can (1) enter its own G1 phase of the cell cycle, (2) become an inactive resting cell (G0), or (3) die. Most chemotherapy inhibits proliferating cells by either inhibiting a specific phase of the cell cycle (phase-specific agents) (Table 15-1) or acting on any phase of the proliferating cell cycle (non–phase-specific) (Table 15-2). Thus, nonproliferating cells in the resting G0 phase are normally not sensitive to the effects of chemotherapy.

MECHANISMS OF RESISTANCE TO CYTOTOXIC CHEMOTHERAPY

Mechanisms of resistance to cytotoxic chemotherapy are shown in Table 15-3.

CELL KINETICS

Log Kill Hypothesis

Cytotoxic chemotherapy is believed to follow first-order kinetics, in which, rather than a specific number of cells, a constant fraction (%) of cells are killed for each course of chemotherapy, regardless of the size of the tumor. Therefore, a given course of chemotherapy that results in a one-log kill would reduce the number of cells by 90% (Fig. 15-2). In this example, a course of chemotherapy would reduce a 10^8 cell tumor to 10^7 cells or a 10^5 cell tumor to 10^4 cells. A 99% cell kill may be achieved using multidrug chemotherapy, in which a one-log kill by one drug reducing the tumor burden by 90% and a one-log kill by a second drug of an additional 90% would result in a two-log kill. Thus, resistance to chemotherapy is increased by using single agents that kill a smaller fraction (log) of tumor cells. Increased (log) cell kill can also be achieved by increasing the dose intensity—the amount of drug per unit time calculated as the total dose of individual drugs in mg/m^2/week.

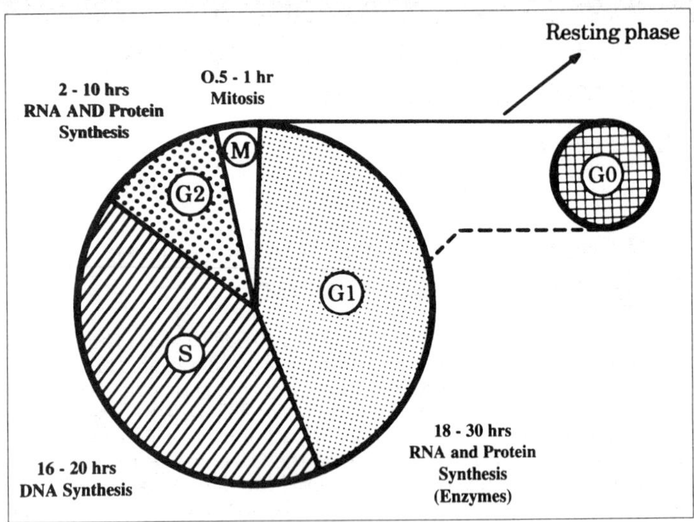

Fig. 15-1. Cell cycle. (M = mitosis; S = DNA synthesis; G1 = gap phase between M and S; G2 = gap phase between S and M; G0 = resting phase.)

Gompertzian Growth Hypothesis

Human tumors do not follow a logarithmic or exponential growth. Rather, they approximate a sigmoid Gompertzian growth with proliferating cells continuing to divide; resting, nonproliferating (G0) cells increasing in number; and other tumor cells ceasing to proliferate and dying. When tumors are small in the initial phase of the Gompertzian growth curve, the relatively small number of tumor cells initially divide and accumulate slowly, then enter a rapid growth phase (log) and finally a slower rate of growth (plateau) phase when the tumor is large and able to kill the host. A large tumor is more resistant to chemotherapy because the growth fraction is small and more cells are in their resting, nonproliferating G0 phase. Also, with increased tumor size comes increased resistance; when a tumor outgrows its blood supply, inadequate circulation results in inadequate diffusion of oxygen and nutrients to the center of the tumor.

CELL MUTATIONS

Goldie-Coldman Hypothesis

Using a mathematical model, Goldie and Coldman have calculated that spontaneous resistant mutation occurs within a tumor at a specific frequency. Therefore, the longer a malignancy is allowed to double, the greater the frequency of spontaneous resistant mutated cells. Based on this model, (1) surgical resection of large tumors prior to chemotherapy reduces the number of spontaneously mutated-resistant cells; (2) treating tumors early prevents the emergence of more mutated-resistant cells; and (3) multiple drugs will be less likely than single-drug therapy to be resistant to spontaneous mutated cells.

Table 15-1. Chemotherapy used for gynecologic malignancies: Effect on cell cycle primarily phase-specific

Agent	*Class*	*Mechanism*	*Phase*
Vincristine	Plant (vinca alkaloid) product	Inhibits mitosis	M
Vinblastine	Plant (vinca alkaloid) product	Inhibits mitosis	M
Etoposide	Plant (epipodophyllo-toxins) product	Inhibits topoisomerase II	G2
Bleomycin	Antitumor antibiotic	Strand scission of DNA	G2
Taxol	Plant (diterpene) product	Arrests mitosis by microtubule assembly and stabilization of tubulen polymer formation	G2
Hydroxyurea	Antimetabolite	Inhibits ribonucleotide reductase	S
Cytarabine	Antimetabolite (pyrimidine nucleoside analogue)	Inhibits DNA polymerase	S
5-Fluorouracil	Antimetabolite (pyrimidine antagonist)	Blocks thymidylates synthesis	S
Methotrexate	Antimetabolite (folate antagonist)	Blocks dihydrofolate reductase	—

Table 15-2. Chemotherapy for gynecologic malignancies: Effect on cell cycle primarily non–phase-specific

Agent	*Class*	*Type*	*Mechanism*
Chlorambucil	Alkylating agent	Nitrogen mustard	1. Binds to DNA by covalent alkyl group 2. Cross-link chains of DNA
Cyclophosphamide	Alkylating agent	Nitrogen mustard	1. Binds to DNA by covalent alkyl group 2. Cross-link chains of DNA
Ifosfamide	Alkylating agent	Nitrogen mustard	1. Binds to DNA by covalent alkyl group 2. Cross-link chains of DNA
Melphalan	Alkylating agent	Nitrogen mustard	1. Binds to DNA by covalent alkyl group 2. Cross-link chains of DNA
Thiotepa (triethylene-thiophosphoramide)	Alkylating agent	Ethylenimine	1. Binds to DNA by covalent alkyl group 2. Cross-link chains of DNA
Cisplatin	Alkylating agent	Metal salt	1. Binds to DNA by covalent alkyl group 2. Cross-link chains of DNA
Carboplatin	Alkylating agent	Metal salt	1. Binds to DNA by covalent alkyl group 2. Cross-link chains of DNA
Dacarbazine	Miscellaneous	Miscellaneous	1. Alkylation 2. Inhibits purine nucleoside
Hexamethylmelamine	Miscellaneous	Miscellaneous	Inhibits incorporation of precursors into DNA and RNA
Dactinomycin	Antitumor Antibiotic	Antitumor Antibiotic	Binds to DNA
Mitoxantrone	Antitumor Antibiotic	Antitumor Antibiotic	Strand scission of DNA
Adriamycin (doxorubicin)	Antitumor Antibiotic	Antitumor Antibiotic	Binds to DNA

Table 15-3. Mechanisms of resistance to chemotherapy

Cell kinetics
- Log kill hypothesis
- Gompertzian growth hypothesis

Cell mutations
- Goldie-Coldman hypothesis

Biochemical
- Multidrug resistance
  - P170 glycoprotein
  - Topoisomerase II
- Increased drug inactivation
- Decreased drug activation
- Increased normal cellular enzymes

Increased DNA repair

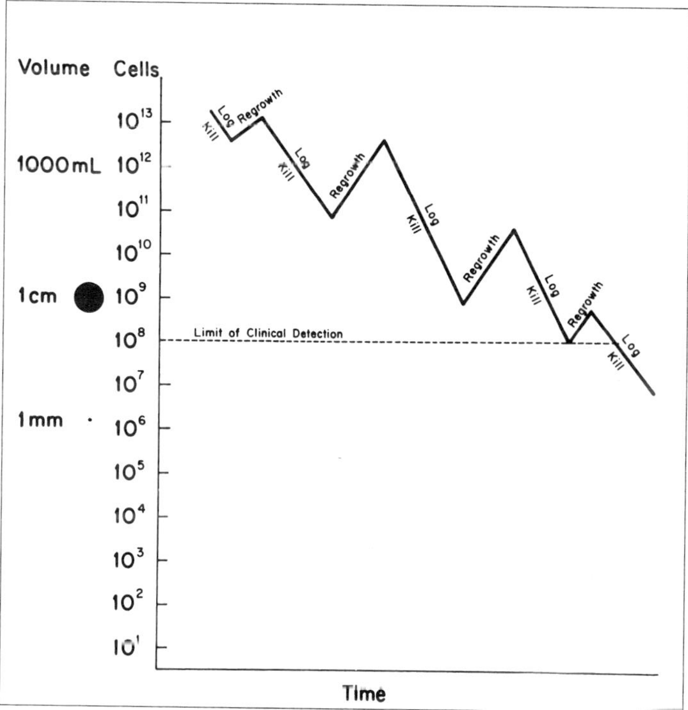

Fig. 15-2. Log kill hypothesis of cytotoxic chemotherapy.

BIOCHEMICAL

Multidrug Resistance

Increased P170 Glycoprotein

Some tumor cells resistant to one class of cytotoxic chemotherapy are also resistant to nonrelated other classes of chemotherapy. This multidrug resistance (MDR) can be caused by increased levels of P170 glycoprotein, a cell-surface membrane that functions as a cellular pump to extrude toxic material out of the cell, resulting in lower intracellular drug concentration. Increased levels of MDR1 gene responsible for the P170 glycoprotein product is one mechanism of resistance to the vinca alkaloids, etoposide, and the antitumor antibiotics.

Change in Levels of Topoisomerase II Enzyme

The MDR phenotype may also arise from cellular changes in topoisomerase II, a nuclear enzyme involved in the regulation of DNA topology. Resistance to topoisomerase II inhibitor drugs, Adriamycin, vinca alkaloids, and etoposide results from qualitative changes in topoisomerase II.

Increased Drug Inactivation

Increased levels of glutathione, an intracellular, nonprotein thiol molecule present in all cells as a mechanism to detoxify anticancer drugs, has been associated with increased resistance to alkylating agents/cisplatin and Adriamycin in vitro.

Decreased Intracellular Drug Activation

Many antimetabolites (5-fluorouracil and cytarabine) require conversion to active forms before they are cytotoxic. Decreased intracellular activation into the corresponding nucleoside or nucleotide would result in drug resistance.

Increased Normal Cellular Enzymes

Increased levels of dihydrofolate reductase (or a variant of it) would inhibit methotrexate due to the decreased free cellular methotrexate concentration that results when methotrexate binds to all of the available dihydrofolate reductase.

INCREASED DNA REPAIR

Since many cancer drugs damage DNA, a tumor cell's ability to repair sustained sublethal damage by chemotherapy will eventually result in resistance to that drug. Increased DNA repair has been observed in cisplatin-resistant ovarian cancer cell lines.

Classification of Chemotherapeutic Agents

Chemotherapeutic agents are classified (Fig. 15-3) as (1) alkylating agents that act primarily by breakage and cross-linkage of double-stranded DNA to prevent DNA replication and transcription of RNA; (2) antimetabolites that interact with intracellular enzymes; (3) antitumor antibiotics that act primarily by complexing with DNA to inhibit DNA, RNA, and protein synthesis; (4) plant products that act primarily by inhibiting mitosis by binding to microtubular proteins to inhibit mitotic spindle formation; (5) hormones that form steroid receptor complexes; and (6) miscellaneous agents. For those drugs listed as miscellaneous, the mechanism of action is either not known or the drug acts by a different mechanism than any of the other five classes. Due to their mechanism of action, platinum analogues are classified here as alkylating agents, rather than miscellaneous. The classification of these individual agents in primary use in gynecologic malignancies is listed in Table 15-4.

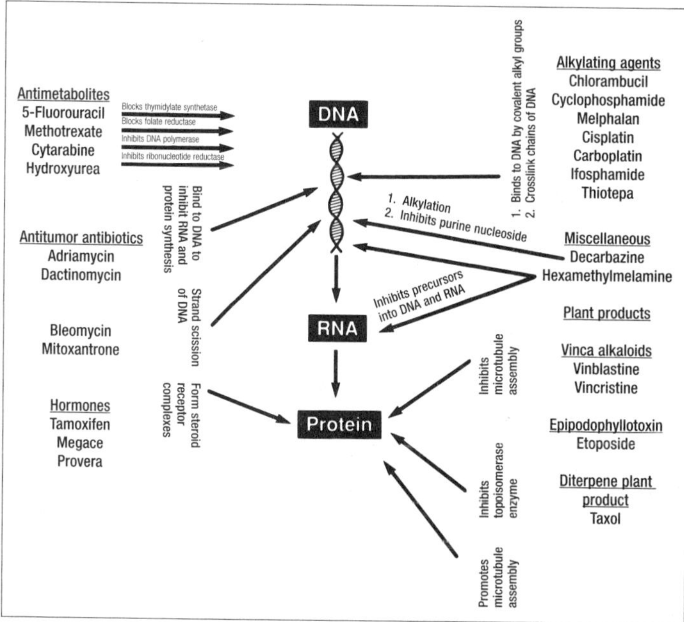

Fig. 15-3. Mechanism of action of anticancer drugs used for gynecologic malignancies.

Chemotherapeutic Agents Used for Gynecologic Malignancies

ALKYLATING AGENTS

Chlorambucil (Leukeran)

Usual dosage: 3–4 mg/m^2 for 3–6 weeks; then adjust dose for maintenance at 1–2 mg/m^2/day.
Special precautions: None.
Adverse reactions: Nausea and vomiting, myelosuppression, infertility, acute nonlymphocytic leukemia in high cumulative doses.

Cyclophosphamide (Cytoxan)

Usual single dose: 1,000–1,500 mg/m^2 IV every 3 weeks. 500–1,000 mg/m^2 in combination with cisplatin or carboplatin.
Special precautions: Ensure significant hydration to prevent hemorrhagic cystitis.
Adverse reactions: Alopecia, pulmonary fibrosis (rare), nausea and vomiting, hemorrhagic cystitis, infertility, myelosuppression, acute nonlymphocytic leukemia in high cumulative doses.

Melphalan (Alkeran)

Usual single dose: 8 mg/m^2 PO days 1–4 every 4 weeks.
Special precautions: None.
Adverse reactions: Nausea and vomiting, myelosuppression, infertility, acute nonlymphocytic leukemia in high cumulative doses.

Table 15-4. Classification and primary use of chemotherapy used for gynecologic malignancies

Classification	*Drug*	*Primary use*
Alkylating agents	Chlorambucil	Epithelial ovarian cancer (EOC)
	Cyclophosphamide	EOC, gestational trophoblastic disease (GTD)
	Melphalan	EOC
	Cisplatin	EOC, ovarian germ cell tumors, cervix and endometrial cancer
	Carboplatinum	EOC
	Ifosfamide	Cervix cancer and sarcomas
	Thiotepa	EOC
Antimetabolites	Methotrexate	GTD
	5-Fluorouracil	Cervix cancer (radiation sensitizer)
	Cytarabine	EOC (intraperitoneal)
	Hydroxyurea	Cervix cancer (radiation sensitizer)
Plant products	Vinblastine	Ovarian germ cell tumors
	Vincristine	Ovarian germ cell tumors, GTD
	Etoposide	Ovarian germ cell tumors, EOC, GTD, endometrial cancer
	Taxol	EOC
Antibiotics	Dactinomycin	GTD
	Adriamycin	EOC, endometrial cancer
	Bleomycin	Ovarian germ cell tumors, cervix cancer
	Mitoxantrone	EOC (intraperitoneal)
Miscellaneous	Dacarbazine	Sarcomas
	Hexamethylmelamine	EOC
Hormones		
Antiestrogens	Tamoxifen	EOC
Progesterones	Medroxyprogesterone acetate (Depo-Provera)	Endometrial cancer
	Megestrol acetate	Endometrial cancer

Thiotepa (Triethylenethiophosphoramide)

Usual single dose: 12 mg/m^2 every 3 weeks.
Special precautions: None.
Adverse reactions: Alopecia, nausea and vomiting, myelosuppression.

Cisplatin (Cisdiamminedichloroplatinum II)

Usual dose: 50–120 mg/m^2 IV every 3–4 weeks.
Special precautions: Maintain hydration and diuresis. Avoid in patients with renal failure. If creatinine is more than 1.5 dg/liter, administer in hypertonic saline.
Adverse reactions: Nausea and vomiting, nephrotoxicity, peripheral neuropathy, myelosuppression, ototoxicity (high tone, significant hearing loss in vocal frequencies is rare), hypomagnesemia, hypocalcemia, hypokalemia.

Carboplatin (Paraplatin)

Usual dose: 300–400 mg/m^2 every 3–4 weeks.
Special precautions: Less need for hydration and diuresis.
Adverse reactions: Nausea and vomiting, myelosuppression (especially thrombocytopenia), hypomagnesemia, hypocalcemia, hypokalemia.

Ifosfamide

Usual single dose: 5 g/m^2 or 1.0–1.2 g/m^2 daily × 5.
Special precautions: Mesna and hydration to prevent hemorrhagic cystitis. Mesna dose: administer in same total dose (g/m^2) as ifosfamide. Administer 20% as a 1-hour infusion prior to ifosfamide, 60% during ifosfamide, and the remaining 20% of the total dose as a 1-hour infusion after ifosfamide.
Adverse reactions: Alopecia, nausea and vomiting, myelosuppression, hemorrhagic cystitis, central nervous system toxicity (confusion, somnolence, and rarely seizures).

ANTIMETABOLITES

Methotrexate

Usual single dose: 15–30 mg PO or IM days 1–5 every 2 weeks (gestational trophoblastic disease) or 40–80 mg/m^2 IV or PO every 2 weeks (other carcinomas).
Special precautions: For more than 80 mg/m^2, administer with leucovorin rescue. Avoid aspirin, sulfonamides, and tetracycline, as they can decrease the effectiveness of methotrexate. Also exercise caution when using the anticoagulant warfarin, which can potentiate the toxicity of methotrexate. In patients with renal insufficiency, the dose needs to be reduced or discontinued.
Adverse reactions: Alopecia, interstitial pneumonitis, nausea and vomiting, stomatitis, gastrointestinal ulceration, diarrhea, hepatotoxicity, myelosuppression, and renal tubular necrosis.

5-Fluorouracil (5-FU)

Usual single dose: 400–500 mg/m^2 IV daily days 1–4, every 4 weeks.
Special precautions: Reduce dose if there is impaired liver function.
Adverse reactions: Alopecia, nausea and vomiting, stomatitis, gastrointestinal ulceration, diarrhea, myelosuppression.

Cytarabine (Cytosine Arabinoside)

Usual single dose: 200 mg/m^2 *intraperitoneal* in combination with cisplatin every 4 weeks.
Special precautions: None.
Adverse reactions: Alopecia, nausea and vomiting, stomatitis, gastrointestinal ulceration, myelosuppression, fever, cerebellar neurotoxicity, hepatic dysfunction (rare).

Hydroxyurea (Hydrea)

Usual single dose: 80 mg/kg every 3 days during radiation therapy for a total of 12 weeks from day 1 of radiation therapy.
Special precautions: Do not administer unless white blood cell count is less than 2,500/mm^3.
Adverse reactions: Myelosuppression, nausea and vomiting.

PLANT PRODUCTS

Vinblastine (Velban)

Usual dose: 4–6 mg/m^2 IV in combination chemotherapy every 3–4 weeks.
Special precautions: Skin necrosis if extravasation. Decrease dose in patients with liver disease.
Adverse reactions: Alopecia, tissue necrosis if extravasation, nausea and vomiting, stomatitis, constipation, ileus, peripheral neuropathy (loss of deep tendon reflexes and parasthesia), myelosuppression.

Vincristine (Oncovin)

Usual dose: 1–2 mg/m^2 IV; maximum dose 2.0–2.4 mg/m^2.
Special precautions: Skin necrosis if extravasation. Reduce dose if liver disease is present. Neurotoxicity is cumulative.
Adverse reactions: Alopecia, tissue necrosis if extravasation, nausea and vomiting, stomatitis, constipation, ileus, diarrhea, peripheral neuropathy.

Etoposide (VP-16)

Usual single dose: 50–100 mg/m^2 IV days 1–5 or 100 mg/m^2 IV days 1, 3, 5 every 3–4 weeks (with other drugs). 100 mg daily PO for 14 days every 3 weeks.
Special precautions: Administer over 30–60 minutes to avoid severe hypotension. Avoid extravasation.
Adverse reactions: Myelosuppression, nausea and vomiting, alopecia, orthostatic hypotension, anaphylaxis.

Paclitaxel (Taxol)

Usual single dose: 135 mg/m^2/24 hours every 3 weeks. 175–250 mg/m^2/24 hours every 3 weeks with granulocyte–colony-stimulating factor (G-CSF) or granulocyte-macrophage–colony-stimulating factor (GM-CSF).
Special precautions: Hypersensitivity reaction may lead to severe hypotension.
Adverse reactions: Alopecia, nausea and vomiting, cardiac arrhythmia, hypersensitivity reaction, tissue necrosis if extravasation, peripheral neuropathy.

ANTIBIOTICS

Dactinomycin (Actinomycin-D)

Usual single dose: 0.4–0.5 mg/m^2 IV days 1–5 every 2–3 weeks (for gestational trophoblastic disease).
Special precautions: Avoid extravasation.
Adverse reactions: Alopecia, skin necrosis if extravasation, nausea and vomiting, stomatitis, gastrointestinal ulceration, diarrhea, myelosuppression, hypocalcemia.

Doxorubicin (Adriamycin)

Usual dose: 50–75 mg/m^2 IV every 3 weeks.
Special precautions: Avoid extravasation. Reduce dose if impaired liver function. Do not exceed lifetime cumulative dose of more than 550 mg/m^2 unless electrocardiogram (ECG) and cardiac ejection fraction are normal.
Adverse reactions: Alopecia, tissue necrosis if extravasation, cardiotoxicity including congestive heart failure, transient ECG changes (sinus tachycardia, T wave flattening, ST segment depression, voltage reduction, and arrhythmia), nausea and vomiting, stomatitis, diarrhea, myelosuppression.

Bleomycin

Usual single dose: 10–20 U/m^2 IV or IM daily × 3 every 3–4 weeks or 20–25 U/m^2/24 hours as a continuous infusion.
Special precautions: Keep total dosage to less than 400 IU. Reduce dose if creatinine is elevated. Continuous infusion is associated with less pulmonary toxicity.
Adverse reactions: Alopecia, pneumonitis progressing to pulmonary fibrosis and death, nausea and vomiting, stomatitis, fever.

Mitoxantrone

Usual single intraperitoneal dose: 10–15 mg/m^2 every 3–4 weeks.
Special precautions: Risk of cardiotoxicity after 160 mg/m^2, but 100 mg/m^2 if previous adriamycin.
Adverse reactions: Myelosuppression, alopecia, nausea and vomiting, cardiotoxicity.

MISCELLANEOUS

Dacarbazine (Imidazole carboximide)

Usual dose: 200–250 mg/m^2 IV days 1–5 every 3–4 weeks.
Special precautions: Avoid extravasation.
Adverse reactions: Alopecia (rare), nausea and vomiting, myelosuppression, flulike syndrome, fever.

Hexamethylmelamine (Hexalen)

Usual dose: 200–300 mg/m^2 PO daily for 14 days every 4 weeks; 150–200 mg/m^2 PO daily days 1–14 when used in combination.
Special precautions: None.
Adverse reactions: Myelosuppression, nausea and vomiting, alopecia, peripheral neuropathy, bone marrow depression.

HORMONES

Antiestrogens

Tamoxifen (Nalvodex)
Usual dose: Loading dose: 40 mg bid × 30 days then 20 mg bid.
Special precautions: None.
Adverse reactions: Nausea and vomiting, abnormal uterine bleeding, hot flashes, ophthalmic changes.

Progesterones

Hydroxyprogesterone Caproate (Delalutin)
Usual dose: 1,000 mg IM weekly.
Special precautions: None.
Adverse reactions: Fluid retention, phlebitis.

Medroxyprogesterone Acetate (Depo-Provera)
Usual dose: 100 mg IM weekly.
Special precautions: None.
Adverse reactions: Fluid retention, phlebitis.

Megestrol Acetate (Megace)
Usual dose: 160 mg/day.
Special precautions: None.
Adverse reactions: Fluid retention, phlebitis.

Toxicity to Chemotherapy

Cytotoxic drugs have their primary effect on rapidly dividing or multiplying cells that frequently include tumor cells. However, the rapidly multiplying normal cells of the bone marrow and mucous membranes of the gastrointestinal tract may also be affected, leading to significant toxicity among these agents.

The most common toxicity is to the bone marrow. White blood cell (WBC) and platelet nadirs usually occur 7–14 days after administration of most chemotherapy. WBC count nadirs of 1,000/mm^3 significantly limit the patient's ability to withstand any systemic infection. Absolute granulocyte counts of less than 500/mm^3 for greater than 5 days may result in fatal sepsis. Prophylaxis with antibiotics for WBC less than 1,000/mm^3 and administration of colony-stimulating factors (G-CSF and GM-CSF) have significantly reduced these episodes of potential life-threatening sepsis. Because of the importance of dose intensity to increased remission rates and disease-free survival, the use of colony-stimulating factors after a WBC nadir of less than 1,000/mm^3 may be more appropriate than the reduction of the dose of individual drugs. Platelet count nadirs of less than 20,000/mm^3 can be associated with significant bleeding. Evidence suggests that prophylactic platelet transfusions in afebrile, nonbleeding patients can be limited to platelet counts of less than 5,000/mm^3 rather than historically accepted counts of less than 20,000 mm^3. Guidelines for dose modifications are shown in Table 15-5. One must always be aware of the major limiting or life-threatening toxicity of all agents used (Table 15-6). Important examples include the pulmonary fibrosis and death associated with bleomycin in cumulative doses of more

Table 15-5. Dose reduction in the presence of myelosuppression*

	Percent of initial dose administered
Leukocyte (WBC nadirs)	
$<1,000/mm^3$	75% or 100% with colony-stimulating factors
$<500/mm^3$	50% or 100% with colony-stimulating factors
Platelet nadirs	
$\leq 50,000/mm^3$	75%
$<25,000/mm^3$	50%

WBC = white blood cell.
*If values have not returned to a WBC count of ≥ 3,000/ml and a platelet count of ≥ 75,000/ml on days 21–28 of a given course, withhold treatment until these minimal counts are reached.

Table 15-6. Major limiting or life-threatening toxicities of antitumor agents used for gynecologic malignancies

Agent	*Toxicity*
Actinomycin-D	Myelosuppression, necrosis if extravasation
Adriamycin	Myelosuppression, cardiomyopathy, necrosis if extravasation
Bleomycin	Pulmonary fibrosis
Carboplatin	Myelosuppression
Cisplatin	Myelosuppression, nephrotoxicity, peripheral neuropathy, ototoxicity
Cyclophosphamide	Myelosuppression, hemorrhagic cystitis, acute nonlymphocytic leukemia in high cumulative doses
Cytarabine	Myelosuppression
Dacarabazine	Myelosuppression
Etoposide	Myelosuppression, hypotension, necrosis of skin if extravasation
5-Fluorouracil	Myelosuppression, gastrointestinal mucositis
Hexamethylmelamine	Myelosuppression, peripheral neuropathy
Hydroxyurea	Myelosuppression
Ifosfamide	Hemorrhagic cystitis, central nervous system toxicity, myelosuppression
Melphalan	Myelosuppression, acute nonlymphocytic leukemia in high cumulative doses
Methotrexate	Myelosuppression, gastrointestinal mucositis
Mitoxantrone	Myelosuppression, cardiotoxicity
Taxol	Myelosuppression, hypersensitivity causing hypotension, cardiac arrhythmia, necrosis of skin if extravasation
Thiotepa	Myelosuppression
Vinblastine	Myelosuppression, peripheral neuropathy, necrosis of skin if extravasation
Vincristine	Myelosuppression, peripheral neuropathy, necrosis of skin if extravasation

than 400 units, the irreversible cardiomyopathy seen with Adriamycin in total cumulative doses of more than 500 mg/m^2, and the potential for acute tubular necrosis and renal failure associated with cisplatin chemotherapy. Moreover, special precautions must be taken with the antitumor antimetabolites and the agents derived from plant alkaloids that can cause severe skin and subcutaneous necrosis with extravasation from the vein.

Modifications of the Gynecologic Oncology Group (GOG) common toxicity criteria for grading toxicity are presented in Table 15-7.

Evaluating the Effectiveness of Chemotherapy: Response and Survival

The clinical effectiveness of chemotherapy (Table 15-8) in the treatment of gynecologic cancer is evaluated by reviewing clinical or surgical measurements of reduced tumor size and the duration of survival. Tumor response is classified as complete (100%) response, partial response, stationary disease, or progression of disease. Complete clinical response to chemotherapy is the complete disappearance of all palpable and radiographic (x-ray, computed tomography scan) evidence of tumor. Partial response is defined as a 50–99% decrease in the product of diameters of measurable tumors, usually lasting a specified time (1–3 months). Surgical responses consist of complete, partial, stationary disease, or progression of disease as judged by second-look exploratory laparotomy. In general, patients who achieve a complete response to chemotherapy live significantly longer than those who exhibit lesser responses or have progression of disease. In contrast, most patients with partial responses to therapy do not live significantly longer than those with stationary disease or progression. However, quality of life may be improved with a partial response with resolution of effusions or significant regression of tumor masses. From clinical observation, it is apparent that patients with improved performance status are able to tolerate appropriate doses of chemotherapy better than those with poor performance status (Table 15-9).

It can be argued that survival from initiation of therapy is an inferior barometer of the effectiveness of specific treatment. However, progression-free survival—the length of survival from primary therapy until last evaluation or progression of disease—is a more accurate assessment of the effect of a specific therapy. The Kaplan-Meier method for calculating progression-free survival and survival time curves is commonly used to adjust for variations in length of follow-up (from initiation of chemotherapy) and end point outcome characteristic of patient populations in clinical trials.

Potential for Improving Response and Survival to Chemotherapy for Gynecologic Malignancies

In truth, most results obtained in treating gynecologic malignancies have been primarily empirical, and to this day, remain primarily empirical trial and error. In the 1960s, the limited number of avail-

Table 15-7. Modified GOG common toxicity criteria

		Grade				
	Toxicity	*0*	*1*	*2*	*3*	*4*
Blood/bone marrow	WBC	≥ 4.0	3.0–3.9	2.0–2.9	1.0–1.9	<1.0
	PLT	WNL	75.0–normal	50.0–74.9	25.0–49.9	<25.0
	Hgb	WNL	10.0–normal	3.0–10.0	6.5–7.9	<6.5
	Granulocytes/bands	≥ 2.0	1.5–1.9	1.0–1.4	0.5–0.9	<0.5
	Lymphocytes	≥ 2.0	1.5–1.9	1.0–1.4	0.5–0.9	<0.5
	Infection	None	Mild	Moderate	Severe	Life-threatening
Gastro-intestinal	Nausea	None	Reasonable intake	Intake significantly decreased	No significant intake	—
	Vomiting	None	1/24 hours	2–5/24 hours	6–10/24 hours	>10/24 hours or parenteral support
	Diarrhea	None	Increase of 2–3 stool/day	Increase of 4–6 stools/day	Increase of 7–9 stools/day	Increase of ≥ 10 stools/day or need for parenteral support
Liver	Bilirubin	WNL	—	<1.5 × N	1.6–3.0 × N	>3.0 × N

Table 15-7 *(continued)*

		Grade				
	Toxicity	*0*	*1*	*2*	*3*	*4*
	Transaminase (SGOT, SGPT)	WNL	≤ 2.5–N	2.6–5.0 × N	5.1–20.0 × N	>20.0 × N
	Alkaline phosphatase or 5-nucleotidase	WNL	≤ 2.5 × N	2.6–5.0 × N	5.1–20.0 × N	>20.0 × N
Kidney						
	Creatinine	WNL	≤ 1.5 x N	1.5–3.0 × N	3.1–6.0 × N	>6.0 × N
Heart						
	Pulmonary	None or no change	Asymptomatic with abnormality in PFTs	Dyspnea on significant exertion	Dyspnea at normal level of activity	Dyspnea at rest
	Cardiac dysrhythmias	None	Asymptomatic, transient, requiring no therapy	Recurrent or persistent, no therapy required	Requires treatment	Requires monitoring or hypotension, or ventricular tachycardia or fibrillation
	Cardiac function	None	Asymptomatic, decline of resting ejection fraction by less than 20% of baseline value	Asymptomatic, decline of resting ejection fraction by more than 20% of baseline value	Mild CHF responsive to therapy	Severe or refractory CHF

	Cardiac ischemia	None	Nonspecific T wave flattening	Asymptomatic, ST and T wave changes suggesting ischemia	Angina without evidence for infarction	Acute myocardial infarction
Neurologic						
	Neurosensory	None or no change	Mild paresthesias, loss of deep tendon reflexes	Mild or moderate objective sensory loss; moderate paresthesias	Severe objective sensor loss or paresthesias that interfere with function	—
	Neuromotor	None or no change	Subjective weakness; no objective findings	Mild objective weakness without significant impairment	Objective weakness with impairment	Paralysis

Table 15-8. Response and survival criteria

Clinical criteria	
Complete response (CR)	100% disappearance of all objective signs of cancer, both clinical and radiologic
Partial response (PR)	Tumor regression of 50–99% in the product of the diameters of measurable tumor and the absence of appearance of new lesions or tumor progression elsewhere
Stationary disease (SD)	≤ 25% increase in size and ≤ 0–49% regression
Progressive disease	≥ 25% increase in size of measurable tumor
Surgical response	
Complete response	Regression of all tumor at second-look laparotomy with histologically negative biopsies from all previous sites of metastatic cancer
Partial response	See above
Stationary disease	See above
Progressive disease	See above
Survival criteria	
Survival	From start of therapy to (1) death or (2) last follow-up
Progression-free survival	Survival from start of therapy to progression of disease or last evaluation

Table 15-9. Performance status score

ECOG (or Zubrod) scale		*Karnofsky score (%)*
0	Asymptomatic and fully active	100
1	Asymptomatic; fully ambulatory; restricted in physically strenuous activity	80–90
2	Symptomatic; ambulatory; capable of self-care; more than 50% of waking hours are spent out of bed	60–70
3	Symptomatic; limited self-care; spends more than 50% of waking hours in bed, but not bedridden	40–50
4	Completely disabled; no self-care; bedridden	20–30

able drugs led to the treatment of most metastatic tumors with single-agent, alkylating-agent chemotherapy to achieve less than satisfactory overall results. In the 1970s, the discovery of Adriamycin (antitumor antibiotic) and cisplatin (platinum compound) led to combination therapy in which a combination of the drugs was used with the belief that the drugs' different mechanism of action might result in improved response and increased survival of patients with gynecologic malignancies. Currently, with the exception of a small percent increase in survival documented primarily by meta-analysis of a large number of studies, this hypothesis remains largely unproven.

Table 15-10. Criteria for selection of multidrug chemotherapy to overcome drug resistance

Demonstrated individual single-agent activity against the tumor
Demonstrated in vitro synergy
Demonstrated different dose-limiting toxicities
Used at maximum-tolerated doses. Dose intensity
Minimize time interval between courses
Combination of cell cycle phase-specific with cell cycle non–phase-specific
Combination drug therapy to prevent development of resistant clones to single agent
Have tumor reduced (surgery or radiation) to their smallest possible size prior to chemotherapy

Notwithstanding, our better understanding of the development of resistance to chemotherapy does allow for a rational approach to the development of multiple-drug regimens for women with advanced gynecologic malignancies (Table 15-10).

Selected Readings

Beutler E. Platelet transfusions: The 20,000/ul trigger. *Blood* 81:1411, 1993.

Bradley G. P-glycoprotein expression in multi-drug resistant human ovarian carcinoma cells. *Cancer Res* 49:2790, 1989.

Goldie JH, Coldman AJ. A mathematical model for relating the drug sensitivity of tumors to their spontaneous mutation rate. *Cancer Treat Rep* 63:1727, 1979.

Hamilton TC. Augmentation of Adriamycin, Melphalan and Cisplatinum cytotoxicity in drug-resistant and sensitive human ovarian cancer cell lines by buthionine sulfoximine mediated glutathione depletion. *Biochem Pharmacol* 34:25, 1985.

Hryniuk W. The Importance of Dose Intensity in Outcome of Chemotherapy. In S Hellman, V DeVita, S Rosenberg (eds), *Important Advances in Oncology*. Philadelphia: Lippincott, 1988. Pp 121–141.

Kaplan EL, Meier P. Non-parametric estimation from incomplete observations. *J Am Stat* 53:457, 1958.

Lai GM. Enhanced DNA repair and resistance to cisplatin in human ovarian cancer. *Biochem Pharmacol* 37:4597, 1988.

Markman M. Why does a higher response rate to chemotherapy correlate poorly with improved survival? *J Cancer Res Clin Oncol* 119:700, 1993.

Norton L, Simon R. The Norton-Simon hypothesis revisited. *Cancer Treat Rep* 70:163, 1986.

Skipper HE. Laboratory models: The historical perspective. *Cancer Treat Rep* 70:3, 1986.

Tannock IF. The relationship between proliferation and the vascular system in a transplanted mouse mammary tumor. *Br J Cancer* 22:258, 1968.

van der Zee AGJ, Hollema H, deJong S et al. P-Glycoprotein expression and DNA Topoisomerase I and II activity in benign tumors of the ovary and in malignant tumors of the ovary, before and after platinum/cyclophosphamide chemotherapy. *Cancer Res* 51:5915, 1991.

16

Principles of Radiation Therapy

James Orner, Kyu Shin, and Anthony Ho

Radiation Biology

MECHANISM OF ACTION

Radiation mediates its damage inside the cell through either direct or indirect action. The most critical target of radiation is DNA. Radiation may interact directly with the target structure, causing atoms to be ionized or excited, thus starting the chain of events that results in cell death. This mechanism, referred to as *direct action*, involves the ionization of atoms within the critical target molecules themselves. *Indirect action* involves radiation interacting with other molecules (other than the target structure), such as water, with the resultant production of free radicals. These highly unstable molecules then interact with the target molecule by stripping electrons and breaking chemical bonds. The majority of damage caused to a cell by photon and electron irradiation is by indirect action. Heavy-charged particle irradiation (such as alpha particles) and neutrons produce a dense cloud of ionization in their path and are less dependent on indirect action.

Linear Energy Transfer

Linear energy transfer (LET) is the amount of energy deposited per unit length of the track of the radiation beam. It is expressed as kiloelectron volts (kev) per micron. LET values depend on factors other than radiation energy; however, the LET value is used as a simple indicator of the radiation quality, with low values for x-rays and high values for heavy-particle irradiation.

Relative Biological Effectiveness

Relative biological effectiveness is the ratio of the dose of 250-kV x-rays to that given by another kind of radiation to produce the same biological effect.

Fractionation of Radiation Therapy

The dose of radiation required to eradicate a tumor is usually given in small increments over a period of days or weeks. The dose given daily is called a *fraction*. The rationale for fractionation is determined by four factors that contribute to differential dose response between normal tissues and tumors: (1) repopulation, (2) repair of sublethal cellular damage, (3) reoxygenation, and (4) redistribution of cells within the cell cycle. Conventional regimens with radiation have been determined because they permit normal tissues to repair sublethal damage and repopulate between fractions. At the same time, they increase tumor damage because of reoxygenation and redistribution of cells into the more sensitive phases of the cell cycle.

TARGET MOLECULE

The target molecule of radiation damage that results in cell death is believed to be DNA. By both direct and indirect action, radiation causes bonds to be broken in the DNA molecule. This, in turn, results in translocations, cross-linkages, double-strand break, and deletions, which ultimately result in loss of genetic material in subsequent cell divisions and in cell death.

THE OXYGEN EFFECT

For photons and electrons, which require indirect action to mediate the majority of their damaging effects, oxygen plays an important role and is necessary to finalize the damage caused by indirect action. The *oxygen enhancement ratio* (OER) is the dose of radiation required to create a given effect without oxygen divided by the dose required in the presence of oxygen. For photons this value is 2 at doses near 2 Gy and 3 at higher doses. The OER is 1.6 for neutrons and approaches unity for heavy-charged particles.

THE CELL CYCLE EFFECT

The sensitivity of mammalian cells to radiation varies with the point in the cell cycle. The most sensitive phases are late G2 and mitosis. The most resistant phases are late S and G0. Early S phase and late G1 are intermediate in sensitivity.

REPAIR OF CYCLE EFFECT

Not all damage inflicted on a cell's DNA (at doses typically used in radiation therapy) results in cell death. Much of it can be repaired if cells are given sufficient time and the proper conditions before administration of more radiation. *Potentially lethal damage* can be modified by manipulating the postirradiation conditions. If cells in culture are placed from culture medium into saline or are prevented from dividing in a plateau phase for 6 hours after irradiation, much of this damage can be repaired and increased cell survival is seen. *Sublethal damage* can be repaired by giving cells time to repair after receiving radiation before giving more radiation. It is believed to represent repair of DNA strand breaks prior to the formation of chromosomal aberrations. Both sublethal and potentially lethal damage repair are significant for photon and electron irradiation but are almost nonexistent for neutrons and heavy-charged particles. In practice a minimum of 6 hours should be given between radiation fractions to ensure maximum repair of sublethal damage in normal late-reacting tissue.

REPOPULATION AND DURATION OF TREATMENT

As cells are lost during a protracted course of radiation, surviving clonogens continue to divide and repopulate. This must be considered in planning a course of radiation. An additional 60 cGy per day is required to eradicate the tumor cells accounted for by repopulation. Because early-reacting normal tissue also reacts similarly, it might seem attractive to extend treatment time by adding planned treatment breaks to reduce early effects. This should be avoided at all costs due to the added tumor burden caused by repopulation. Treatment delays in the range commonly encountered in cancer treatment have virtually no effect on late-reacting tissue and thus do not decrease the incidence of late effects.

THE SINGLE FRACTION CELL SURVIVAL CURVE

When the log of surviving mammalian cells is plotted against an increasing single fraction dose, the resultant curve has an initial linear slope that proceeds to bend or become more "curvy" at higher doses. This initial "flatter" portion of the curve is known as the "shoulder" of the curve. This shoulder may represent a dose region of the curve where sublethal damage has occurred, and given sufficient time, the majority of this may be repaired. As the dose increases, the curve begins to drop more steeply, possibly representing a range at which the cell is overwhelmed and cannot repair enough damage to maintain reproductive viability. Late-reacting tissues such as muscle exhibit a broad shoulder on their survival curve, whereas early-reacting tissues, such as mucosa of the gastrointestinal tract and mouth, exhibit a small or almost no shoulder.

THE LINEAR QUADRATIC FORMULA

The mammalian cell survival curve is well described by the formula $S = e^{-1D-BD2}$ (where S = fraction surviving, D = dose, and e and B are constants for the cells in question) at fraction sizes that are typically used clinically. Looking at this formula, one can see that at low doses the curve is dominated by the portion of the curve that is linear due to its dependence on dose to the single power. As the dose increases, the equation becomes dominated by the beta (quadratic) portion, which is dependent on dose squared, and the curve begins to bend more sharply and become more "curvy." It is believed that the linear portion of the curve represents cell killing that requires a single event, and the quadratic component of the curve represents cell killing that is dependent on the occurrence of two separate events.

Basic Radiation Physics

In radiation therapy treatment planning, a simulator reproduces the geometric setup of the patient on the radiation therapy machine or reproduces the positions of the brachytherapy sources with nonradioactive dummy sources placed inside the brachytherapy applicator.

PRODUCTION OF IONIZING RADIATION

X-Ray Tubes

Radiation therapy equipment in the 50- to 150-kV (kilovolts = 1,000 volts) range is used for superficial treatment. The x-ray is produced by accelerating the electrons through a large voltage difference and hitting the target of the x-ray tube. There are two mechanisms by which x-rays are produced: (1) bremsstrahlung x-rays (braking radiation) are the result of the interaction between a high-speed electron and a nucleus and (2) characteristic x-rays are the result of an outer orbital electron filling an electron vacancy that is caused by the interaction of the high-speed incident electron with the atoms of the target.

The difference between diagnostic x-rays and x-rays for therapy is the amount of radiation produced per unit time. The simulator such as the Varian Ximatron uses a diagnostic x-ray tube, while radiation

Table 16-1. Skin dose and maximum depth dose versus energy source

		Depth where percentage of maximum dose occurs			
Energy	*Skin dose (%) (of max. dose)*	*dmax (cm)*	*d_{80} (cm)*	*d_{50} (cm)*	*d_{10} (cm)*
6-MV photon	50	1.5	7.0	15.0	>50
18-MV photon	40	3.0	10.0	22.0	>50
6-MeV electron	78	1.2	2.0	2.3	2.9
9-MeV electron	82	2.0	3.1	3.5	4.3
12-MeV electron	88	2.6	4.3	5.1	6.1
16-MeV electron	94	2.8	5.8	6.8	8.2
20-MeV electron	96	2.8	6.9	8.4	10.4

therapy equipment such as the Oldelft superficial unit uses an x-ray tube that produces much more radiation per unit time. The dose rate of the superficial unit is in the range of 200–500 cGy per minute at the end of the applicator cone.

For x-rays produced by a superficial radiation therapy unit, the maximum dose is delivered to the skin surface of the patient, with a rapid fall off of dose with increasing depth—e.g., for a 50-kV x-ray, 80% of the maximum dose (d_{80}) occurs at 1 cm, d_{50} at 3 cm, and d_{10} at 10 cm.

Linear Accelerator

The method of accelerating electrons through voltage differences may be used up to approximately 300 kV. A medical linear accelerator (linac), using microwave technology, can accelerate electrons up to 18 MV (million volts) or more. The electrons may be used directly for patient treatment, or the electrons may be directed at a target to produce a high output of x-rays. These high-energy x-rays have the ability to penetrate a greater depth of tissue.

Linacs such as the Varian Clinac 600C produces 6-MV photons only, while the Varian Clinac 2100C provides a choice of 6-MV photons, 19-MV photons, and five different electron energies of 6, 9, 12, 16, and 20 MeV (million electron volts). Table 16-1 gives an approximate range of skin dose, depth of maximum dose (dmax), d_{80}, d_{50}, and d_{10}.

In general, there is more skin sparing for higher-energy photon beams, and the skin dose increases with increasing electron energies. The dose increases with depth initially until dmax is obtained. Beyond the dmax region, the dose falls gradually with depth for higher-energy photon beams, and it falls rapidly with depth for electron beams.

Radionuclides

All radionuclides decay to stable nonradioactive isotopes at a rate characteristic of their internal nuclear structure. The rate of decay is constant, which is usually characterized as *half-life*, the time required for the radionuclide to decay to half of its initial activity. The traditional unit of activity is a curie (Ci), which is equal to 3.7 x 10^{10} disintegrations per second (dps). A lower activity may be given as mCi, which is 0.001 Ci. The Systems International d'Unites (SI) unit of activity is the becquerel (Bq), which is equal to 1 dps.

Table 16-2. Radionuclides used for brachytherapy

Radionuclide	*Half-life*	*Photon energy (MeV)*
Radium (Ra-226)	1,600 yrs	0.83 (average)
Radon (Rn-222)	3.83 days	0.83 (average)
Cobalt (Co-60)	5.26 yrs	1.17, 1.33
Cesium (Cs-137)	30 yrs	0.662
Iridium (Ir-192)	74.2 days	0.38 (average)
Iodine (I-125)	60.2 days	0.028 (average)

Another unit of activity is the mgRaeq, which is milligram radium equivalent or equivalent mass of radium. For example, a cesium-137 (Cs-137) source used for gynecologic purposes may be listed as equivalent to so many milligrams of radium filtered with 1 mm platinum (Pt). The equivalence is determined by equal dose rates at equal distances from the sources.

Teletherapy ("Long-Distance" Therapy)

Cobalt-60 (Co-60) is used in teletherapy, such as in the Theratronics Cobalt unit. A typical Co-60 teletherapy source is a cylinder of 1–2 cm in diameter by 1–3 cm long, with an activity of about 5,000 Ci. The Co-60 source is mounted on a metal drawer that slides horizontally in a large shielding material. The source faces an aperture for treatment in the "beam on" position and moves to its shielding location in the "beam off" position.

Since Co-60 has a half-life of 5,261 years, the radiation output has to be adjusted at monthly intervals. The output is approximately 1% lower per month. The average energy of the Co-60 gamma rays is 1.2 MeV. There is some skin-sparing effect, and dmax is 0.5 cm below the surface. Beyond the dmax region, the dose falls off faster than that of the 6-MV photon beam; d_{50} occurs at approximately 12 cm.

Brachytherapy ("Short-Distance" Therapy)

Brachytherapy is a method of radiation treatment in which sealed radioactive sources are used to deliver a high dose locally by intracavitary, interstitial, or surface application, resulting in a rapid dose fall-off in the surrounding normal tissue. The most commonly used radioactive sources and their characteristics are illustrated in Table 16-2.

Inverse Square Law

Radiation exposure or intensity is inversely proportional to the square of the distance from a point source. The concept of a point source allows a simple mathematical calculation of exposure at a distance. Non–point source may be considered as approximate point source at large distances. The gynecologic use of Cs-137 tubes and other linear sources involves calculations near the non–point source. The exposure at these points requires an evaluation of an integral equation, which is more complicated than the simple equation used for a point source. However, computers are routinely used for the calculation of dose and dose distribution (Figs. 16-1 and 16-2).

Radium-226

Radium-226 (Ra-226) became the most commonly used radionuclide in brachytherapy since its discovery in 1898. Ra-226 disintegrates

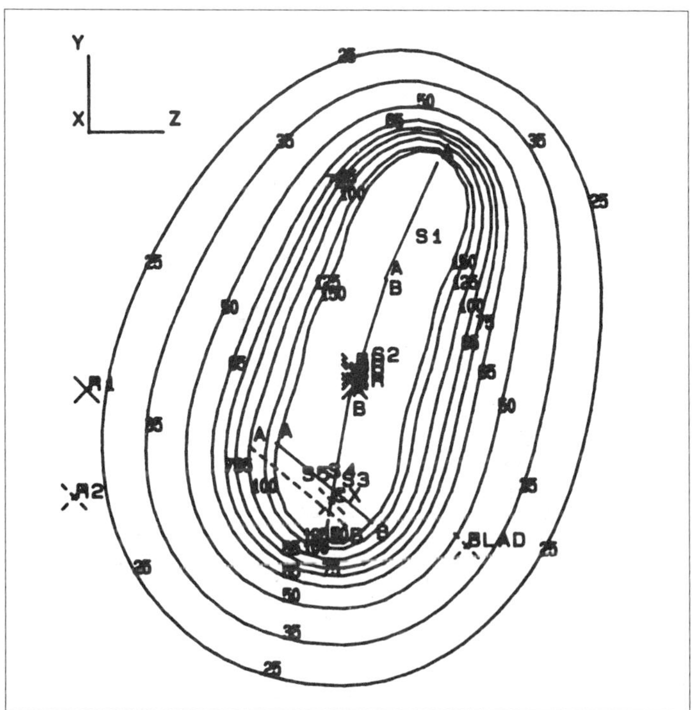

Fig. 16-1. Computerized plan (lateral view) for intracavitary implant consisting of a tandem and vaginal colpostats. The numbers on each line indicate the dose rate per hour.

with a half-life of 1,600 years to form radon, a radioactive gas. The average energy of the gamma rays is approximately 1 MeV, which is a combination of about 50 gamma rays ranging from 0.2 to 2.0 MeV. Because of radiation safety concerns when working with Ra-226, it has been replaced with radionuclides such as Cs-137.

Cesium-137

Cs-137 has a 30-year half-life and a gamma ray energy of 0.66 MeV. Since it has a long half life, Cs-137 may be reused for different patients over many years. The traditional low-dose rate (LDR) Cs-137 tube source has a physical length of about 20 mm, and the usual range of the activity is 5–25 mgRaeq. Most brachytherapy is now practiced with "afterloading" devices that allow loading of radioactive sources after the applicators or catheters are placed inside the patient and have been checked radiographically for proper positioning using dummy sources. Afterloading techniques may require either handling the radioactive sources manually or using a remotely controlled afterloading device for loading of radioactive sources into the previously inserted applicators. A remote afterloader such as the Nucletron Selectron-LDR unit uses a spherical Cs-137 source of 2.5 mm in diameter. Typical activity of the LDR source is 20 mCi. For the Selectron-LDR unit, the Cs-137 sources and the inactive

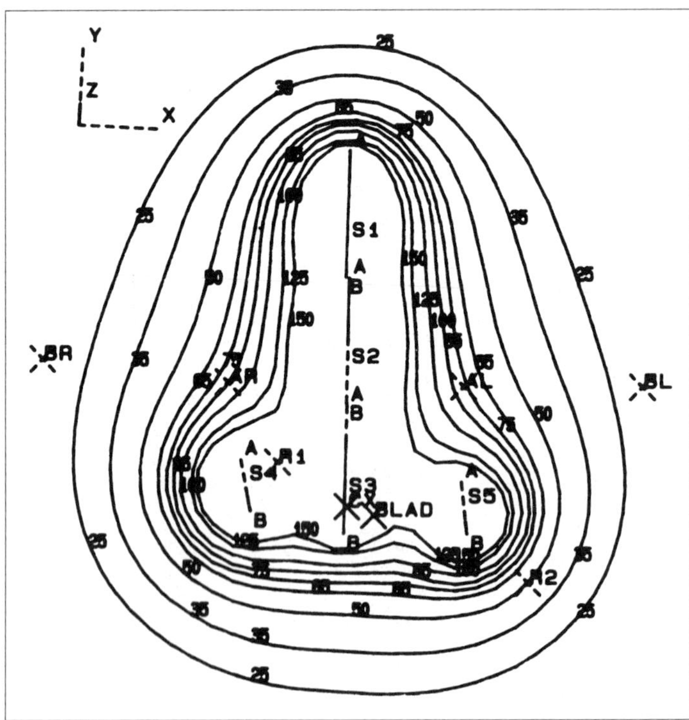

Fig. 16-2. Computerized plan: "Anterior view" of an intracavitary implant using a tandem and colpostats. There are three radioactive cesium sources in the tandem and two sources in the colpostats.

spacers are moved by a microprocessor-controlled pneumatic system. Typical application uses either one or three channels. The sources are contained in a storage shield when not in use or when the door of the patient's room is opened.

Iridium-192

Iridium-192 (Ir-192) has a half-life of approximately 74 days, and the average energy of the many gamma rays is 0.34 MeV. Because of the lower energy, Ir-192 sources require less shielding for personnel protection than either Ra-226 or CS-137. Ir-192 may be used for either LDR or high-dose rate (HDR) applications. For LDR applications, nylon ribbons containing the iridium metal encased in small stainless steel seeds are placed in catheters that have been surgically implanted in the tumor. The 3 mm long, 0.5 mm diameter Ir-192 sources are usually ordered for each procedure after preliminary treatment planning is done to determine the activity and number of seeds and ribbons required. The activity per seed is approximately 1 mgRaeq. LDR Ir-192 sources may also be fabricated in the form of thin flexible wires that can be cut to desired length. For remote afterloading HDR applications such as the Nucletron microSelec-tron-HDR unit, one Ir-192 source of 4.5 mm long and an activity of approximately 10 Ci are used.

The source steps through different dwell positions in a catheter to achieve a uniform dose. The HDR Ir-192 source is welded to the end of a flexible cable, which is microprocessor-controlled and may be programmed for one or many channels. The source is contained in a storage safe when not in use.

Both sources mentioned above—Cs-137 and Ir-192—are left in the patient for a limited time and then removed and stored or disposed of. For the HDR unit, the Ir-192 source is typically replaced every 3 months, at which time the old source is taken out from the shielding of the unit and a new source is installed.

There are some short half-life radionuclides used for permanent implant. Radioactive gold seeds, Au-198, with a half-life of 2.7 days, emit both beta particles and gamma rays with an energy of about 0.41 MeV. Iodine (I-125) in a metal-encased seed is also used for permanent implants. It has a half-life of 60 days and emits gamma rays for low energy of approximately 0.03 MeV.

INTERACTION OF IONIZING RADIATION

When radiation, either electromagnetic (i.e., x-ray or gamma ray) or charged particles (e.g., electron) is absorbed in tissue, both ionization and excitation of the media result. *Ionization* means the atom is ionized by removing an electron from a neutral atom. When the energy is not sufficient to eject an electron from the atom but is used to raise the electron to a higher energy level, the process is called *excitation*. The particular type of interaction between the radiation and the atom of the median depends on variables such as the energy, type of radiation, and composition of tissue at the interaction site.

Electromagnetic

Photoelectric Effect

For the superficial units or as the megavoltage photon beam is attenuated and scattered, more lower-energy photons are produced. The lower-energy photons are more likely to interact through the photoelectric effect, where the low-energy photon transfers all its energy to an orbital electron (photoelectron), resulting in its ejection. The photoelectric effect varies strongly with the atomic number (Z) of the scattering media, approximately proportional to Z^3. Low-energy photon beams produced by superficial machines cause high absorption of x-ray energy in bone because of this Z^3 dependence. As the photon energy (E) increases, the probability of photoelectric effect decreases approximately as $1/E^3$.

Compton Scattering

The most probable means of interaction between x-ray or gamma ray photon and an atom within the megavoltage energy range used in radiation therapy is Compton scattering. The incident photon interacts with free electrons in the absorbing median and is scattered. The result is a recoil electron and a photon of less energy than the original photon. Compton effect is independent of Z. It depends only on the number of electrons per gram, which is about the same for most body tissues. The Compton effect also decreases with increasing photon energy.

The recoiled electron from the Compton effect and the photoelectron from the photoelectric effect, along with the secondary ionization these electrons produce, cause the biological damage to the tissue.

Pair Production

The third process, pair production, requires a photon energy of at least 1.02 MeV. In this interaction, a pair of electrons, one positive and one negative, are produced after the photon is absorbed. Both electrons produce ionization and excitation, but the positive electron soon combines with an electron in the medium to produce a pair of photons that produces more ionization. The probability of pair production varies approximately linearly with the atomic number of the medium. For photons below 10 MV, only a small fraction of the interactions are pair production.

Charged Particles

The particle of importance in radiation therapy is the *energetic electron*. It may be produced by electromagnetic radiation or by the linac. The electrons "collide" with other electrons or atoms in tissue. The electron-electron interaction is one means of transferring energy and producing ionization. For an energetic electron, this process leaves a track of ionization until all the electrons have expended their energy. An energetic electron may also be scattered by the nucleus of an atom; bremsstrahlung radiation is produced in this process.

The electron may interact with the electron of the medium atom and cause excitation. The relative proportion of the interactions depends on the electron energy and the tissue composition. The radiation effect on the tissue is a result of the ionization and excitation produced by these processes.

MEASUREMENT OF IONIZING RADIATION

Radiation Exposure

Roentgen (R) is a unit of exposure and the SI unit is coulomb per kilogram (C/kg). Exposure is a measure of ionization produced in air by photons. When photons interact with air through the process of photoelectric effect, Compton effect, and pair production, electrons are produced. With the presence of an air-filled ionization chamber (ion chamber), the positive charges move toward the negative electrode and the negative charges move toward the positive electrode because of the voltage applied between the two electrodes of the ion chamber. Either the positive or negative charges may be collected and measured by an electrometer.

Absorbed Dose

Radiation-absorbed dose is defined as the average amount of energy deposited in a small volume of medium. The SI unit of absorbed dose is the gray (Gy), and 1 Gy = 1 joule/kilogram, where joule is a unit of energy and kilogram is the mass of material where the dose is deposited. A *centigray* (cGy) is equivalent to 0.01 Gy. An "old" unit of absorbed dose is the rad, and 1 Gy = 100 rad or 1 cGy = 1 rad.

Absorbed dose is measured with different dosimeters. The most common dosimeter is the ion chamber. The calibration of the ion chamber is traceable to the National Institute of Standards and Technology. Medical physicists use the ion chamber to calibrate the output of linacs, cobalt teletherapy units, superficial units, and radionuclides. The ionization produced in the small cavity of the ion chamber may be used to determine the absorbed dose in a medium such as water or muscle.

Thermoluminescent dosimeters (TLDs) are crystals such as lithium fluoride (LiF) used as radiation detectors. When LiF is irradiated by ionization radiation, some of the electrons are trapped in an excited state. Subsequent heating of these crystals releases the trapped electrons, and the crystal emits light as a result. The TLD reader is used for heating and detecting the light, which provides information on the dose the crystal has received. Once the TLD and TLD reader are calibrated, the absorbed dose may be determined.

Other types of dosimeters include (1) calorimeters, in which a rise in temperature of an irradiated object is measured and converted to absorbed dose; (2) film, in which the optical density of the exposed film may be calibrated for absorbed-dose determinations; (3) diodes, in which the charge collected may be related to absorbed dose once it is calibrated; and (4) chemical dosimeter, in which the ferrous ions, Fe^{2+}, are oxidized by radiation to ferric ions, Fe^{3+}, the yield of which may be converted to absorbed dose.

Radiation Therapy for Cervix Cancer

GENERAL PRINCIPLES OF TREATMENT

Radiation therapy is an effective treatment for stages I–IVA cervix cancer and is the preferred treatment for all disease except stage I and early stage IIA. The optimal treatment of cervix cancer with radiation requires the use of both external beam radiation and brachytherapy. The proportion of dose delivered by brachytherapy and external beam treatment varies with both stage and bulk of disease and from institution to institution, with some institutions preferring to give a greater proportion of the central dose for a given stage with brachytherapy.

In general, the larger the bulk of disease, the greater the proportion of dose delivered by external beam treatments. The usual dose is 50 Gy for microscopic disease. The dose can be increased to 60 Gy by reducing the field size or to 70 Gy by further reduction. Because of the steep fall-off of dose from brachytherapy, external beam treatments are used to shrink the volume of bulky disease before brachytherapy. This allows the isodose lines of the implant to better encompass the volume of residual disease and often improves the geometry of the implant to allow better dose distribution.

Data from the Patterns of Care Study indicate that two or more brachytherapy implants are superior to a single insertion. The improvement in local control, rate of distant metastases, and survival is believed to be related to the ability to administer a higher paracentral dose with multiple implant insertions.

EXTERNAL BEAM TREATMENT

The use of external beam radiation in the treatment of cervix cancer requires megavoltage equipment. Treatment planning computers are used to calculate and optimize radiation doses within the patient. The use of four fields (Fig. 16-3) is preferable to two fields (Fig. 16-4), especially when using lower-energy photons (^{60}Co or 4–6 MV) or in thick patients, because it decreases the total dose delivered to the peripheral normal tissues and allows some shielding of the bowel and distal rectum and anus.

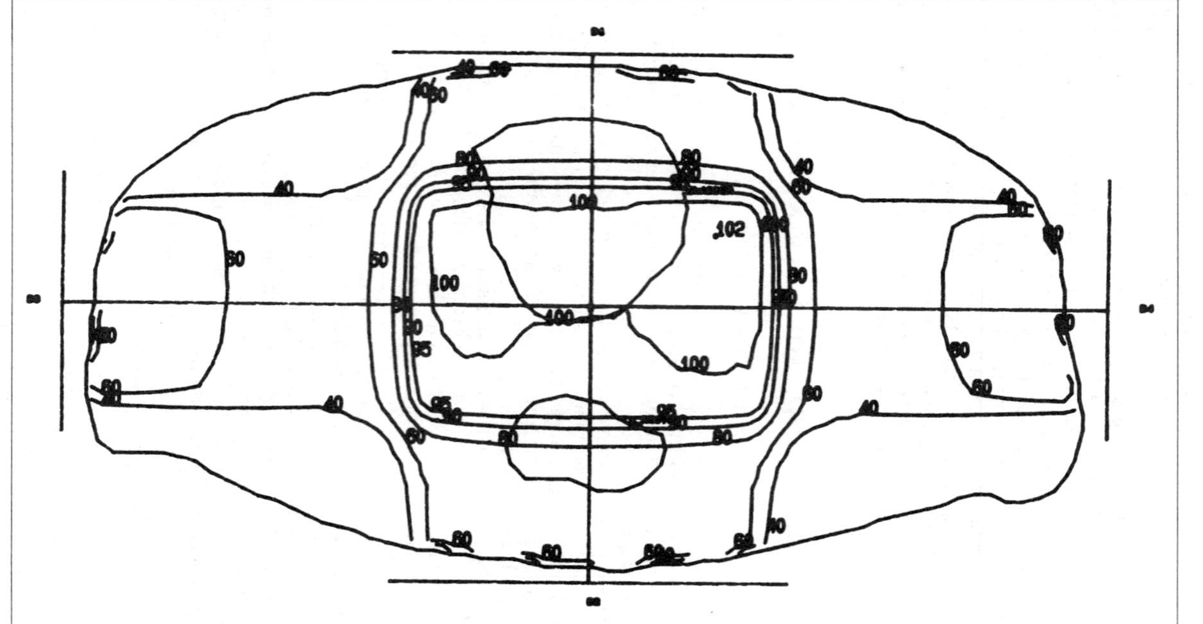

Fig. 16-3. Computerized plan for the four-field technique. It involves an anterior, a posterior, and two lateral fields. This technique is commonly used to treat the pelvis with cobalt 60 machines.

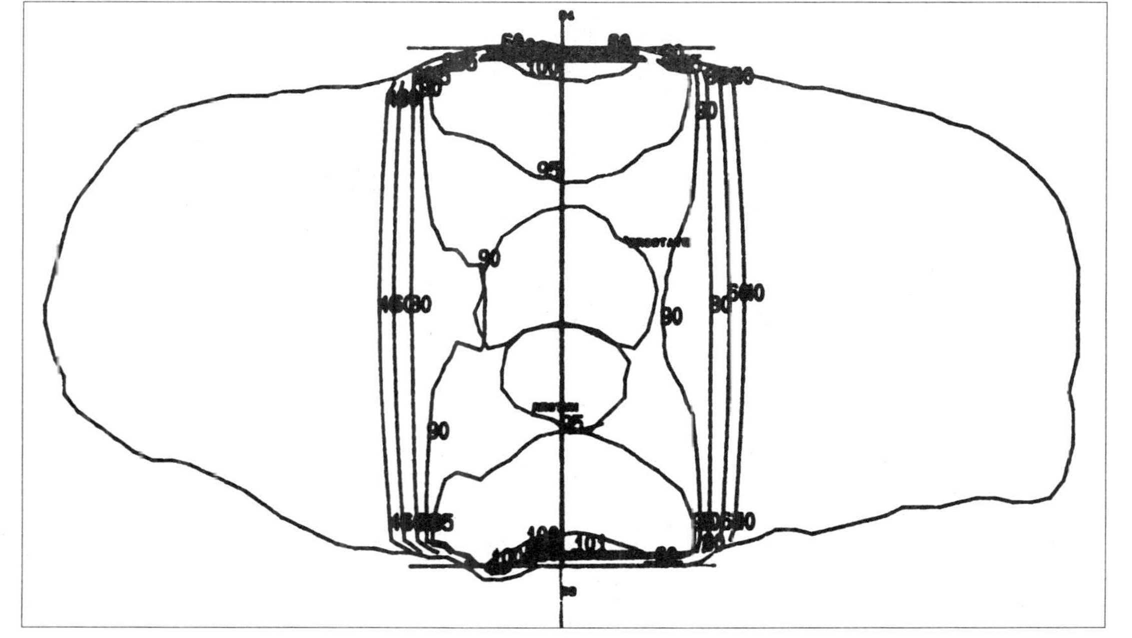

Fig. 16-4. Isodose distribution of a treatment plan involving two fields. The fields are opposed: anterior and posterior. The "90 line" encloses the volume of tissue that received 90% of the applied dose.

The purpose of external beam radiation is to treat the parametrium and draining lymphatics as well as to shrink bulky central disease before brachytherapy to achieve optimal implant geometry and dose distribution. Daily doses are typically 170–200 cGy. Higher daily doses are associated with increased complications.

Field Size

The field borders for the treatment of the pelvis are (1) below the obturator foramen inferiorly, (2) 1.5–2.0 cm lateral to the sidewall of the bony pelvis laterally, and (3) two-thirds the way up the sacroiliac (SI) joint if coverage is to include the external iliac nodes or the top of L5 if coverage of the common iliac nodes is required superiorly. If there is vaginal involvement, the inferior border is generally extended to cover the most distal extent of disease with a 2-cm margin.

If lateral fields are to be treated, the posterior border should include the entire anterior sacral silhouette to ensure adequate coverage of the uterosacral and cardinal ligaments. The anterior border should be 1 cm anterior to the pubic symphysis to give adequate coverage to the external iliac nodes. Shielding may be added to protect the anus and some bowel.

Split Pelvis Field

To bring the dose to structures located laterally and superiorly in the pelvis (and thus receiving only a small contribution of dose from the brachytherapy insertions) to a desired dose level (typically 50–60 Gy) without increasing the dose to the centrally located dose-limiting structures (i.e., bladder and rectum), a *split pelvis* field is used for part of the treatment. This is accomplished with an AP/PA pelvic field with a central block measuring 4.0–4.5 cm in width. At some institutions, the central block is custom-designed to match the isodose distribution of the implant in a stepwise manner.

INTRACAVITARY BRACHYTHERAPY

Intracavitary brachytherapy is the placement of radioactive material inside a body cavity and in close approximation to the tumor. Because the dose delivered by a point source of radiation falls off by the square of the distance, a high dose of radiation is delivered to the adjacent area while normal tissue a short distance away receives a significantly lower dose.

Inverse Square Law

Cervix cancer should never be treated with colpostats alone. Due to the rapid fall-off of dose, the majority of dose is delivered at the vaginal surface with a steep dose gradient and underdosage in the cervix and parametrium. If patient anatomy will not allow placement of a tandem, the patient is better served by an interstitial implant or external beam radiation alone.

Technique

After the applicator is placed, usually under general anesthesia, localization films are taken to ensure proper placement. The implant applicator is then afterloaded with radioactive sources. Traditionally, this has been done by hand, with resultant exposure to medical personnel. Computerized remote afterloading systems are now available that introduce the sources to the applicator through cables. These systems prevent the radioactive exposure of others who must enter the room because they automatically remove the sources when the room is entered and replace them when it is exited.

Radium Versus Cesium

Ra-226 was traditionally used as the isotope of choice in intracavitary brachytherapy. It has largely been replaced by Cs-137, which has the advantage of almost identical dosimetry, lesser shielding requirements, and no problem of possible radon gas leakage.

Manchester System Versus Milligram-Hour System

Manchester System

The Manchester system is based on prescribing a dose to a series of set points. Point A was originally defined as 2 cm above the top of the lateral vaginal fornix and 2 cm lateral to the middle of the cervical canal. Point B was described as 3 cm lateral to point A. The definition was later revised to place the vertical origin of point A 2 cm above the cervical os instead of the vaginal fornix.

Typical dose rates used at point A are 50–60 Gy/hour. Higher dose rates have been shown to be associated with increased complications and should be avoided. The total dose at point A (including external beam irradiation) is typically 8,000–8,500 cGy, although this can vary with disease extent. The dose rate at point B is typically in the range of 15 cGy/hour with standard recommended loadings. Dose is also typically monitored at the bladder with a Foley catheter balloon and in the rectum by using a point 0.5 cm posterior to the colpostats or by using a radiopaque marker.

A major problem with the use of point A is that it bears no constant relationship to patient anatomy. It will vary in location dependent on patient size, disease extent, geometry of implant, and anatomic variance.

Milligram-Hour System

The M.D. Anderson Cancer Center milligram-hour system uses standard specified loadings of radioactive sources, with the duration of the implant being specified by the total milligram-radium-equivalent contained in the implant. Dose is specified by milligram-hours, which is simply the duration of the implant in hours multiplied by the total milligram-radium-equivalent contained in the implant. The proportion of dose given by implant and external beam varies with the extent of disease and is based on clinical experience.

It is important that if Cs-137 is used with the milligram-hour system, a cesium correction factor of 1.07 should be used to multiply the total milligram-hours. This is because modern cesium sources are standardized against radium sources with 0.5-mm platinum filtration, whereas the clinical experience of M.D. Anderson (which the milligram-hour system is based on) used radium tubes with 1-mm platinum filtration.

Fletcher-Suit Applicator

The most commonly used applicator is the afterloading Fletcher-Suit colpostats and tandem (Fig. 16-5). It consists of a pair of barrel-shaped colpostats designed to sit in the lateral fornices at the apex of the vagina at the end of long, hollow handles. The colpostats have

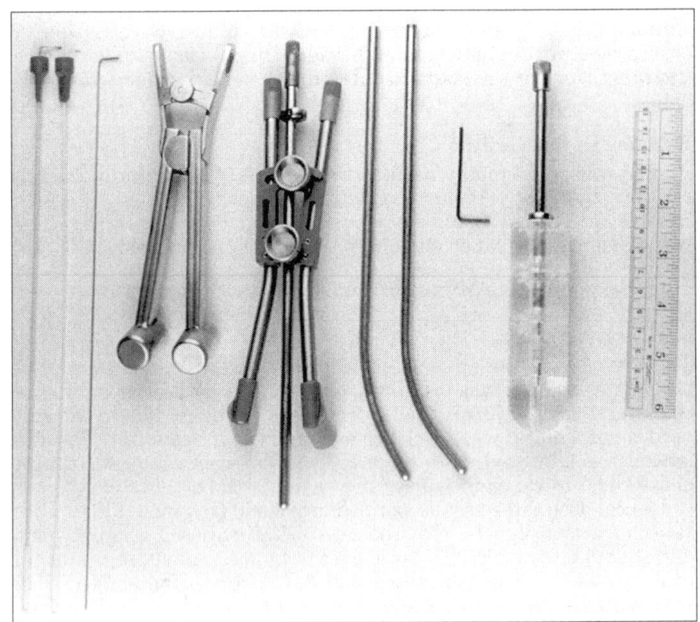

Fig. 16-5. Common applicators used for intracavitary irradiation of gynecologic tumors. Right to left: Simon's capsules, Fletcher colpostats, Delclos colpostats, and a tandem combination (two tandems and a vaginal cylinder).

tungsten shielding at each end to protect the bladder and rectum and hold one radioactive source each. They are 2 cm in diameter and may be fitted with plastic caps to increase their diameter to 2.5–3.0 cm. The size of the colpostat chosen should be as large as will be permitted, yet still lie in the lateral fornices. This places the vaginal mucosa as far as possible from the source and toward the shallow portion of the dose-distance curve. This, in turn, produces a lesser gradient between the dose delivered at the vaginal surface and that delivered in the parametrium (i.e., improved depth-dose). The intrauterine tandem is designed to fit within the corpus of the uterus and hold several radioactive sources in a linear array. The tandems are available in one curvature of four different lengths to fit differing uterine anatomies. A flange or cervical collar is placed on the tandem and sits flush against the cervical os.

When properly placed, the flange should be seen at two-thirds the height of the colpostats on the anterior localization film. The tandem should be midline and the system should not be skewed to either side. On lateral view, the tandem should bisect the midpoint of the colpostats and sit mid-distance between the sacral promontorium and the pubis.

High-Dose Brachytherapy

High–dose rate brachytherapy uses a high activity source to deliver in minutes doses that would typically take hours to deliver with typical low–dose rate implants. The potential benefits of this treatment are the ability to perform implants in the outpatient setting and the use of remote afterloading equipment that eliminates exposure to hospital personnel. Potential disadvantages of this treatment are the theoretical concerns of increased complications due to the predicted decreased therapeutic ratio for a given dose of high–dose rate compared to low–dose rate, the need to do multiple implants (typically 4–6), and the uncertainty as to what is the best dose and schedule to ensure the best treatment results with the lowest risk of complications. In a review of the literature, Orton showed that similar 5-year survival and complication rates have been reported with the use of high–dose rate brachytherapy in the treatment of carcinoma of the cervix.

INTERSTITIAL BRACHYTHERAPY

Interstitial brachytherapy is the placement of radioactive sources directly into the substance of the tumor and surrounding tissue. This may be accomplished by inserting "live" radioactive sources in the shape of needles (most commonly radium) or by placing hollow needles into the area to be implanted, either free-hand or with a template, and afterloading them with a radioactive source (most commonly iridium-197 ribbons). This technique is particularly well-suited for cases in which extensive disease will not allow good intracavitary implant placement and in cases of central disease recurrence.

Syed-Neblett Templates

The most common commercially available templates are the Syed-Neblett templates. These are made in a "butterfly" arrangement and allow hollow needles to be placed transperineally into the parametrium. They also allow placement of an intrauterine tandem and/or vaginal cylinder in the center of the template. Minimum dose rates are typically 40–80 cGy/hour at the periphery of the implant volume and are determined by multiple-level computer-generated isodose diagrams.

COMPLICATIONS AND NORMAL TISSUE TOLERANCE

Complications

Radiation tolerance of normal tissue is a function of total dose delivered, fraction size (or dose rate for brachytherapy), and volume of organ irradiated. In the treatment of cervix cancer, we are most concerned with the late-occurring complications involving the bladder, rectum, small bowel, vagina, and, in cases where extended-field radiotherapy is used, spinal cord. The most serious complications include fistulas, bowel obstruction, vaginal ulceration, rectal stenosis, and ulceration and transverse myelitis.

Tolerance Dose

The dose tolerance of an organ is typically expressed as the $TD_{5/5}$ or the dose that causes a given complication in 5% of those treated in 5 years. The $TD_{5/5}$ for late complications with fractionated radiation is 65 Gy for bladder, 65 Gy for rectum, 50 Gy for bowel, and 50 Gy for spinal cord.

Typically, doses to the rectum and bladder are kept at a maximum of 70–80 Gy delivered to a single maximum-dose reference point. Dose to the spinal cord is typically limited to 45–50 Gy (a dose range in which transverse myelitis is almost never seen). Perez has shown that doses of 75–80 Gy to limited volumes result in an approximately 5% incidence of grade 2 and 3 complications of the bladder and rectum, with the incidence rising to over 10% at higher doses. He also noted an increase in injury to the small bowel with doses of over 60 Gy to the pelvic sidewall.

TREATMENT AND RESULTS

Carcinoma in Situ and Stage I

Carcinoma in Situ and Stage IA

Most lesions of carcinoma in situ (CIS) and stage IA are successfully treated by surgical procedures. In the few patients in whom surgery is contraindicated or who show diffuse CIS with involvement of the vagina, radiation can be used with excellent results.

Stage IB

Stage IB lesions can be treated either by radical hysterectomy and bilateral pelvic lymphadenectomy or radiation therapy with excellent results. The size of the primary cervical tumor affects survival and should be considered in deciding on optimal therapy.

SURVIVAL. The worldwide average 5-year survival rate for patients treated with radiation for stage I cervix cancer (mostly stage IB) is about 80%; however, large institutions with extensive experience have shown survival and disease-free survival approaching 85–90% and greater for stage IB. Locoregional control obtained with radiation is in the range of 90% for stage IB.

SITES OF FAILURE. In the classic analysis of failure from M.D. Anderson Cancer Center, the most common cause of central failure in stages IB and IIA disease was a skewed radium system that caused underdosage to the parametrium. Other causes included the use of a vaginal cylinder in place of colpostats, which also underdosed the parametrium.

Stage II

Stage IIA

With the exception of limited stage IIA, radiation is the treatment of choice for stage II disease. The factors that go into choosing between surgery and radiation for early stage IIA disease are similar to those listed above for stage IB.

SURVIVAL. Survival and disease-free survival range from 75% to 80%, and locoregional control is approximately 85–90%.

Stage IIB

The treatment of choice for stage IIB is pelvic radiation and a minimum of two brachytherapy applications. Patients who undergo pretherapy surgical staging and para-aortic lymph node biopsy or para-aortic lymphadenectomy are treated with extended-field irradiation if there is histologic documentation of para-aortic lymph node metastasis (see section on para-aortic radiation).

SURVIVAL. Survival and disease-free survival range from 60% to 65% and locoregional control approximates 75%.

SITES OF FAILURE. The most common cause of locoregional failure in stage IIB disease is bulky central disease causing an unsuitable anatomy for implant. Skewing of the radium system away from the side of recurrent disease without compensation from external beam irradiation was the most common reason for parametrial failure.

Stage III

Radiation therapy is the treatment of choice for stage III and consists of external pelvic radiation with two or more brachytherapy applications. Patients who undergo pretherapy surgical staging and para-aortic lymph node biopsy or para-aortic lymphadenectomy are treated with extended field irradiation if there is histologic documentation of para-aortic lymph node metastasis (see section on para-aortic radiation).

Survival

Several large series show long-term survival and disease-free survival in the range of 40%. Locoregional control in stage III treated with radiation is 50–60%.

Stage IVA

Radiation is the treatment of choice in stage IVA disease. Five-year survival for stage IVA disease is in the range of 15–20% but may be higher in those with limited parametrial involvement.

Stages IB, II, III, and IVA with Metastasis to the Para-Aortic Lymph Nodes

Patients with small-volume para-aortic lymph node metastasis in what is thought to be controllable pelvic disease can be cured by pelvic and extended field pelvic radiation. Aggressive surgical debulking of lymph node metastasis in conjunction with pelvic and extended field irradiation improves local control and overall survival. Treatment of unresected para-aortic lymph node metastasis with pelvic and extended field radiation prolongs survival but most likely does not lead to cure. The role of prophylactic para-aortic radiation in locally advanced cervical cancer remains controversial.

Concurrent Chemotherapy and Radiation Therapy

Hydroxyurea

There have been several randomized trials comparing hydroxyurea (HU) as a radiation potentiator to radiation alone or radiation and misonidazole in cervix cancer. These trials demonstrate an increase in survival for the HU arm compared to the control arm or the misonidazole arm.

Cisplatin

Wong reported on a randomized trial of stage IIIB and III patients in which patients were assigned to receive either radiation alone, radiation and weekly cisplatin, or radiation and twice weekly cisplatin. Survival, relapse free survival, and response were similar in all three groups.

Unusual Cervical Anatomy

Carcinoma of the Cervical Stump

Carcinoma of the cervical stump poses the challenge of poor anatomy for intracavitary brachytherapy due to the inability to place a full intrauterine tandem. Results have been similar to those obtained in the treatment of cervical carcinoma with an intact uterus.

The Barrel-Shaped Cervix

Several institutions have reported their results with radiation alone versus radiation and surgery for bulky stage I and II disease. M.D. Anderson Cancer Center reported that when all patients treated were reviewed, there appeared to be a significant effect of adjuvant hysterectomy on outcome. However, it was difficult to draw conclusions because of the patient selection factors, which put more patients with poor prognostic factors (i.e., tumors ≥ 8 cm, positive lymphangiogram, palpable disease after external beam irradiation, and stage IIB) in the radiation-alone group. When patients with tumors of 8 cm or more were removed from the analysis, no significant differences were seen in survival or pelvic control between the two treatment groups.

Radiation Therapy for Endometrial Cancer

STAGE I

Adjuvant Treatment

Postoperative radiation therapy is recommended for most surgically resected stage I endometrial cancers. Patients with a high probability of pelvic lymph node metastasis (grade 3 tumors or deep [≥ 50%] invasion of the myometrium) require pelvic field radiation, while those with very low probablity of lymph node metastasis (grades 1 and 2 and tumor invading the myometrium <50%) frequently require only vaginal radiation to lower the incidence of vaginal recurrence. Vaginal implants are given with either colpostats or vaginal cylinders. Colpostats have the advantage of stretching the mucosa of the vaginal apex and thus improving depth-dose distribution. Vaginal cylinders offer the advantage of no variation of dose rate at a given depth for a given loading from patient to patient and the ability to treat a greater length of vaginal mucosa if desired.

Vaginal Radiation

Piver and associates randomized stage I patients to total abdominal hysterectomy and bilateral salpingo-oophorectomy (TAH/BSO) alone, preoperative intrauterine and cervical implant delivering 5,000–6,000 cGy at 2 cm depth followed by TAH/BSO, or TAH/BSO followed by intravaginal implant using a vaginal cylinder and prescribing 3,000 cGy at 0.5 cm depth. In the group receiving postoperative intravaginal radiation, there were no vaginal recurrences compared to 5% vaginal recurrence in the preoperative implant group and 8% vaginal recurrence in the TAH/BSO alone group.

Vaginal Radiation with or without Pelvic Radiation in Nonsurgically Staged Patients

Aalders reported on a randomized prospective trial for stage I patients. Following TAH/BSO, patients received an intravaginal implant delivering 6,000 cGy to the vaginal surface. They were then randomized to receive either no further treatment or 2,000 cGy of whole pelvis external beam radiation followed by 2,000 cGy of split pelvis irradiation. Although a decrease in local regional failure was seen in the pelvic irradiation group, it was offset by an increase in distant metastases, and there was no improvement in overall survival in patients who received pelvic radiation.

Radiation Therapy in Surgically Staged Patients
Although postoperative radiation decreases the incidence of local and pelvic recurrence in patients who underwent selective pelvic and para-aortic lymph node biopsy at the time of TAH/BSO, improved survival has not been proven in this group of patients. However, in a report of patients with histologically negative para-aortic lymph node metastasis with grade 3 or deeply invasive tumors treated with postoperative pelvic radiation, the 5-year disease-free survival was 88%.

Treatment in Medically Inoperable Patients
In medically inoperable patients, carcinoma of the endometrium can be successfully treated with intracavitary brachytherapy or a combination of external beam irradiation and intracavitary brachytherapy. An update of data from M.D. Anderson showed a 5-year disease-specific survival of 87% for stage I patients. Intrauterine recurrence was 14% for stages I and II combined.

STAGE II

Approaches to the treatment for stage II endometrial cancer are similar to those discussed for stage I. Most authors recommend surgical staging laparotomy and TAH/BSO, followed by irradiation.

In patients who are medically inoperable, radiation is the treatment of choice. Survival rates in the range of 50–60% with pelvic control and in the range of 65–80% have been reported for clinical stage II patients treated with radiation alone. An update of data from M.D. Anderson showed 5-year disease-specific survival rates of 88% for stage II patients treated with radiation alone.

STAGE III

Treatment for patients with stage III disease must be individualized by both the extent and location of disease as well as the resectability. In patients with resectable disease, radiation is usually given in the postoperative setting. Patients with inoperable disease are treated with irradiation as their primary modality. Survival is generally poor in stage III patients treated primarily with irradiation and in the range of 10–30%.

STAGE IV

For patients with large pelvic disease, radiation therapy consisting of pelvic radiation and intrauterine vaginal cesium is used to control local disease.

Radiation Therapy for Vulvar Cancer

INGUINAL FEMORAL RADIATION

Irradiation of the lymphatic drainage of the vulva must include the inguinofemoral nodes with or without the pelvic nodes. The anterior field should extend laterally to the anterior superior iliac spine and inferiorly to 2 cm below the ischial tuberosities. If the vulvar region is not to be treated in these fields, a midline block is placed to shield this area or separate fields are used to treat each side individually. It is important to use computed tomography (CT) scans in treatment planning because the depth of the femoral vessels varies greatly from individual to individual, and significant underdosing can occur, particularly when a significant portion of the dose is being delivered with anterior electron beam fields.

PELVIC NODE RADIATION

When the pelvic nodes are being treated, either parallel opposed AP/PA (in thin patients) or four-field technique can be used. In either case, it may be necessary to give a portion of the dose to the inguinal region (particularly the lateral inguinal region if the femoral heads are to be spared) with anterior electron beam fields, and computer dosimetry must be used. Because of the anterior nature of the draining nodal regions, the AP/PA fields are often weighted anteriorly or mixed beam energies may be used (with lower-energy anterior to shift the isodoses anteriorly). The use of extensive pelvic fields has been questioned because of the poor prognosis of those with pelvic adenopathy and the increased incidence of complications associated with increasing field size.

VULVAR, INGUINAL, AND PELVIC RADIATION

In cases of advanced or unresectable disease, it may be necessary to treat the vulva in continuity with the inguinal and pelvic region for at least the first 45–50 Gy. In this case, the daily treatment dose should not exceed 160–180 cGy due to the already poor tolerance of the vulvar mucosa and the increased reaction caused by the tangential incidence of photons in the inferior-most regions. It is recommended that the patient be treated with her legs spread apart to avoid a bolus effect from the thighs in the vulva and groin creases.

In many cases it is not necessary to treat the entire vulva, and radiation to the vulva can be delivered with an en face perineal electron field of appropriate energy with tissue-equivalent bolus if necessary. Daily doses should be kept in the range of 160–180 cGy and total doses should be kept below 65 Gy when possible to avoid late complications such as fibrosis, ulceration, atrophy, telangiectasia, and necrosis.

PELVIC LYMPHADENECTOMY VERSUS PELVIC RADIATION

Because of the morbidity associated with radical vulvectomy and inguinal lymphadenectomy, attempts have been made to lessen the amount of surgery and combine irradiation for subclinical residual disease, as well as to improve on the results achieved with surgery alone. The Gynecologic Oncology Group (GOG) reported on a trial in which all patients underwent a radical vulvectomy and bilateral inguinal node dissection. Patients with positive inguinal adenopathy were then randomized between pelvic lymph node dissection or 4,500–5,000 cGy to the pelvic and inguinal nodal regions. A significant improvement in survival, disease-free survival, and groin control rates were seen in the radiation group. This effect was most pronounced in patients with more than one positive node and those with palpable suspicious (N2), fixed, or ulcerated nodes (N3). Multivariate analysis showed the most important prognostic factors to be clinical nodal status (N0, N1 versus N2, N3), number of positive nodes (1 versus $\geq$ 2), and pelvic radiation.

INGUINAL RADIATION VERSUS INGUINAL LYMPHADENECTOMY

A second GOG study examined the use of elective groin irradiation compared to groin dissection in patients with clinically nonsuspicious inguinal nodes (N0, N1). Radiation consisted of 50 Gy in 200-cGy fractions prescribed to 3 cm depth below skin surface. Those in the groin dissection group found to have positive nodes were also given ipsilateral groin and hemipelvic radiation (50 Gy) to the affected side. The study was closed prematurely due to an excessive number of groin recurrences in the groin radiation group (18.5% versus 0%). The groin dissection group also showed a significantly better progression-free interval as well as survival. Unfortunately, it appears that this trial had major flaws in the calculation and delivery of dose to the femoral nodes.

RADIATION FOR ADVANCED DISEASE

In advanced disease, radiation therapy has been successfully used preoperatively to reduce the extent of required surgery or make inoperable lesions operable. Doses in the range of 4,500–5,400 cGy were most often used.

RADIATION THERAPY WITHOUT SURGERY

For patients unable for medical reasons to undergo radical vulvectomy and inguinal lymphadenectomy who have very advanced disease, high-dose radiotherapy may result in long-term survival rates.

COMPLICATIONS

Because of its thin mucosa and moistness and the constant friction caused by walking, the vulva tolerates radiation poorly. Painful desquamation is a common side effect during treatment and often causes undesirable treatment breaks. Late complications include atrophy, fibrosis, telangiectasia, painful ulceration, and necrosis. The incidence of these side effects can be minimized by avoiding large fraction sizes and limiting the total dose when possible.

Radiation Therapy for Ovarian Cancer

EPITHELIAL CANCER

Although there are data to support the use of radiation in the treatment of ovarian epithelial cancer, particularly in limited disease, its role in the United States has been limited. Nevertheless, radiation therapy is still used routinely in the treatment of early-stage epithelial ovarian cancers in Canada and outside North America. To date, there has been no randomized trial comparing state-of-the-art radiation to modern standard chemotherapy and showing one to be superior to the other in the adjuvant setting.

Technique

The two most common techniques of whole abdominal irradiation are the moving strip and the open field techniques.

Moving Strip

The moving strip technique is seldom used because of its increased technical complexity, increased time required, and inferiority to the open field technique and is mainly of historical interest. The technique uses a 10-cm field that is moved in 2.5-cm daily increments so that each 2.5-cm "strip" of abdomen receives 8–10 treatments.

Open Field

The open field technique treats the entire abdominal cavity with a single pair of parallel opposed fields. The inferior border of the field is below the obturator fields. The inferior border of the field is below the obturator foramen. The lateral borders must include the lateral peritoneal fat strip by several centimeters as seen radiographically to ensure adequate inclusion of the peritoneal reflections. Superiorly, the borders must extend a minimum of 1 cm above the domes of the diaphragm as seen on exhalation. It is important to pick a beam energy that will provide a homogeneous dose distribution throughout the abdomen without underdosing the anterior and posterior surfaces of the peritoneum.

The Toronto technique uses 100- to 120-cGy daily treatments to treat the abdomen to a total dose of 22.5–28.0 Gy. Posterior renal shielding (5 HVL) is added as treatment progresses to maintain the total renal dose at 18–20 Gy with the lower-dose limit preferred if chemotherapy is also to be given. Commonly, patients are treated to a total of 2,250 cGy with posterior renal shielding being added at 1,500 cGy. At the completion of treatment to the abdomen, the pelvis is then treated to a total dose (including the contribution of whole abdominal irradiation) of 4,500 cGy in 180- to 200-cGy fractions. Other authors have advocated treating the abdominal cavity to higher doses using partial liver shielding and boost doses to the para-aortic and diaphragmatic areas, while others have advocated limiting doses delivered to the upper abdomen to 2,000 cGy and not using any visceral shielding.

Complications

The dose-limiting organs of concern in the treatment of ovarian cancer with radiation are the kidneys, liver, spinal cord, lungs, bone marrow, and bowel. The $TD_{5/5}$ for late complications (5% complications at 5 years) is approximately 2,000 cGy for kidney, 3,500 cGy for liver, 5,000 cGy for spinal cord, and 2,000 cGy for lung with conventionally fractionated radiation. In practice, renal dose is usually kept below 2,000 cGy, and the majority of the liver parenchyma below 2,800 cGy.

Many patients will suffer transient fatigue, nausea, and diarrhea during treatment, especially if fractions exceeding 120 cGy are used for whole abdominal treatments. These symptoms are usually easily controlled by conservative means, seldom requiring treatment interruption, and resolve soon after completion of therapy. Thrombo-cytopenia and leukopenia may occur due to the large volume of marrow eradicated, but platelets fall below $50 \times 10^9/1$ in only about 10% of patients and usually recover shortly after completion of treatment.

Serious bowel complications have been reported in 4–7% of patients treated after first staging laparotomy. Higher fraction size and total doses have been associated with increased bowel complication rates. Increased incidence of hematologic toxicity and late bowel complications have been reported in patients receiving radiation for consolidation and salvage and is probably due to previous chemotherapy and multiple surgical procedures.

Serious late renal and hepatic complications are rare if care is taken to limit the dose to these organs to acceptable levels. The majority of serious hepatic toxicity reported involves treatment with the moving strip technique.

Consolidation Radiation Therapy After Chemotherapy for Advanced Disease

Radiation has been used in an attempt to either consolidate or salvage patients with advanced disease after chemotherapy and second-look laparotomy. Four randomized trials have been published comparing radiotherapy to chemotherapy for consolidation in patients with complete response or minimal residual disease after second-look laparotomy. These trials showed radiotherapy to be either equivalent or inferior to chemotherapy.

Radiation Therapy for Vaginal Cancer

Except for very early stage I disease, vaginal cancer is usually treated with a combination of external beam and intracavitary or interstitial implant. Because of the potential multifocality of this disease, radiation therapy is the treatment of choice in most cases. The M.D. Anderson Cancer Center has published excellent results treating small stage I tumors with local irradiation using brachytherapy with or without transvaginal irradiation. For lesions 5 mm and less in thickness, a vaginal cylinder or ovoids may be used to deliver dose to the primary lesions, but for thicker lesions, interstitial therapy should be added to ensure adequate dose at depth without unnecessary dose at the vaginal mucosa. The proximity of the bladder and rectum to the vagina increases complications while decreasing treatment options.

Stages II–IV are best treated with a combination of external beam radiotherapy and brachytherapy. External beam radiotherapy should include the entire vagina including the introitus, pelvic nodes, and paravaginal and parametrial tissues, and in tumors that involve the lower third of the vagina, the inguinal nodes as well. The proportion of brachytherapy and external beam dose given to the central disease varies from institution to institution, but a midline block is generally used for part of treatments to reduce the dose to central structures as in the treatment of cervical cancer.

Selected Readings

Alder JG, Abeler V, Kolstad P. Postoperative external irradiation and prognostic parameters in stage I endometrial carcinoma: Clinical and histopathologic study of 540 patients. *Obstet Gynecol* 56:419, 1980.

Cunningham MJ, Vigliotti AP, Wen BC et al. Extended field radiation for carcinoma of the uterine cervix with positive paraaortic nodes. *Int J Radiat Oncol Biol Phys* 23:501, 1992.

Dancuart F, Delclos L, Wharton JT et al. Primary squamous cell carcinoma of the vagina treated by radiotherapy. A failures analysis—the MD Anderson Hospital experience 1955–1982. *Int J Radiat Oncol Biol Phys* 14:745, 1988.

Delgado G, Bundy B, Zaino R et al. Prospective surgical-pathological study of disease-free interval in patients with stage IB squamous cell carcinoma of the cervix: A Gynecologic Oncology Group study. *Gynecol Oncol* 38:352, 1990.

Dembo AJ. Epithelial ovarian cancer: The role of radiotherapy. *Int J Radiat Oncol Biol Phys* 22:835, 1992.

Downey GO, Potish RA, Adcock LL et al. Pretreatment surgical staging in cervical carcinoma. Therapeutic efficacy of pelvic lymph node resection. *Am J Obstet Gynecol* 160:1055, 1989.

Feder BH, Syed AMD, Neblett D. Treatment of extensive carcinoma of the cervix with the "transperineal parametrial butterfly." *Int J Radiat Oncol Biol Phys* 47:735, 1978.

Grigsby PW, Perez CA, Kuske RR et al. Results of therapy analysis of failures and prognostic factors for clinical and pathological stage III adenocarcinoma of the endometrium. *Gynecol Oncol* 27:44, 1987.

Homesley HD, Bundy BN, Sedlis A et al. Radiation versus pelvic node resection for carcinoma of the vulva with positive groin nodes. *Obstet Gynecol* 68:733, 1988.

Homesly HD, Bundy BN, Sedlis A et al. Prognostic factors for groin node metastasis in squamous cell carcinoma of the vulva. A Gynecologic Oncology Group study. *Gynecol Oncol* 49:279, 1993.

Jampolis S, Andras EJ, Fletcher GH. Analysis of sites and causes of failure of irradiation in invasive squamous cell carcinoma of the intact uterine cervix. *Radiology* 115:681, 1975.

Johns HE, Cunningham JR. *The Physics of Radiology*. Springfield, IL: Charles C Thomas, 1983.

Koh WJ, Chiu M, Stelzer KJ et al. Femoral vessel depth and the implications for groin node radiation. *Int J Radiat Oncol Biol Phys* 27:969, 1993.

Kovalic JJ, Grigsby PW, Perez CA et al. Cervical stump carcinoma. *Int J Radiat Oncol Biol Phys* 20:933, 1991.

Kupelian PA, Eifel PJ, Tornos C. Treatment of endometrial carcinoma with radiation therapy alone. *Int J Radiat Oncol Biol Phys* 27:817, 1993.

Lambert HE, Rustin GJ, Gregory WM et al. A randomized trial comparing single-agent carboplatin with carboplatin followed by radiotherapy for advanced ovarian cancer. A North Thames Ovary Group study. *J Clin Oncol* 11:440, 1993.

Marcial LV, Marcial VA, Krall JM et al. Comparison of 1 vs 2 or more intracavitary brachytherapy applications in the management of carcinoma of the cervix with irradiation alone. *Int J Radiat Oncol Biol Phys* 20:81, 1991.

Morrow CP, Bundy BN, Kurman RJ et al. Relationship between surgical-pathological risk factors in outcome of clinical stage I and II carcinoma of the endometrium. A Gynecologic Oncology Group study. *Gynecol Oncol* 40:55, 1991.

Orton CG. High dose rate versus low dose rate brachytherapy for gynecological cancer. *Semin Radiat Oncol* 3:232, 1993.

Perez CA, Breaux S, Bedwinick J et al. Radiation therapy alone in treatment of the uterine cervix. II. Analysis of complications. *Cancer* 54:235, 1984.

Piver MS. Invasive cervical cancer in the 1990s. *Semin Surg Oncol* 6:359, 1990.

Piver MS, Hempling RE. A prospective trial of postoperative vaginal radium/cesium for grade 1–2 less than 50% myometrial invasion and pelvic radiation for grade 3 or deep myometrial invasion in surgical stage I endometrial adenocarcinoma. *Cancer* 66:1133, 1990.

Piver MS, Yazigi R, Blumenson L et al. A prospective trial comparing hysterectomy, hysterectomy plus vaginal radium, and uterine radium plus hysterectomy in stage I endometrial carcinoma. *Obstet Gynecol* 54:85, 1979.

Stehman FB, Bundy BN, DiSaia PJ et al. Carcinoma of the cervix treated with radiation therapy. I. A multivariate analysis of prognostic variables in the Gynecologic Oncology Group. *Cancer* 67:2776, 1991.

Stehman FB, Bundy BN, Thomas G et al. Groin dissection versus radiation in carcinoma of the vulva. A Gynecologic Oncology Group study. *Int J Radiat Oncol Biol Phys* 24:389, 1992.

Thomas WW, Eifel PJ, Terry LS et al. Bulky endocervical carcinoma: A 23-year experience. *Int J Radiat Oncol Biol Phys* 23:491, 1992.

Wong LC, Chao YC, Choy D et al. Long-term follow up of potentiation of radiotherapy by cisplatinum in advanced cervical cancer. *Gynecol Oncol* 35:541, 1987.

17

Principles of Tumor Immunology

Kenneth A. Foon

The immune system involves the interaction of lymphocytes, monocytes/macrophages, dendritic cells, endothelial cells, and other cells throughout the body.

Lymphocytes

B-lymphocytes likely develop in the bone marrow. Immunoglobulin on the surface of B cells act as antigen receptors. B cells also have receptors for lymphokines. B cells require the presence of antigen and help from antigen-specific T cells to generate antibodies.

T-lymphocytes require the thymus for normal differentiation. In the thymus they differentiate into a variety of subpopulations. T cells are involved in cellular immune reactions and recognize antigens via receptors on their cell surface membrane. The T cell receptor is similar to immunoglobulin in that it is generated from a combination of germ line genes to produce a large number of receptors that can bind antigen in concert with major histocompatibility complex (MHC) molecules. The T cell receptor is associated with the CD3 complex. While B cells can recognize antigens alone, the T cell requires association with MHC molecules.

There are two major subsets of T cells:

1. CD8 T cells: MHC class I molecules (serologically defined as human leukocyte antigen [HLA] A, B, or C) are involved in the presentation of precessed antigens to this subset. CD8 T cells function as cytotoxic/suppressor cells.
2. CD4 T cells: MHC class II molecules (DP, DQ, and DR) present antigens to this subset. CD4 T cells function as helper cells.

Null cells are lymphocytes that express neither T cell nor B cell surface markers. Natural killer (NK) cells and lymphokine-activated killer (LAK) cells are derived from this population. NK cells lyse cultured cell lines without prior exposure. LAK cells develop the ability to kill cell lines and fresh tumor cells following incubation with interleukin-2 (IL-2). One of the cell subsets that mediate antibody-dependent cellular cytotoxicity (ADCC) is derived from the null cell population.

Other Cells in the Immune System

Monocytes are circulating cells that develop into tissue macrophages. These cells are capable of presenting antigens to lymphocytes. Monocytes kill tumor cells by phagocytosis and ADCC.

Other cells that are antigen-presenting cells include Langerhans' cells, dendritic cells, and endothelial cells.

Immune Effector Systems

There are a variety of immune effector systems that destroy tumor cells. Antibodies may mediate cell destruction (1) by binding complement, (2) by opsonizing cells to facilitate phagocytosis by phagocytic cells that have Fc receptors (i.e., monocyte/macrophage), or (3) by ADCC.

Cytotoxic T-lymphocytes interact with cell surface antigens via the T cell receptor and a class I or II MHC molecule. Lysis involves direct contact and occurs within minutes. Cytotoxic T-lymphocytes may bind to antibody on cells via their Fc receptors and mediate cell death by ADCC.

NK cells lyse without prior sensitization. They lyse cultured tumor cells, but their role in vivo is not clear.

LAK cells kill tumor cells in a non–MHC-restricted fashion. LAK cells acquire the ability either in vitro or in vivo to destroy a variety of tumor cells following incubation with IL-2. LAK cells are unique in that they lyse tumor cells but not normal fresh target cells in in vitro assays.

Cytokines may be secreted by immunocytes that destroy tumor cells (i.e., interferon-alpha, interferon-gamma, and tumor necrosis factor).

Cytokines

Cytokines are soluble proteins produced by immunocytes that have a variety of regulatory actions on other cells of the immune system. Cytokines are proteins or glycoproteins with a molecular weight in the range of 15,000–40,000. A list of the various cytokines and interleukins is shown in Table 17-1. Each cytokine reacts with receptors specific for that cytokine on the cell surface.

Growth Factors

Hematopoietic cells are derived from self-renewing pluripotent stem cells. Pluripotent stem cells are able to differentiate into committed progenitor cells, which eventually give rise to discrete cells lineages (Table 17-2).

Tumor Antigens

CELLULAR IMMUNE RESPONSES FOR DETECTING HUMAN TUMOR ANTIGEN

T cell receptors recognize processed peptides on the surface of tumor cells.

1. CD4+ T-lymphocytes recognize small peptides bound to MHC class II molecules (HLA-DR).
2. CD8+ T-lymphocytes recognize peptides bound to MHC class I molecules (HLA-A, -B, -C).

Table 17-1. Cytokines and interleukins

Molecules	*Synonyms*	*Molecular weight (kD)*	*Activity*
IL-1, alpha	Hemotopoietin-1	14–17	Synergy with G-CSF, GM-CSF, M-CSF, IL-3, and IL-8 Radioprotectant Numerous immunologic activities
IL-2	TCGF	15	Costimulates T cells and LAK cells Differentiation and maturation of B cells Stimulates T cells, B cells, NK cells, and monocytes
IL-3	Multi-CSF	14–18	Stimulates CFU-GM, CFU-GEMM, CFU-G, GFU-M, BFU-E, and CFU-MK Growth of B and T cells
IL-4	BSF-1	15–20	Activates B cells, T cells, and macrophages Synergy with G-CSF, EPO, and IL-1 Costimulates IL-2–induced LAK in mice
IL-5	BCGF-II, TRF	12–18	Synergy with GM-CSF or IL-3 to stimulate CFU-Eo and IL-2 to generate T killer cells Stimulates B cells Stimulates eosinophils
IL-6	BSF-2	21–29	Synergy with IL-1, IL-3, GM-CSF in CFU-GEMM assays Stimulates platelets in primates (±IL-3)
IL-7	pBCGF		Stimulates B cells, T cells CTL, NK, and LAK cells Synergy with IL-2 and stimulates B and T cells
IL-8 (PF4 super family)	NCF, TCF		Chemotactic for basophils, neutrophils, T and B cells
IL-9	p40	20–30/14	Stimulates megakaryocyte cell line, BFU-E, CD4-T cells and mast cells
IL-10	CSIF	17–21 (murine)	Suppression of IFN-γ production by macrophages Stimulates CD4-T and CD8-T cells, mast cells, and B cells

IL-11		24	Stimulates plasmacytoma and BFU-MK
IL-12	CLM/NKSF	75	Stimulates CD4-T and CD8-T cells, LAK cells, NK cells, lymphoblasts (synergy with IL-2)
IFN-α or -β		15–26	Antiproliferative to certain tumors
			Enhances expression of surface molecules including MHC class I antigens and tumor-associated antigens
			Augments NK and monocyte-macrophage function
IFN-γ		15–25	Antiviral activity, augments NK activity, induces expression of MHC class I and II molecules, activates macrophages, enhances tumor-associated antigen expression
TNF-α		17	Stimulates T cell proliferation, enhances NK activity, induces macrophage tumoricidal activity, directly cytotoxic to some tumor cells, activates granulocytes, enhances expression of class I and II molecules

G-CSF = granulocyte colony-stimulating factor; GM-CSF = granulocyte-monocyte colony-stimulating factor; M-CSF = monocyte colony-stimulating factor; CFU-GM = colony forming unit granulocyte-monocyte; CFU-GEMM = colony-forming unit granulocyte-erythrocyte-monocyte-megakaryocyte; CFU-G = colony-forming unit granulocyte CFU-M = colony-forming unit monocyte; BFU-E = burst-forming unit erythrocyte; CFU-MK = colony-forming unit megakaryocyte; EPO = erythropoietin; CFU-EO = colony-forming unit eosinophil; BFU-MK = burst-forming unit megakaryocyte; CSIF = cytokine synthesis inhibitor factor; CLMF/NKSF = cytotoxic lymphocyte maturation factor-natural killer–stimulating factor.

Table 17-2. Hematopoietic growth factors

Molecules	*Synonyms*	*Molecular weight (kD)*	*Activity*
Erythropoietin		34–39	Stimulates CFU-E, CFU-MK Increases red blood cells in vivo
Multi-CSF	IL-3	14–28	Stimulates CFU-GM, CFU-GEMM, CFU-G, CFU-M, BFU-E, and CFU-MK Increases neutrophils in vivo
GM-CSF	CSF-alpha	18–30	Stimulates CFU-GM, CFU-MK Activates neutrophils, eosinophils, and monocytes Increases neutrophils in vivo
G-CSF	CSF-beta	20–25	Stimulates CFU-G Activates neutrophils Increases neutrophils in vivo
M-CSF	CSF-1	45–70	Stimulates monocyte progenitors and differentiates and activates monocytes
MGF/SCF/KL		28–35	Stimulates multi- and committed stem cells, mast cells, megakaryocytes, and melanocytes
PIXY321	GM-CSF/IL-3	35	Stimulates CFU-GEMM, CFU-GM, CFU-MK, BFU-MK, BFU-E Increases neutrophils and platelets in monkeys

CFU-E = colony-forming unit erythrocyte; CFU-MK = colony-forming unit megakaryocyte; CFU-GM = colony-forming unit granulocyte-monocyte; CFU-GEMM = colony-forming unit granulocyte-erythrocyte-monocyte-megakaryocyte; CFU-G = colony-forming unit granulocyte; CFUM = colony-forming unit monocyte; BFU-E = burst-forming unit erythrocyte; CFU-MK = colony-forming unit megakaryocyte; EPO = erythropoietin; CFU-EO = colony-forming unit eosinophil; BKU-MK = burst-forming unit megakaryocyte; MGF/SCF/KL = mast cell growth factor, stem cell factor, kit ligand.

3. LAK cells kill tumor cells in a non–MHC-restricted fashion. They are generated in vivo or in vitro by IL-2.
4. Tumor-infiltrating lymphocytes (TILs) recognize tumor antigens and directly lyse tumor cells by release of cytokines. TILs are derived directly from the tumor and are expanded in vitro with IL-2.

All of these tumor antigens are specifically reactive with the patients' tumor cells and are MHC-restricted.

ANTIBODIES FOR DETECTING TUMOR ANTIGEN

Antibodies detect specific epitopes on antigenic molecules by recognition and binding via the variable region.

Immunoglobulins consist of two polypeptide chains, the light chains with a molecular weight of approximately 23,000 and the heavy chains with a molecular weight of 55,000–70,000.

Five different classes of immunoglobulins have been identified based on the structural differences within the heavy-chain constant region: IgM, IgG, IgA, IgD, and IgE. IgG is the predominate immunoglobulin in the sera. IgM constitutes about 5–10% of serum immunoglobulin and is the largest molecule. IgA is the predominate immunoglobulin in exocrine secretions, and IgE immunoglobulins are involved in allergic reactions. The function of IgD immunoglobulin is unknown.

Polyclonal antibodies have historically identified antigens such as the carcinoembryonic antigen (CEA).

The development of monoclonal antibodies has significantly improved the ability to detect tumor-associated antigens. By this technology, mice are immunized against a specific antigen and their splenocytes are fused with a mouse myeloma cell line. It is now possible to make recombinant chimeric monoclonal antibodies that contain the variable region of murine origin and the constant region of human origin. There is an enormous number of monoclonal antibodies available that identify tumor-associated antigens. Virtually all monoclonal antibodies have at least some reactivity with normal tissues, although the degree of cross-reactivity can be minimal.

Clinical Applications of Cytokines, Growth Factors, and Monoclonal Antibodies

CYTOKINES

Interferons

Interferons are a family of closely related proteins and glycoproteins that have antiviral activity and are potent regulators of cell gene expression, structure, and function. They also have direct antiproliferative activity. These properties underlie the current interest in interferons as anticancer agents. All of the interferons are available as recombinant molecules.

Cell Origin of Interferons

Interferon-alpha is produced by B cells, T cells, null cells, and macrophages following exposure to B cell mitogens, viruses, foreign cells, or tumor cells. Interferon-beta is produced by fibroblasts after exposure to viruses or foreign nucleic acids. Interferon-gamma is produced by T-lymphocytes after stimulation of T cell mitogens, specific antigens, or IL-2.

Clinical Applications of Interferons

Clinical uses of interferon-gamma and interferon-beta are quite limited. Interferon-alpha has a somewhat broader applicability. In addition to its approved uses for hairy cell leukemia, Kaposi's sarcoma, and venereal warts, it is also active in a variety of hematologic malignancies including low-grade non-Hodgkin's lymphoma and chronic myelogenous leukemia. There is very limited applicability for solid tumors, although in combination with 5-fluorouracil there appears to be an improved response for patients with colon cancer. Perhaps combined with other chemotherapy agents such as cisplatin, there will be a broader applicability for other solid tumors including ovarian cancer. This is currently under investigation. Toxicity of interferon-alpha includes fever, chills, fatigue, and malaise.

Interleukin-2

IL-2 is released after antigen recognition and presentation to T cells and causes T cell proliferation. It was originally referred to as T cell growth factor. It is currently available as a recombinant molecule and is being used in many clinical trials. As mentioned above, IL-2 activates lytic mechanisms of LAK cells for fresh tumors and appears to activate cytolytic T cells. IL-2 as a single agent with or without ex vivo cultured LAK cells is active in renal cell cancer and, to a lesser degree, melanoma. Toxicities of IL-2 include fever, chills, nausea, vomiting, diarrhea, hypotension, and fluid retention. IL-2 currently has no role in the treatment of gynecologic tumors.

Growth Factors

Granulocyte colony-stimulating factor (G-CSF) (Filgrastim, Neupogen) is a recombinant molecule and has been approved for the treatment of neutropenia secondary to chemotherapy. The recommended dose of G-CSF is 5 μg/kg/day by subcutaneous bolus or intravenous injection (15–30 minutes) every 24 hours. G-CSF should begin 24 hours after the completion of chemotherapy. Vials come in 300 μg and 480 μg, and to prevent waste, a single vial is often used for daily therapy. G-CSF leads to a rapid rise in granulocyte counts. It may decrease the period of neutropenia as well as the incidence of febrile neutropenia. G-CSF may also allow for higher doses of drugs in the situation in which the major drug toxicity is bone marrow suppression. The increased dose could lead to better and more durable responses. Clearly, the toxicity of other organs will limit how high a dose can be given. Toxicity secondary to G-CSF is primarily limited to mild bone pain that is dose-dependent.

Granulocyte-monocyte colony-stimulating factor (GM-CSF) (Sargramastim, Leukine) is a recombinant molecule and increases and activates neutrophils, eosinophils, and monocytes. GM-CSF has been released for use in neutropenia secondary to bone marrow transplantation but may also increase neutrophils following chemotherapy. The recommended dose is 250 $\mu g/m^2$/day as a 2-hour infusion beginning 2–4 hours after transplant or 24 hours after chemotherapy. It is also given subcutaneously. The vials come as 250 or 500 μg, which are often used as the total dose to prevent waste.

Side effects include capillary leak syndrome, edema, renal and hepatic toxicity, low-grade fever, myalgias, phlebitis, and flushing. Like G-CSF, it is typically very well tolerated, with minimal toxicity.

Erythropoietin (Epoetin alfa, Procrit, Epogen) is a recombinant molecule indicated for anemia secondary to renal failure and HIV-infected patients who are on zidovudine (AZT) with endogenous serum erythropoietin levels of 500 mU/ml. It may also be effective in anemic cancer patients undergoing chemotherapy. The patients who tend to respond have low baseline serum erythropoietin levels (≤ 200 mU/ml). Doses begin at 150 U/kg SC three times weekly. The dose may be increased up to 300 U/kg total ideal weight. Side effects are mild and typically limited to mild fever, diarrhea, and edema.

Recombinant IL-3 has the potential to increase platelets as well as white blood cells; however, in vivo trials have not demonstrated an increase in platelets with any consistency.

PIXY321 is a recombinant fusion product of GM-CSF and IL-3 and increases neutrophils and platelets in nonhuman primates. In early clinical trials, it appears to have promise in increasing platelets as well as neutrophils.

Recombinant IL-6 is in clinical trials and also has the potential for increasing platelets.

MONOCLONAL ANTIBODIES

A number of monoclonal antibodies have been used for therapy and diagnosis for a variety of tumors including ovarian carcinoma. The only approved monoclonal antibody for tumor imaging is B72.3 conjugated with indium-111 (Satumomab pendetide, OncoScint CR/OV). This antibody reacts with a variety of tumors including gastrointestinal cancer and ovarian cancer.

Critical Factors for Successful Monoclonal Antibody Therapy

Most antibodies are directed against tumor-associated antigens rather than tumor-specific antigens. The most effective of these antibodies should minimally cross-react with antigens on normal tissues, or at least the antigen density should be less than on tumors.

Ideally, the antigen should be dense and homogeneous on the tumor cell surface. The antibody should bind to the antigen with high affinity. It is important that the antigen-antibody complex not disassociate from the cell membrane, although internal incorporation of the antigen-antibody complex by pinocytosis might be advantageous when immunoconjugates with drugs, toxins, or isotopes are used.

Some tumor-associated antigens are shed from the tumor cells and are present in the blood and may bind up the antibody and prevent tumor localization. Ideally, one should choose antibodies selective for noncirculating antigens.

Intact immunoglobulin can be broken down into various fragments. Intact murine IgG has a half-life of approximately 24 hours, $F(ab')_2$ 10 hours, and Fab 90 minutes. The choice of the appropriate form of antibody varies for the tumor antigen system and the conjugate. For unlabeled antibody therapy, fragments of antibody would not be useful, as the Fc portion is critical for activating human effector systems.

For antibody to react with tumor cells, the tumor must be vascular. The number of blood vessels in the tumor decreases proportionally as the tumor enlarges. In addition, as the tumor enlarges, the diameter of the capillaries increases, leading to a decrease in the total vascular cross-sectional area of the tumor. It is not unusual for the outer, better profused, and more viable portions of tumors to concentrate more antibody than the less vascular, more necrotic interior portions.

Human Antiglobulin Response

One major problem in clinical trials using murine monoclonal antibodies is the development of human antimouse antibodies (HAMAs or antiglobulin response). These antibodies alter the clearance and organ distribution of injected antibodies by neutralizing the antibodies and preventing them from binding to tumor cells. While there are a number of putative approaches to prevent the development of HAMAs, most have not been very successful. The most successful approach is the humanization of the murine monoclonal antibody so that the antibody is entirely human except for the specific binding region of the antibody, which remains murine. Humanized antibodies have generally been shown to have decreased immune responses in clinical trials.

Clinical Trials with Unlabeled Antibodies

Clinical trials with unlabeled antibodies (not bound to drugs, toxins, or isotopes) result in only minor responses in humans. This is not surprising, because most murine antibodies do not activate human effector systems or have direct cytotoxic effects. The most impressive clinical responses of unlabeled antibodies have been with anti-idiotypic antibodies for B cell lymphoma patients, in melanoma patients treated with an antibody that activates human complement and effector cells, and in breast cancer patients treated with antibodies that bind to the her-2/neu receptor (also on ovarian cancer).

Immunoconjugates with Toxins

Several potent plant and bacterial toxins have been coupled to antibodies. The most common plant toxin used is ricin. The most commonly studied bacterial toxins are diphtheria toxin and *Pseudomonas* exotoxin. All of these immunotoxin conjugates demonstrate specific antitumor cytotoxicity in in vitro and in vivo animal models. Thus far, clinical trials have only demonstrated modest responses, primarily reported in patients with B cell lymphoma and malignant melanoma. This approach is limited because tumor cell killing requires binding to all tumor cells.

Immunoconjugates with Cytotoxic Drugs

Another approach to generate immunoconjugates is by attaching cytotoxic drugs such as doxorubicin, methotrexate, and vinblastine to antibody. The advantages of using drugs is that their antitumor activity and toxicity are well-defined. The disadvantage of drugs is they are not as potent as toxins and cannot kill cells other than the single cell the antibody binds (similar to toxins). Clinical trials with immunoconjugates with cytotoxic drugs have not demonstrated activity in humans.

Immunoconjugates with Radioisotopes

The major limitation of diagnostic imaging techniques is the lack of specificity. The attractive feature of radiolabeled monoclonal antibodies is the potential to specifically localize to tumor cells. Similarly, conventional radiation therapy is not specific for tumor cells. The field that can be radiated is only limited. Radiolabeled antibodies should be able to radiate tumor deposits throughout the body with minimal radiation to normal tissues.

Diagnostics with Monoclonal Antibodies

Several radionuclides can be linked to monoclonal antibodies for diagnostic purposes. The choice is governed by radionuclide energy, half-life, technical requirements for conjugation, conjugate stability, safety, and cost. The most popular isotopes for imaging with monoclonal antibodies have been technetium-99m (Tc-99m), which has a half-life of 6 hours and has optimal energy for gamma cameras currently in use. Because of its short half-life, it is typically conjugated to a Fab fragment of a monoclonal antibody. The other popular isotope for imaging has been indium-111, which has a 3-day half-life and also has optimal energies for current gamma camera imaging. Because of its longer half-life, it is typically conjugated to the whole immunoglobulin. The disadvantage of Tc-99m has been rapid excretion with localization in the kidney. The major problem with indium-111 has been nonspecific localization in the liver and spleen. The only product marketed in the United States for imaging is B72.3 labeled with indium-111. B72.3 reacts with approximately 80% of colorectal cancer, 95% of ovarian cancer, and the majority of breast, non–small cell lung, and gastrointestinal cancers. It is approved for colorectal cancer.

Therapy with Monoclonal Antibodies

Radioisotopes such as ^{32}P and ^{131}I have been used to treat malignancies such as polycythemia vera and thyroid carcinoma. A reasonable extension of this approach is to link isotopes to antibodies. The choice of the appropriate radioisotope for therapy is complex. Longer particle length radionuclides such as ^{90}Y and ^{188}Re are preferred for tumors with heterogeneous antibody binding. This should allow for destruction of nonlabeled tumor cells but also may increase toxicity to normal tissues. Shorter–particle length radionuclides are preferred where there is uniform antibody binding. Electron capture or internal conversion decay radionuclides such as ^{125}I would be optimal in such a situation; other choices include alpha emitters such as ^{211}Astatine. There have been a number of clinical trials, primarily with ^{131}I in humans. Antiferritin antibody labeled with ^{131}I has demonstrated activity in hepatomas and Hodgkin's disease. Therapy with ^{131}I-labeled antiovarian antibody injected into the peritoneum demonstrated responses in nine of 24 patients. Only patients with small volume (<2 cm) disease responded. The most impressive responses have been for patients treated with B cell lymphomas with ^{131}I-labeled CD20 antibodies. Complete responses have been reported from two studies in more than 50% of patients.

TUMOR VACCINES

Another potential antitumor strategy is activation of host defenses against tumor-associated antigens. This is referred to as *active specific immunotherapy* and attempts to boost the host's immune response.

Nonspecific Vaccines

Agents such as bacillus Calmette-Guérin (BCG) and *Corynebacterium parvum* have been used for the treatment of a variety of solid tumors with little to no activity. These agents activate the immune system nonspecifically, and early studies of leukemia and malignant melanoma demonstrated responses. These have not been reproducible.

Tumor Cell Vaccines

A variety of vaccines using autologous or allogeneic tumor cells or cell lines or tumor cell extracts have been used either alone or mixed with agents such as BCG. Studies of renal cell carcinoma, lung cancer, and malignant melanoma have demonstrated limited responses but have not necessarily been reproducible. A major problem with tumor vaccines is the inability to standardize the contents of the vaccine, particularly with reference to the tumor-associated antigen of interest.

Anti-Idiotype Vaccines

Tumor-associated antigens are often a part of "self" and evoke a very poor immune response in the tumor-bearing host because of T cell–mediated suppression and tolerance to the antigen. Recent data indicate that a weak antigen can be turned into a strong antigen by simply changing the molecular environment of the haptenic structure. These changes in the haptenic carrier activate T cell help and increase the immune response. In addition, altering the carrier can turn a tolerogenic antigen into an immunogenic antigen. The immune status of cancer patients is often suppressed, and they can respond to only certain T-dependent antigens, not to other antigen forms. These considerations suggest introduction of molecular changes into the tumor antigens before using them as vaccines.

According to the idiotypic network hypothesis, certain anti-idiotype antibodies express three dimensional shapes that resemble the structure of external antigens. The internal antigens are stereochemical copies of external antigens that produce specific immune responses similar to responses induced by external antigen and can compete with normal antigens in binding assays. If a tumor-specific monoclonal antibody is available, then a second monoclonal anti-idiotypic antibody can be made and selected for the structure that represents the tumor antigen. This approach is presented in Fig. 17-1. An antitumor-associated antibody (Ab1) is generated and is used to make a second antibody or anti-idiotypic antibody (Ab2). The Ab2 antibody that is the "internal image" of the tumor antigen is then injected intracutaneously into patients who can then evoke an anti–anti-idiotypic response or Ab3 response. These Ab3 antibodies may cross-react with the tumor-associated antigen identified by the Ab1 antibody. Such studies have been conducted with patients with gastrointestinal cancer, malignant melanoma, and T cell lymphoma with responses reported in each of these patient groups. Anti-idiotypic antibody responses (Ab3), as well as idiotypic-specific T cell responses, were reported in many of these patients.

Immunize mouse with tumor cell to generate Ab1

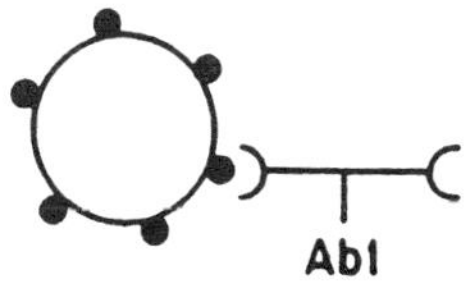

Immunize mouse with Ab1 to generate anti-idiotype (Ab2)

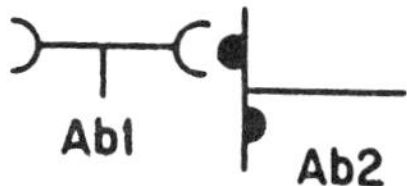

Immunize patients with anti-idiotype to generate Ab3

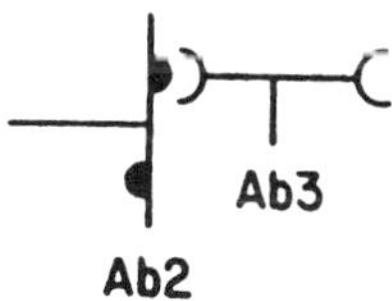

Fig. 17-1. Idiotype tumor network. Concept of monoclonal anti-idiotype vaccines. An Ab1 is generated to a tumor-associated antigen. The Ab1 is used to immunize mice to generate an anti-idiotype monoclonal Ab2. The Ab2 that is the mirror image of the tumor-associated antigen is then used to immunize patients to generate an Ab3 response to the tumor-associated antigen. Note that the Ab3 (or Ab1^{-}) has a binding specificity identical to that of Ab1.

Selected Readings

Bagby GC, Segal GM. Growth Factors and the Control of Hematopoiesis. In R Hoffman, EJ Benz, ST Shattil et al. (eds), *Hematology Basic Principles and Practice*. New York: Churchill-Livingstone, 1991. Pp 97–121.

Fleischman RA. Clinical use of hematopoietic growth factors. *Am J Med Sci* 305:248, 1993.

Foon KA. Biologic response modifiers: The new immunotherapy. *Cancer Res* 49:1621, 1989.

Foon KA. The cytokine network. *Oncology* 7(Suppl):11, 1993.

Rosenberg SA. Principles and Applications of Biologic Therapy. In VT DeVita, S Hellman, SA Rosenberg (eds), *Cancer Principles and Practice of Oncology*. Philadelphia: Lippincott, 1993. Pp 293–324.

VI
Diagnostic Modalities

18

Pathology of Gynecologic Malignancies

Yoshiaki Tsukada

The basics of pathology of malignant gynecologic tumors are presented in this chapter. For more comprehensive review, the reader is referred to textbooks of gynecologic pathology, a chapter on the female genital tract in major surgical pathology textbooks, and the original references in this chapter. The Armed Forces Institute of Pathology (AFIP) tumor fascicles are also good sources of information on pathology of gynecologic tumors.

Common Epithelial Tumors of the Ovary

The term *common epithelial tumor* comes from the fact that this tumor arises from the epithelium covering the surface of the ovary or its inclusions and that it is the most common tumor of the ovary. Approximately 90% of ovarian cancers are common epithelial carcinoma.

CLASSIFICATION

The common epithelial tumors are classified according to cell types. Each of the subtypes is subclassified into benign, borderline (or carcinoma of low malignant potential), and carcinoma (e.g., serous adenoma, serous tumor of borderline malignancy or serous carcinoma of low malignant potential, and serous carcinoma). Both borderline tumor and carcinoma microscopically show atypical proliferative activity and are architecturally and cytologically abnormal. The only difference between the two is absence of destructive stromal invasion in borderline tumor (minor modification exists in mucinous tumor). The diagnosis of borderline tumor is based solely on the histologic appearance of the primary tumor, and presence of peritoneal implant or metastasis does not change the diagnosis. Common epithelial carcinoma is graded based on degree of gland formation and nuclear atypia (well-, moderately, and poorly differentiated, or grades 1–3).

SEROUS TUMOR

The relative frequency of serous tumors among common epithelial cancers is 50–60%. Approximately 30% of the serous tumors are malignant. Grossly, both borderline tumors and carcinomas are cystic and papillary. Papillary excrescences may be on the inner surface of cysts or on the external surface. In carcinoma, papillary areas are mixed with solid areas, and often tumor extends to the external surface. Microscopically, the tumor cells resembling tubal epithelial cells form a complex papillary pattern (Fig. 18-1). In borderline tumors, there is no stromal invasion. The prognosis of borderline tumors is influenced by patterns of peritoneal implants. Those with an invasive pattern or severe cytologic atypia behave less favorably. In poorly differentiated carcinoma, the tumor cells form solid areas as well as a papillary pattern. Psammoma bodies are commonly seen

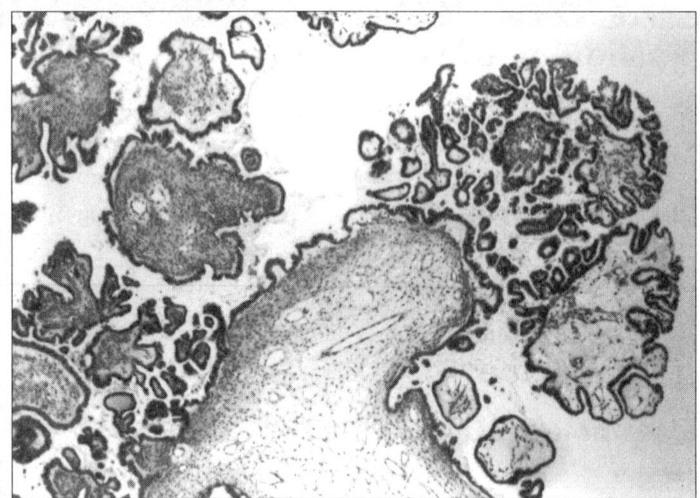

Fig. 18-1. Serous papillary tumor of borderline malignancy. Complex papillary tumor composed of atypical cells resembling tubal epithelial cells. There is no stromal invasion.

in both borderline tumor and carcinoma. This structure is also seen in benign serous tumor.

MUCINOUS TUMOR

The relative frequency of mucinous tumors among common epithelial cancers is 10–15%. Approximately 15% of the mucinous tumors are malignant. Grossly, both borderline tumors and carcinomas are cystic, with multiple locules containing mucinous fluid. Solid areas between cysts are common in carcinomas. Microscopically the tumor is composed of mucinous cells resembling those of endocervical or colonic glands. Diagnosis of carcinoma is made when there is stromal invasion. In addition, when the tumor cells are stratified in more than three layers or form cribriform patterns or stroma-free papillae, the tumor is considered to be carcinoma. A recently described variant of borderline mucinous tumor is borderline müllerian mucinous tumor. Microscopically this tumor has a papillary architecture similar to that of borderline serous tumor and is composed exclusively of endocervical-type cells. Its behavior is similar to that of serous borderline tumor.

A rare complication of mucinous tumor (benign, borderline, or carcinoma) is pseudomyxoma peritonei. In this condition, the vermiform appendix is frequently involved by a similar mucinous tumor. In such a case, ovarian tumor is most likely metastatic from the appendix.

ENDOMETRIOID TUMOR

The relative frequency of endometrioid tumors among common epithelial cancers is 20–25%. The benign form of this tumor does not exist, and borderline tumor is rare. The latter is mostly in a form of endometrioid adenofibroma.

Endometrioid carcinoma is grossly cystic or solid. Endometriosis is seen in about 10% of patients. Microscopically the tumor resembles endometrioid adenocarcinoma of the endometrium. Focal squamous differentiation is not uncommon. Fifteen to 30% of the patients with endometrioid adenocarcinoma of the ovary have simultaneous endometrial hyperplasia or adenocarcinoma.

Malignant müllerian mixed tumor is also included in this group. It is uncommon in the ovary. Histologically it is similar to that occurring in the endometrium.

CLEAR-CELL TUMOR

The relative frequency of clear-cell tumors among common epithelial cancers is 5–10%. Benign and borderline tumors are rare. Clear-cell carcinoma is frequently associated with pelvic endometriosis and sometimes arises in endometriotic cysts. Microscopically the tumor is composed of clear cells and hob-nail cells forming a diffuse, papillary, or tubulocystic pattern. The histology is similar to clear-cell carcinoma occurring in other sites (e.g., vagina, endometrium).

TRANSITIONAL CELL (BRENNER) TUMOR

The majority of tumors in this group are benign; malignant forms are rare. Borderline Brenner tumor histologically resembles grade 1 transitional cell carcinoma without stromal invasion. No malignant behavior has been recorded in this tumor, and some prefer the term *proliferating Brenner tumor* for this lesion. There are few cases reported in which noninvasive carcinoma is grade 3 transitional cell carcinoma or squamous cell carcinoma in situ (Brenner tumor of low malignant potential). Invasive tumor is subdivided into malignant Brenner tumor (tumor in which invasive transitional cell carcinoma or squamous cell carcinoma coexists with benign Brenner tumor) and transitional cell carcinoma (no coexisting Brenner tumor).

UNDIFFERENTIATED CARCINOMA AND SMALL-CELL CARCINOMA

The majority of these tumors are most likely poorly differentiated adenocarcinoma (serous or endometrioid). Small-cell carcinoma of pulmonary type is a rare primary ovarian cancer and histologically similar to small-cell carcinoma of the lung. The tumor occurs in older women (average age is 59), often affects both ovaries, and frequently coexists with common epithelial tumor. Thus, this tumor most likely belongs to the common epithelial group. Small-cell carcinoma of the hypercalcemic type, however, occurs mostly in young women (average age is 22) and affects one ovary. It is composed of small cells forming a follicle-like structure. Two-thirds of these tumors are associated with hypercalcemia. Its histogenesis is unknown.

PRIMARY PERITONEAL CARCINOMA

The female pelvic and lower abdominal peritoneum has müllerian potential and can give rise to a variety of tumors histologically similar to common epithelial tumor. The most common malignant tumor is serous papillary carcinoma of the peritoneum. The ovaries of the patient with this tumor are normal or show only microscopic surface involvement.

PROGNOSTIC FACTORS

Degree of differentiation (or grade) of the tumor is more important than cell type in predicting prognosis. High mitotic rate, high-grade nuclei, and nuclear DNA aneuploidy are associated with aggressive behavior.

Sex Cord–Stromal Tumors of the Ovary

Sex cord–stromal tumors of the ovary include tumors composed of specialized sex cord–stromal cells or nonspecific stromal fibroblasts of the ovary. The tumors consisting of specialized cells are divided into the tumors composed of ovarian-type cells (granulosa cell tumor and thecoma) and testicular-type cells (Sertoli-Leydig cell tumor). These tumors are capable of steroid hormone production. An extremely rare tumor composed of both ovarian- and testicular-type cells is gynandroblastoma. A clinically malignant form of sex cord–stromal tumors accounts for approximately 2% of ovarian cancer.

GRANULOSA CELL TUMOR

Granulosa cell tumor is hormonally active in approximately two-thirds of patients (mostly estrogenic). It is solid or cystic, and the cut surface is often yellow. Microscopically the tumor is composed of granulosa cells with a characteristic nuclear groove. They typically form a microfollicular pattern with Call-Exner bodies (Fig. 18-2). They may also form macrofollicular, insular, trabecular, diffuse, or watered silk patterns. An important variant is juvenile granulosa cell tumor (less than 5% of granulosa cell tumors). This tumor occurs mostly in children and is characterized by nodular arrangement of tumor cells with irregular large follicles. The tumor cells are larger, with greater cytologic atypia and mitotic activity than those in usual granulosa cell tumors (adult granulosa cell tumor). Luteinization of the tumor cells is common.

The granulosa cell tumor is, in general, of low-grade malignancy and in about 90% of patients, the tumor is stage I at diagnosis. Recurrence may occur after a long interval. Pathologic factors that may influence prognosis adversely are large size, nuclear atypia, and high mitotic rate.

THECOMA AND FIBROSARCOMA

Thecoma is almost always benign. Most of the fibroblastic tumors are benign (fibroma). Those with significantly atypical nuclei or with four or more mitotic figures per 10 high-power fields (HPFs) are malignant (fibrosarcoma).

SERTOLI-LEYDIG CELL TUMOR (ANDROBLASTOMA, ARRHENOBLASTOMA)

Androblastoma or arrhenoblastoma may be composed purely of Sertoli cells (Sertoli cell tumor) or may contain both Sertoli and Leydig cells (Sertoli-Leydig cell tumor). The tumor composed of Leydig cells only (Leydig cell tumor) is usually classified under steroid cell tumor.

Sertoli Cell Tumor

Approximately two-thirds of Sertoli cell tumors are estrogenic. The tumor is usually well differentiated, with hollow or solid tubules formed by Sertoli cells. Tumor cells may contain abundant lipid in their cytoplasm (lipid-rich Sertoli cell tumor or folliculoma lipidique). Malignant forms are very rare.

Sertoli-Leydig Cell Tumor

Sertoli-Leydig cell tumor is androgenic in about 40% of cases. Histologically the tumor shows various degree of differentiation.

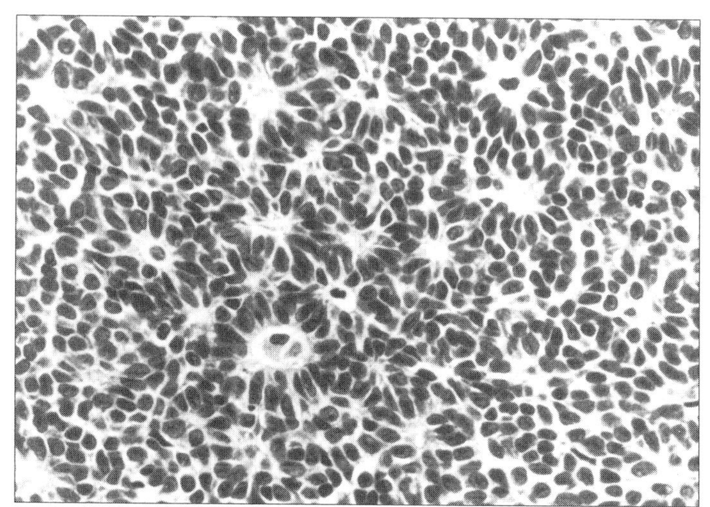

Fig. 18-2. Granulosa cell tumor. Tumor cells with a nuclear groove surround small round spaces (Call-Exner bodies).

Well-differentiated tumor is composed of Sertoli cells forming tubules and cells resembling normal Leydig cells. Poorly differentiated tumor is composed of spindle cells with sarcomatoid appearance. Well-differentiated tumor is benign. Some of the tumors of intermediate and poor differentiation are clinically malignant with extraovarian spread (11% and 59%, respectively). Approximately 20% of the tumors contain heterologous elements; this occurs in tumors of intermediate or poor differentiation. The heterologous element may be endodermal (benign glands or cysts composed of gastrointestinal-type epithelium) or mesodermal (skeletal muscle or cartilage, which is often malignant). One variant is retiform Sertoli-Leydig cell tumor, in which the tumor cells form a pattern similar to the rete testis.

SEX CORD TUMOR WITH ANNULAR TUBULES

Sex cord tumor with annular tubules is considered a variant of Sertoli cell tumor by some authors and is characterized by sex cord cells forming annular tubules that contain hyaline material. When it occurs with Peutz-Jehgers syndrome, the tumor is microscopic, multifocal, and benign. In an isolated form, it is often large and may be malignant (20% of patients).

STEROID CELL TUMOR (LIPID CELL TUMOR)

Steroid cell tumor is composed of cells resembling Leydig, lutein, or adrenal cortical cells. The tumor made up of cells containing Reinke crystals (Leydig cells) is a Leydig cell tumor and is benign. Stromal luteoma is a small, well-circumscribed tumor composed of lutein cells in the ovarian stroma and is benign. All other tumors are classified as steroid cell tumor, not otherwise specified. This is the most common in the group, and about 40% are androgenic. Approximately one-fourth are clinically malignant. Large size, severe nuclear atypia, and mitotic rate of two or more per 10 HPFs suggest malignancy.

Germ Cell Tumors of the Ovary

Malignant germ cell tumors account for approximately 3% of the ovarian cancers. The majority of these tumors are composed of primitive cells (primitive germ cell tumors; see below) and usually occur in young women (average age is 21). The other type is the germ cell tumor composed of adult (mature) cells and includes mature cystic teratoma with malignant transformation and some of the monodermal teratomas.

DYSGERMINOMA

The relative frequency of dysgerminomas among primitive germ cell tumors is 50%. The tumor is composed of cells similar to primordial germ cells (equivalent of seminoma of the testis). It is bilateral in 20% of patients (grossly, 10%; microscopically, another 10%). Bilaterality is less than 1% in all the other malignant germ cell tumors. Grossly, the tumor is usually solid with a smooth or nodular surface. The cut surfaces are tan and fleshy. Microscopically, the tumor cells are uniform and form diffuse sheets, nests, and trabeculae (Fig. 18-3) with stroma that often contains lymphocytic infiltration and/or granulomatous reaction. In approximately 3% of cases, the tumor contains isolated syncytiotrophoblasts. In these patients, elevated serum human chorionic gonadotropin (hCG) may produce hormonal manifestation (estrogenic or occasionally androgenic).

ENDODERMAL SINUS TUMOR (YOLK SAC TUMOR)

Endodermal sinus tumors are primitive germ cell tumors showing differentiation toward the yolk sac. The relative frequency of endodermal sinus tumors among primitive germ cell tumors is 20%. Grossly, the tumor is solid and cystic, often with hemorrhage and necrosis. Microscopically, the most common feature is microcystic and papillary patterns. Schiller-Duval bodies (small papillae with a fibrous core containing a central blood vessel) are not always present but are characteristic of this tumor. PAS (+) hyaline bodies are also common. Polyvesicular-vitelline or hepatoid patterns may be present. Immunohistochemical stain for alpha-fetoprotein is positive.

EMBRYONAL CARCINOMA

Embryonal carcinomas are primitive germ cell tumors that are the least differentiated. The relative frequency of embryonal carcinomas among primitive germ cell tumors is 3%. In the past, the term *embryonal carcinoma* was used for ovarian endodermal sinus tumor, and most of the cases reported as ovarian embryonal carcinoma in the old literature are actually endodermal sinus tumors. However, it has been shown that embryonal carcinoma similar to that of the testis does exist in the ovary and is different histologically and clinically from ovarian endodermal sinus tumor.

Grossly, tumor is solid, with frequent hemorrhage and necrosis. Microscopically, the tumor resembles embryonal carcinoma of the testis and is composed of large atypical cells with vesicular nuclei showing a prominent nucleolus. They form solid, glandular, or papillary patterns. A characteristic feature is presence of isolated syncytiotrophoblasts. Serum hCG and alpha-fetoprotein are elevated in patients with this tumor.

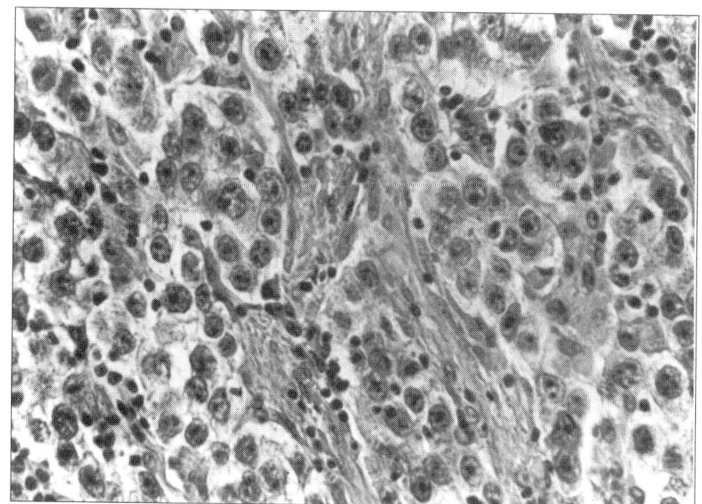

Fig. 18-3. Dysgerminoma. Uniform tumor cells resembling primordial germ cells form solid nests.

CHORIOCARCINOMA

Although isolated syncytiotrophoblasts are found in some of the primitive germ cell tumors, pure nongestational choriocarcinoma is very rare in the ovary. The relative frequency of choriocarcinomas among primitive germ cell tumors is less than 1%. To make a diagnosis of choriocarcinoma, it is required that syncytiotrophoblasts form the characteristic biphasic pattern with cytotrophoblasts.

IMMATURE (EMBRYONAL) TERATOMA

Immature (embryonal) teratomas are primitive germ cell tumors that contain immature (or embryonic) tissue from three germ layers. The relative frequency of immature teratomas among primitive germ cell tumors is 19%. Grossly, the tumor is mostly solid, but cysts are also present. Soft, fleshy, solid areas with hemorrhage and necrosis usually correspond to histologically malignant areas. Microscopically, immature (malignant) tissue is predominantly a neural tissue forming neuroepithelial tubules. Often other types of immature tissue, both epithelial and mesenchymal types, are also present. The immature tissue is often mixed with mature (benign) tissue. Based on the degree of immaturity and the relative quantity of immature tissue, the tumor is graded into three grades. The grade of the tumor correlates well with prognosis. Immature teratoma or solid mature teratoma is rarely associated with peritoneal implants of mature glial tissue (peritoneal gliomatosis). Such implants do not affect prognosis.

One tumor commonly misdiagnosed as immature teratoma is malignant müllerian mixed tumor. Malignant tissue in this tumor is the adult type and is limited to the müllerian kind without a neural component. The tumor occurs in older women, while immature teratoma is seen mostly in young women.

MALIGNANT MIXED GERM CELL TUMOR

Malignant mixed germ cell tumor is a primitive germ cell tumor in which more than one primitive cell type is present. The relative frequency of malignant mixed germ cell tumors among primitive germ cell tumors is 8%.

MATURE CYSTIC TERATOMA WITH MALIGNANT TRANSFORMATION

A variety of malignant tumors can arise in mature cystic teratoma. Its incidence is 1–2%, and it usually occurs in postmenopausal women. The vast majority of such tumors are squamous cell carcinomas.

MONODERMAL TERATOMA

Monodermal teratoma is composed entirely or predominantly of one type of adult tissue. Included in this category are struma ovarii and carcinoid. Some of these tumors are malignant.

The struma ovarii is solely or predominantly composed of thyroid tissue. Criteria for malignancy are similar to those used for thyroid carcinoma. Occasionally benign struma ovarii is associated with peritoneal implant (peritoneal strumosis).

The carcinoid tumor is potentially malignant, but less than 5% develop metastasis, which usually occurs in the insular or mucinous type. Metastatic carcinoid to the ovary is usually bilateral and does not contain other teratomatous components.

Mixed Germ Cell-Sex Cord–Stromal Tumors of the Ovary

GONADOBLASTOMA

Gonadoblastoma almost always occurs in dysgenetic gonads. It is frequently associated with malignant germ cell tumor (60%). The majority of the tumor arising in gonadoblastoma is germinoma (dysgerminoma or seminoma). Less commonly, endodermal sinus tumor, embryonal carcinoma, choriocarcinoma, or immature teratoma is seen.

Gonadoblastoma is bilateral in one-third of patients, and its typical histologic appearance is discrete nests containing primitive germ cells similar to those in dysgerminoma and smaller cells resembling Sertoli or granulosa cells. The stroma may contain cells resembling Leydig or lutein cells. Stromal hyalinization and calcification is common. Gonadoblastoma may be overgrown by associated malignant germ cell tumor, and its presence may be obscured. Presence of calcification suggests gonadoblastoma. Extensive sampling of the tumor and karyotyping of the patient may help establish the diagnosis.

UNCLASSIFIED GERM CELL-SEX CORD–STROMAL TUMOR

Unclassified germ cell-sex cord–stromal tumor is a very rare tumor and is different from gonadoblastoma in that it occurs in females with normal ovaries and normal karyotype (usually children) and that histologically it does not have the distinct nesting pattern of gonadoblastoma. Dysgerminoma or other malignant germ cell tumors may be associated with this tumor.

Sarcoma of the Ovary

Pure sarcomas or mixed tumors containing sarcoma are rare in the ovary. Those specific for the female genital tract include malignant müllerian mixed tumor, adenosarcoma, and endometrial stromal sarcoma. Their histology is similar to that of the uterine counterparts. Involvement of the ovary by malignant lymphoma and leukemia is fairly common, but cases in which an ovarian mass is a presenting symptom are rare except in Burkitt's lymphoma. Malignant lymphoma primarily involving the ovary is mostly B cell lymphoma.

Metastatic Cancer of the Ovary

Some of the metastatic ovarian tumors can mimic primary ovarian cancer pathologically as well as clinically. Metastatic tumor most commonly mistaken for primary ovarian carcinoma is metastatic adenocarcinoma from the colon. Grossly the tumor may be cystic and histologically may resemble mucinous or endometrioid adenocarcinoma. Mucinous adenocarcinoma of the colon or pancreas metastatic to the ovary may produce histologic features similar to mucinous borderline tumor or carcinoma. Metastatic adenocarcinoma from the stomach, in contrast, is usually solid and produces a characteristic histologic feature with signet-ring cells (Krukenberg's tumor). Krukenberg's tumor is almost always metastatic. A primary site is the stomach, but it occasionally occurs in other organs (e.g., colon, breast, appendix). Metastatic breast carcinoma to the ovary is fairly common, but involvement of the ovaries is usually small and clinically silent. Metastatic melanoma can mimic small-cell carcinoma of the hypercalcemic type or granulosa cell tumor. Immunohistochemical stain for S-100 protein and HMB-45 is positive in malignant melanoma and is helpful in differential diagnosis.

Precursors of Cervical Cancer

CERVICAL INTRAEPITHELIAL NEOPLASIA

Cervical intraepithelial neoplasia (CIN) (see Chap. 6) is a spectrum of neoplastic changes confined within the cervical squamous epithelium and is graded according to degree of abnormality (CIN 1 to CIN 3). A classification with dysplasia-carcinoma in situ (CIS) is still used to describe the same changes. However, since these epithelial changes are a spectrum of one disease process rather than two separate entities (dysplasia and CIS), the CIN classification is more appropriate.

Morphology of CIN is characterized by abnormality of maturation and presence of atypical squamous cells with increased nuclear to cytoplasmic (N/C) ratio and with nuclei showing hyperchromasia, abnormal chromatin, and increased mitotic rate. In CIN 1, absence of maturation and presence of atypical cells are limited to the lower one-third of the epithelium. In CIN 2, the changes extend into the middle third. The changes involve more than two-thirds of the thickness of the epithelium in CIN 3 (Fig. 18-4). CIN 1 corresponds to mild dysplasia, CIN 2 to moderate dysplasia, and CIN 3 to severe dysplasia and CIS. The Bethesda system is a new classification that describes abnormality of squamous cells of CIN in cytology specimens. In this system, the term *low-grade squamous intraepithelial*

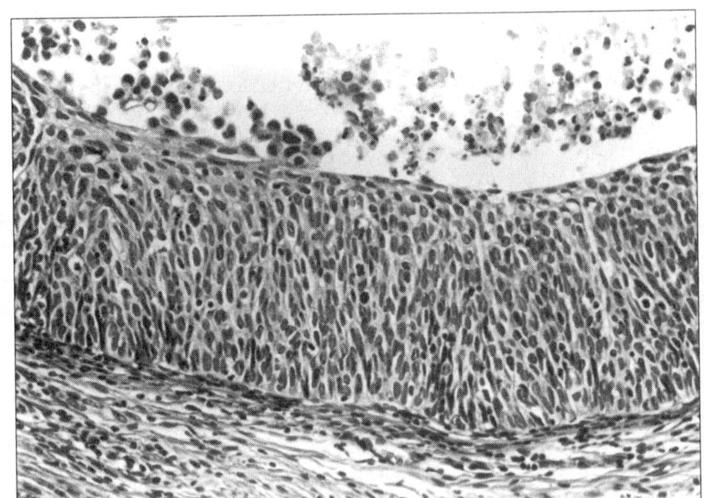

Fig. 18-4. CIN 3 (squamous cell carcinoma in situ). Atypical squamous cells occupy the entire thickness of the epithelium.

lesion (LSIL) is used for CIN 1 and *high-grade squamous intraepithelial lesion* (HSIL) for CIN 2 and CIN 3. Squamous cells showing koilocytosis are also included in LSIL. This terminology is also used to describe histologic changes.

Koilocytosis or koilocytotic atypia of the squamous cells is a histologic hallmark of human papillomavirus (HPV) infection and often coexists with CIN. The change is composed of perinuclear halos and a variety of nuclear changes including anisonucleosis, polychromasia, wrinkling, and binucleation. Types of HPV commonly associated with CIN and related lesions are 6 and 11 (condyloma); 16, 31, 33, and 35 (HSIL; invasive carcinoma); and 18 (invasive carcinoma). A variety of types including those above are seen in LSIL.

ADENOCARCINOMA IN SITU

Adenocarcinoma in situ is an uncommonly diagnosed lesion typically composed of preexisting endocervical glands partially or entirely lined by malignant-appearing glandular cells (Fig. 18-5). There may be an outpouching, cribriform pattern or intraluminal papillary projection. The malignant cells may be of endocervical, intestinal, or endometrioid type. In more than half of the cases, the lesion is accompanied by CIN. A similar glandular lesion but with less degree of atypia is termed *endocervical glandular dysplasia*.

Microinvasive Carcinoma of the Cervix

MICROINVASIVE SQUAMOUS CELL CARCINOMA

According to the International Federation of Gynecologists and Obstetricians (FIGO), microinvasive carcinoma (stage IA2) is a tumor in which depth of invasion is 5 mm or less and horizontal spread is 7

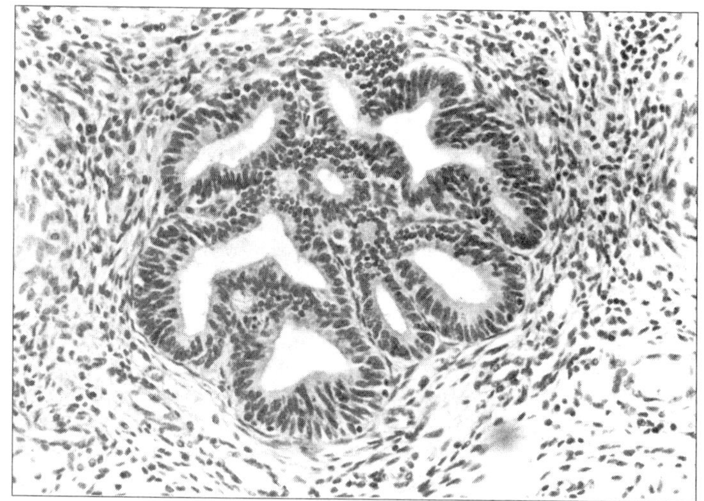

Fig. 18-5. Adenocarcinoma in situ. Endocervical glands lined by stratified atypical columnar cells.

mm or less. Since the tumors with a depth of 3.1–5.0 mm sometimes metastasize to pelvic lymph nodes (1–13%) and those with a depth of less than 3 mm usually do not, most gynecologic oncologists use a definition proposed by the Society of Gynecologic Oncologists. According to this definition, microinvasion is invasion with a depth less than 3 mm. Lesions with vascular-lymphatic invasion are excluded.

The depth of invasion is measured from the nearest and most superficial basement membrane of the overlying squamous epithelium to the deepest point of invasion by a calibrated ocular micrometer. Diagnosis of microinvasive carcinoma should be made only in adequate specimens (cone or hysterectomy specimen), and when there is tumor on the resection margin, the diagnosis is not valid. Glandular involvement by CIS should not be mistaken for early invasion. The former has rounded regular contours and produces no stromal reaction.

MICROINVASIVE ADENOCARCINOMA

Some investigators define microinvasive adenocarcinoma as tumor in which the maximum depth of stromal invasion is less than 5 mm as measured from the mucosal surface. However, one study noted positive lymph nodes in 11.1% (2 of 18) of patients with adenocarcinoma with a depth of invasion of 2–5mm. Until more definite criteria are established for microinvasive adenocarcinoma, one should approach this type of lesion with caution.

Invasive Carcinoma of the Cervix

SQUAMOUS CELL CARCINOMA

About 80% of invasive carcinomas are of squamous type. Most pathologists subdivide squamous cell carcinoma into three grades based on degree of keratinization and nuclear atypicality (well-, moderately, and poorly differentiated, or grades 1–3). A rare variant of squamous cell carcinoma is verrucous carcinoma. This extremely well-differentiated squamous cell carcinoma is pathologically similar to verrucous carcinoma of the vulva.

ADENOCARCINOMA AND ADENOSQUAMOUS CARCINOMA

Adenocarcinomas and adenosquamous carcinomas account for about 18% of invasive carcinomas. The most common tumor in this group is the endocervical type adenocarcinoma (70%). It is composed of cells resembling mucinous cells of the endocervical glands. An important variant of this tumor is adenoma malignum (minimal deviation adenocarcinoma) (10%). This tumor is composed of extremely well-differentiated glands that mimic benign endocervical glands. In spite of the innocuous histology, the prognosis of the tumor is worse than that of usual adenocarcinoma. One subtype is villoglandular papillary adenocarcinoma, which tends to occur in young women and is associated with a relatively favorable prognosis.

Adenosquamous carcinoma is composed of both malignant squamous and glandular cells and is the second most common tumor in this group. Glassy cell carcinoma is a poorly differentiated adenosquamous carcinoma and is composed of tumor cells with ground glass–like cytoplasm and large nuclei showing prominent nucleoli.

Other rare types of carcinoma in this group include endometrioid carcinoma, clear-cell carcinoma, serous carcinoma, mesonephric carcinoma, intestinal type carcinoma, signet-ring cell carcinoma, adenoid basal carcinoma, and adenoid cystic carcinoma.

SMALL-CELL UNDIFFERENTIATED CARCINOMA

Small-cell undifferentiated carcinoma was originally considered to be a variant of squamous cell carcinoma. The majority of the tumors, however, express neuroendocrine differentiation and are currently considered to be small-cell carcinoma equivalent to those occurring in the lung. The tumor probably arises from argyrophilic cells that have been demonstrated within the cervical epithelium. Histologically the tumor is similar to pulmonary small-cell carcinoma. Foci of squamous or glandular carcinoma may be present. The tumor is very aggressive with early dissemination.

Endometrial Hyperplasia

CLASSIFICATION OF ENDOMETRIAL HYPERPLASIA

The most current classification of endometrial hyperplasia is by the International Society of Gynecologic Pathologists (ISGP). In this classification, hyperplasia is divided into simple hyperplasia and complex hyperplasia by degree of gland crowding and complexity. Each of these two types is subdivided into one without atypia and one with atypia (i.e., simple hyperplasia, atypical simple hyperplasia, complex hyperplasia, and atypical complex hyperplasia).

In simple hyperplasia, the glands are not markedly crowded and some of the glands are cystic. Nondilated glands are round to slightly tortuous but lack the complex angularity of complex hyperplasia. In complex hyperplasia, the glands are more closely packed and show increased architectural complexity (Fig. 18-6). The atypia is manifested by changes in glandular epithelial cells including loss of

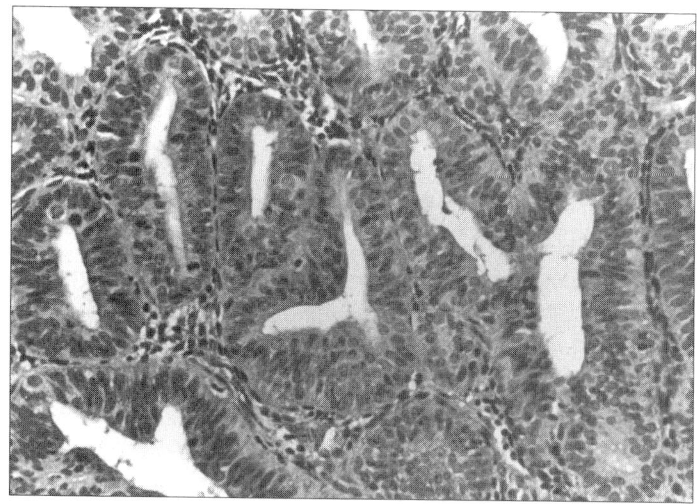

Fig. 18-6. Complex hyperplasia with atypia. Crowded irrregular glands. Stratified glandular cells show enlarged hyperchromatic nuclei.

polarity, stratification, increased N/C ratio, nuclear changes (rounding, enlargement, pleomorphism, and hyperchromasia), nucleoli, and increased mitotic figures. Atypia is the most important factor correlating with further progression to carcinoma.

The term *adenocarcinoma in situ* has been applied to different types of lesions by different authors, but it is best not to use this term to avoid confusion.

DISTINCTION BETWEEN ATYPICAL HYPERPLASIA AND WELL-DIFFERENTIATED ADENOCARCINOMA

Among the proposed criteria for carcinoma, those by Kurman and Norris emphasize evidence of stromal invasion with semiquantitative measurement, and those by Hendrickson et al. stress architectural and cytologic abnormalities. The criteria by Kurman and Norris are useful in predicting the likelihood of myometrial invasion.

Endometrial Carcinoma

ENDOMETRIOID ADENOCARCINOMA

The majority of endometrial carcinomas (80%) are composed of glands that resemble hyperplastic endometrial glands and are termed *endometrioid adenocarcinoma* in the ISGP/World Health Organization (WHO) classification. About one-third of this type show focal areas of squamous differentiation. When the squamous element appears histologically benign, the tumor is termed *adenoacanthoma* or *adenocarcinoma with squamous metaplasia*, and when the squamous element appears histologically malignant, the tumor is called *adenosquamous carcinoma*. WHO prefers the term *endometrioid carcinoma with squamous differentiation* for both lesions because (1) it is sometimes difficult to determine whether the squamous element looks histologically benign or malignant and

(2) prognosis of the tumor depends on the grade of the glandular component rather than the appearance of the squamous element.

Rare variants of endometrioid carcinoma include secretory carcinoma and ciliated carcinoma. In the former, neoplastic glands resemble glands of secretory endometrium, and in the latter, the majority of neoplastic glands are composed of ciliated cells.

OTHER SUBTYPES OF ENDOMETRIAL CARCINOMA

The most important among this group is serous papillary adenocarcinoma. The tumor occurs in older women and is much more aggressive than endometrioid carcinoma. It is histologically similar to serous papillary carcinoma of the ovary and often shows myometrial lymphatic invasion. A tumor that should not be mistaken for serous carcinoma is endometrioid carcinoma with papillary pattern. In this tumor, the tumor cells have an appearance similar to those of endometrioid carcinoma and contain low-grade nuclei.

Clear-cell adenocarcinoma is histologically similar to clear-cell carcinoma of the ovary. Its behavior is similar to serous carcinoma. Mucinous adenocarcinoma is composed of endocervical-type glands, and its behavior is similar to endometrioid carcinoma. Squamous cell carcinoma is rare and sometimes associated with cervical stenosis and pyometra. Undifferentiated carcinoma may be composed of large or small cells and is associated with aggressive clinical behavior. Mixed carcinoma is composed of more than one type of carcinoma, with each component greater than 10%.

GRADING OF ENDOMETRIAL ADENOCARCINOMA

FIGO grading of endometrial adenocarcinoma is based primarily on the histologic architecture. Grade 1 tumor is one in which nonsquamous solid area (versus glandular area) is 5% or less. In grade 2 tumor, it is 6–50%, and in grade 3 tumor, more than 50%. When there is significant nuclear atypia unusual for its grade, the grade is upgraded by one. In serous and clear-cell carcinoma, the tumor is graded by the nuclear grade.

Uterine Sarcoma

The uterine cancer purely or partly composed of sarcoma is not very common and accounts for only about 3% of the uterine tumors. The majority of these tumors occur in the body of the uterus. The most common type according to the AFIP file is malignant müllerian mixed tumor (30%). This is closely followed by leiomyosarcoma (27%) and endometrial stromal sarcoma (26%). Adenosarcoma (8%) and other miscellaneous and unclassified sarcomas complete the list. Leiomyosarcoma and endometrial stromal sarcoma are pure sarcoma, while malignant müllerian mixed tumor and adenosarcoma are mixed epithelial-mesenchymal tumor.

Pure Sarcoma of the Uterus

LEIOMYOSARCOMA OF THE UTERUS

Leimyosarcoma primarily involves the myometrium and forms a fleshy, poorly circumscribed mass, often with necrosis and hemorrhage. It may be intramural, submucosal, or subserosal.

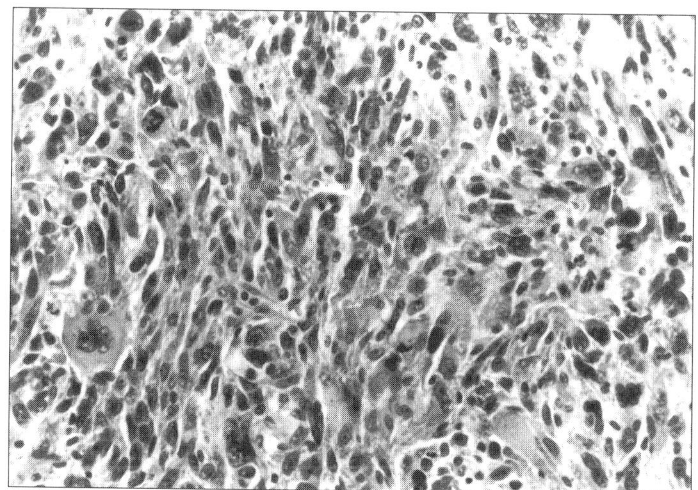

Fig. 18-7. Leiomyosarcoma. Cellular tumor composed of markedly atypical spindle cells with frequent mitotic figures.

Diagnostic Criteria

Leiomyosarcoma is microscopically characterized by hypercellularity, nuclear atypia, and high mitotic activity (Fig. 18-7). The key to the diagnosis is mitotic rate, cellular atypia, and coagulation tumor cell necrosis. A mitotic rate of more than 10 mitotic figures per 10 HPFs for cellular tumors and a mitotic rate of more than five per 10 HPFs for tumors with significant nuclear atypia or epithelioid features are considered diagnostic of leiomyosarcoma (except for myxoid leiomyosarcoma and mitotically active leiomyoma; see below). A tumor with significant atypia and coagulation necrosis is also considered malignant regardless of mitotic rate. Myxoid leiomyosarcoma is a rare variant of leiomyosarcoma and grossly shows a myxoid cut surface. Microscopically the tumor is hypocellular with abundant myxoid background. Mitotic rate is low (0–2 per 10 HPFs), but the tumor has markedly infiltrative borders.

Smooth-Muscle Tumor of Uncertain Malignant Potential

These are smooth-muscle tumors that cannot be diagnosed reliably either as malignant or benign. These include tumors with mild nuclear atypia showing five to nine mitotic figures per 10 HPFs, tumors with significant nuclear atypia or epithelioid features showing two to four mitotic figures per 10 HPFs, tumors with more than 15 mitotic figures per 10 HPFs but without hypercellularity or nuclear atypia, and tumors with abnormal mitotic figures or coagulation necrosis but without other diagnostic requirements for sarcoma.

Leiomyomas Mimicking Leiomyosarcoma

Mitotically active leiomyomas typically occur in young women (<35 years of age) and are usually small and well circumscribed. It shows increased mitotic activity (5–15 per 10 HPFs) but no nuclear atypia. The tumor is often associated with progestational stimulation (exogenous, pregnancy, secretory phase of menstrual cycle, etc.). Atypical (bizarre or symplastic) leiomyoma is composed of cells with bizarre, pleomorphic, or multiple nuclei without increased mitotic activity. Diffuse peritoneal leiomyomatosis (leiomyomatosis peritonealis disseminata) is a condition usually associated with pregnancy or the use of oral contraceptives and is characterized by multiple small leiomyomatous nodules on the peritoneum mimicking metastatic tumor. Benign metastasizing leiomyoma is diagnosed when single or multiple pulmonary benign-appearing smooth-muscle nodules appear in a patient with a history of uterine leiomyoma. These cases represent a true metastasizing uterine leiomyoma or a low-grade leiomyosarcoma inadequately sampled and misinterpreted as leiomyoma. In some cases, pulmonary and uterine tumors may be independent.

ENDOMETRIAL STROMAL SARCOMA

The endometrial stromal tumor is composed of cells resembling the stromal cells of the proliferative endometrium. The tumor is divided into benign and malignant groups based on the appearance of its borders on microscopic examination. Those with circumscribed borders are benign and termed *stromal nodule*. Those with irregular and infiltrating borders are malignant (endometrial stromal sarcoma). Endometrial stromal sarcoma is subdivided into low-grade and high-grade sarcomas.

Low-Grade Endometrial Stromal Sarcoma (Endolymphatic Stromal Myosis)

Low-grade endometrial stromal sarcomas primarily affect the myometrium, forming worm-like masses or multiple small, soft, tan nodules. Microscopically, the tumor is composed of uniform small cells with bland nuclei resembling the stromal cells of the proliferative endometrium. The tumor on microscopic examination has irregular infiltrating borders and often extends into lymphatics or veins. Mitotic figures are scanty and usually less than 10 per 10 HPFs. In some cases they may exceed 10 per 10 HPFs. However, as long as tumor cells show a bland cytologic appearance, behavior of the tumor is similar to those with low mitotic rate.

High-Grade Endometrial Stromal Sarcoma

High-grade endometrial stromal sarcoma primarily involves the endometrium forming a fungating, polypoid, or infiltrating mass, often with hemorrhage and necrosis. Myometrial invasion is frequent. The tumor is composed of spindle cells resembling endometrial stromal cells, but with nuclei showing significant atypia. Mitotic figures are more than 10 per 10 HPFs with frequent atypical forms. When the tumor cells have little or no resemblance to endometrial stromal cells, designation as *undifferentiated endometrial sarcoma* is more appropriate.

Malignant Mixed Epithelial-Mesenchymal Tumor of the Uterus

The tumors in this group are composed of both epithelial and mesenchymal cells. In malignant müllerian mixed tumors, both epithelial and mesenchymal elements are malignant, while in adenosarcoma, the epithelial element is benign and the mesenchymal element is malignant.

MALIGNANT MÜLLERIAN MIXED TUMORS (CARCINOSARCOMA, MALIGNANT MESODERMAL MIXED TUMOR, SARCOMATOID CARCINOMA)

Malignant müllerian mixed tumors primarily involve the endometrium and typically form a large, sessile, polypoid mass, often with hemorrhage and necrosis. The tumors are divided into homologous and heterologous types. In the homologous type, the sarcomatous element is composed of types of cells normally found in the uterus (endometrial stromal sarcoma, leiomyosarcoma, nonspecific spindle cell sarcoma). In the heterologous type, it is composed of types of cells not normally found in the uterus (rhabdomyosarcoma, chondrosarcoma, osteosarcoma, liposarcoma). The epithelial element is usually adenocarcinoma, but squamous cell or undifferentiated carcinoma may be present. Prognosis for homologous and heterologous types is similar.

ADENOSARCOMA

Grossly, an adenosarcoma forms a sessile polypoid or villous endometrial mass. Myometrial extension is uncommon (about one out of six cases). Microscopically, the tumor is composed of a benign glandular component and malignant mesenchymal component. The former is usually proliferative-type endometrial glands. The sarcomatous component usually has an appearance of low-grade endometrial stromal sarcoma or fibrosarcoma. Characteristically, these cells show high concentration around the glands. In about 20% of cases, heterologous elements are seen. A mitotic rate of two or more per 10 HPFs within the stroma or marked stromal cellularity or atypia is a key to diagnosis. The tumor is generally of low-grade malignancy with local recurrence and rare hematogenous spread, except when there is sarcomatous overgrowth.

Gestational Trophoblastic Disease

In normal chorionic tissue, three types of trophoblastic cells are found: cytotrophoblasts (CTs), syncytiotrophoblasts (STs), and intermediate trophoblasts (ITs). These cells are also present in gestational trophoblastic disease (GTD). The normal CTs and STs are mostly found in the chorionic villi (villous trophoblasts), while the ITs are typically found outside the villi (extravillous trophoblasts), especially at the implantation site. The CTs are proliferating stem cells and are hormonally inactive. They are polygonal in shape with a single vesicular nucleus in a clear cytoplasm. The STs are formed by fusion of the mature CTs and produce hCG (highest in the first trimester) and human placental lactogen (hPL) (highest in the third trimester). They are multinucleated with an abundant eosinophilic cytoplasm that is often vacuolated. The ITs are morphologically intermediate between the CTs and STs. They are larger than the CTs and generally mononuclear. Their cytoplasm is dense amphophilic or eosinophilic. They are weakly positive for hCG.

HYDATIDIFORM MOLE

Hydatidiform mole (HM) is an abnormal placental tissue composed of chorionic villi with hydropic swelling and abnormal trophoblastic proliferation. The HM is divided into complete HM, in which all the villi show hydropic change, and partial HM, in which only some of the villi show hydropic change. HM is caused by abnormal fertilization. Most cases of complete HM are formed by fertilization of an "empty egg" with a single sperm resulting in a diploid karyotype (46XX), while in most cases of partial HM, fertilization of an egg with two sperm takes place and its karyotype is triploid (69XXY, 69XXX, or 69XYY).

In complete HM, most of the villi are transformed into grapelike vesicles. Fetal tissue is absent. Microscopically, the enlarged villi show stromal edema with cistern or cavity formation and trophoblastic hyperplasia. The latter occurs all around the villi (circumferential versus polar in normal early villi), and both STs and CTs are seen. Nuclear atypia may be prominent in the CTs. Degree of hyperplasia and nuclear atypia is not predictive of the clinical outcome of the mole.

In the partial HM, the tissue obtained is less voluminous, and not all villi show hydropic swelling. Size of the enlarged villi is smaller (mean size = 0.51 cm versus 0.71 cm in complete mole). Fetal tissue is often identified. Microscopically, the enlarged edematous villi are mixed with small sclerotic villi. The enlarged villi are irregular in shape with scalloped outlines and invagination of trophoblastic cells into the stroma. Trophoblastic hyperplasia is less prominent and generally focal with predominance of the ST. Because of less striking pathologic as well as clinical features, partial HM is often underdiagnosed.

Incidence of persistent GTD is 10–20% in complete HM and less than 5% in partial HM. Postmolar choriocarcinoma occurs in 1–2% of complete HM and is extremely rare in partial HM.

INVASIVE HYDATIDIFORM MOLE (CHORIOADENOMA DESTRUENS)

Invasive mole is an HM that has invaded the myometrium or its vascular spaces. Once vascular invasion takes place, molar villi can spread to the other organs, most commonly to the vagina, vulva, and lung.

GESTATIONAL CHORIOCARCINOMA

Grossly, primary or metastatic choriocarcinoma forms a soft, large hemorrhagic nodule or nodules. Microscopically, the tumor is composed of an alternating arrangement of the CT and ST (biphasic or dimorphic pattern) with a flamelike appearance (Fig. 18-8). The ITs may be present. Villi are not seen except in very rare cases of choriocarcinoma arising in a normal placenta.

PLACENTAL SITE TROPHOBLASTIC TUMOR

Placental site trophoblastic tumor is a rare lesion predominantly composed of ITs. It was previously termed *trophoblastic pseudotumor* since the lesion was thought to represent an exaggerated form of *syncytial endometritis*. However, it became apparent that the lesion represents a true neoplasm with malignant potential, and the current term was adopted.

Grossly, the tumor involves the endometrium and/or myometrium and can be polypoid or infiltrative. Microscopically, the tumor is composed mostly of ITs (monomorphic) with scattered CTs. High mitotic rate (more than four per 10 HPFs) generally correlates with malignant behavior. Immunohistochemical stain for hPL is positive and is useful in differential diagnosis. Production of hCG is variable. Chemotherapy is not effective for this tumor.

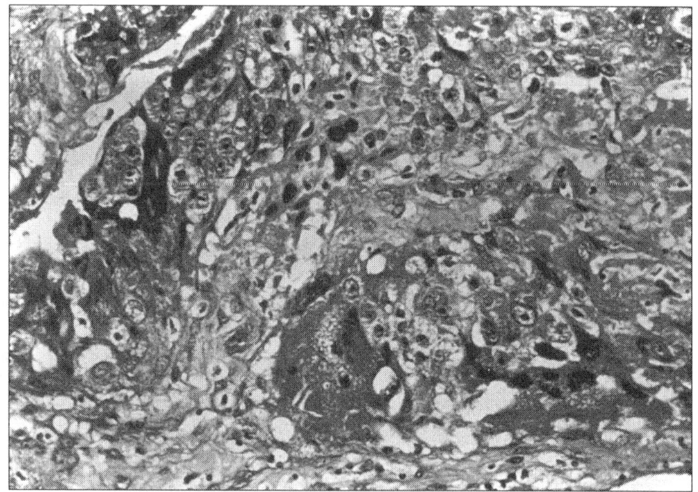

Fig. 18-8. Choriocarcinoma. Tumor is composed of intimately intermixed cytotrophoblasts and syncytiotrophoblasts (biphasic pattern).

Vulvar Dystrophy and Vulvar Intraepithelial Neoplasia

Under the current classification, lesions previously classified as dystrophy are listed under "non-neoplastic epithelial disorders of skin and mucosa," which includes lichen sclerosis (formerly lichen sclerosis et atrophicus or atrophic dystrophy), squamous hyperplasia (formerly hyperplastic dystrophy), and other dermatoses. The dystrophy does not show atypia and is not a precursor of cancer.

Vulvar intraepithelial neoplasia (VIN), in contrast, is a neoplastic epithelial disorder with malignant potential and is histologically characterized by abnormal maturation and presence of atypical cells.

DYSTROPHY

Lichen Sclerosis

Lichen sclerosis is grossly a pale white and plaque-like lesion and in its advanced stage has a wrinkled parchment-like appearance. Histologically, there is thinning of the epidermis with loss of rete ridges and melanin pigment. No atypia is present. Hyperkeratosis is common. The underlying dermis is edematous and hyalinized. Beneath this zone is a band of chronic inflammatory cells.

Squamous Hyperplasia

Most cases of squamous hyperplasia is secondary to chronic irritation and is more common in premenopausal women. Grossly, the lesion is usually plaque-like and may be white or red. It is rarely symmetric, and shrinkage does not occur. Histologically the epidermis is thickened with widening and elongation of the rete ridges. There is no atypia. Hyperkeratosis is frequent. The dermis shows no significant inflammation.

VULVAR INTRAEPITHELIAL NEOPLASIA

The term *VIN* applies the concept of CIN to vulvar squamous intraepithelial lesions. It replaces such terms as atypia, dysplasia, carcinoma in situ (CIS), Bowen's disease, bowenoid papulosis, and erythroplasia of Queyrat. In VIN 1 (mild dysplasia), abnormal maturation and atypical cells are seen in the lower third of the squamous epithelium. In VIN 2 (moderate dysplasia), these changes extend into the middle third, and in VIN 3 (severe dysplasia and CIS), the changes involve more than two-thirds of the thickness of the epithelium. VIN 3 is subclassified into three types: warty (bowenoid or condylomatous), basaloid (undifferentiated), and differentiated (simplex) types.

Squamous Cell Carcinoma of the Vulva

Vulvar cancer accounts for approximately 5% of malignant tumors of the female genital tract. Of these, 80–90% are squamous cell carcinoma.

SUPERFICIALLY INVASIVE (MICROINVASIVE) SQUAMOUS CELL CARCINOMA

Superficially invasive squamous cell carcinoma has a depth of invasion of 1 mm or less and a diameter of 2 cm or less. The depth of invasion is measured from the basement membrane of the epidermis covering the most superficial adjacent normal dermal papilla to the deepest point of invasion by a calibrated ocular micrometer. Risk of lymph node metastasis is zero in this type of tumor.

TYPICAL SQUAMOUS CELL CARCINOMA

Typical squamous cell carcinoma forms a solitary nodular or ulcerated mass. Microscopically, the tumor is nearly always keratinizing. Adjacent skin commonly shows squamous hyperplasia. VIN is infrequent and, if present, is the differentiated (simplex) type. Lichen sclerosis coexists in 15–30% of the cases. The tumor affects elderly women (mean age of 77) and has little association with HPV.

VARIANTS OF SQUAMOUS CELL CARCINOMA

Basaloid Carcinoma

Grossly the tumor is similar to typical squamous cell carcinoma. The tumor is composed of small basaloid squamous cells with scanty cytoplasm. VIN of basaloid type is seen in adjacent skin.

Warty (Condylomatous) Carcinoma

Grossly, the tumor is exophytic and papillary, resembling verrucous carcinoma. Microscopically, however, it is composed of atypical squamous cells forming irregular nests. Cytoplasmic vacuolation similar to koilocytosis is seen. Basaloid and warty carcinomas occur in younger women (mean ages of 54 and 45, respectively) and are etiologically related to HPV (mostly type 16).

Verrucous Carcinoma

Grossly, the tumor forms an exophytic, often papillary mass. Microscopically, it is composed of extremely well-differentiated squa-

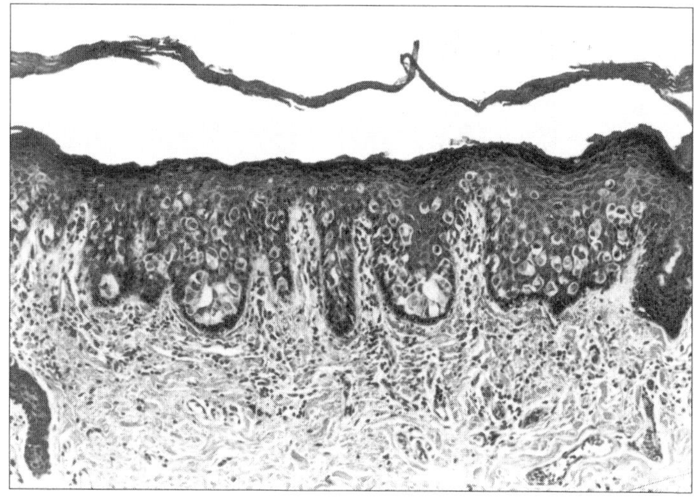

Figure 18-9. Paget's disease. Large, pale Paget's cells are seen in the basal portion of the epidermis.

mous cells that form large bulbous sheets or nests with pushing borders. The tumor is associated with HPV type 6. Giant condyloma of Buschke-Löwenstein most likely represents verrucous carcinoma.

Vulvar Cancer Other Than Squamous Cell Carcinoma

PAGET'S DISEASE

Paget's disease accounts for about 2% of cases of vulvar cancer. Vulvar Paget's disease is different from Paget's disease of the breast in that the latter is almost always associated with underlying ductal carcinoma, while in vulvar Paget's disease, underlying carcinoma is rare. In the majority of cases, vulvar Paget's disease is intraepithelial adenocarcinoma arising from the multipotential cells in the epidermis. It may become invasive, but this is very rare.

Grossly, the disease usually presents as a red eczematous lesion with white areas. Its margin is fairly well demarcated, but the tumor is often found beyond the gross margin on microscopic examination. Microscopically, the lesion is characterized by large cells with pale cytoplasm that is positive with periodic acid–Schiff (PAS) or mucicarmine (Paget's cells) (Fig. 18-9). These cells are seen mostly at the basal portion of the epidermis, sometimes forming glands.

CARCINOMA OF BARTHOLIN'S GLAND

Carcinoma of Bartholin's gland constitutes 2–7% of the cases of vulvar cancer. To make a diagnosis of primary Bartholin's gland carcinoma, the tumor has to be in the right location and extension or metastasis from carcinoma of other sites has to be ruled out. The tumor has a poor prognosis because of an abundance of lymphatics in the area and frequent delay in diagnosis. Main histologic types are adenocarcinoma (40%), squamous cell carcinoma (40%), and adenoid cystic carcinoma (15%). Adenoid cystic carcinoma is composed of basaloid cells with cribriform pattern.

BASAL CELL CARCINOMA

Basal cell carcinoma accounts for 2–4% of the cases of vulvar cancer. It is grossly and microscopically identical to basal cell carcinoma of the skin elsewhere. Grossly, the tumor is usually circumscribed and forms a mass or ulcer. Metastasis is extremely rare.

MALIGNANT MELANOMA

Malignant melanoma comprises about 4% of cases of vulvar cancer. The lesion is slightly elevated or nodular and may be pigmented or nonpigmented. Histologically, melanoma cells may not contain melanin (amelanotic) and may mimic cells of other tumors (e.g., Paget's cells or cells of VIN). Immunohistochemical stain is helpful in differential diagnosis. Melanoma markers (S-100, HMB-45) are negative in Paget's disease and VIN. Melanoma and VIN are nonreactive for carcinoembryonic antigen (CEA), while Paget's disease is reactive.

The level of invasion or thickness of the tumor is the most reliable histologic prognostic indicator. The Clark classification divides the levels of invasion into five levels: I, intraepithelial; II, papillary dermis; III, interface between papillary and reticular dermis; IV, reticular dermis; and V, subcutaneous fat. The thickness of melanoma is defined as vertical measurement from the top of the granular layer of the overlying epidermis to the deepest point of invasion (Breslow). The lesion less than 0.76 mm thick has little or no metastatic risk.

Vaginal Cancer

Eighty to 90% of vaginal cancers are secondary tumors extending or metastatic from the adjacent organs (cervix, vulva, endometrium, ovary, urinary bladder, rectum). Primary vaginal cancer is rare and accounts for only 1–2% of cancers of the female genital tract. The majority of these are of the squamous type.

VAGINAL INTRAEPITHELIAL NEOPLASIA

Vaginal intraepithelial neoplasia (VAIN) encompasses both squamous dysplasia and squamous cell carcinoma in situ. The criteria for grading are similar to those for CIN. VAIN is rarer than CIN and occurs in older women. The majority of VAIN is associated with CIN or cervical carcinoma (earlier, concurrent, or subsequent).

SQUAMOUS CELL CARCINOMA

Diagnosis of primary vaginal carcinoma is made only after extension or metastasis from carcinoma of other sites is excluded. When there is simultaneous involvement of the cervix or vulva, the tumor is considered not primary in the vagina (FIGO staging).

The tumor is most common in the upper third of the vagina and is histologically similar to the cervical squamous cell carcinoma. The majority of the tumors are nonkeratinizing. Verrucous carcinoma is a variant of squamous cell carcinoma and is pathologically similar to the same tumor in the vulva.

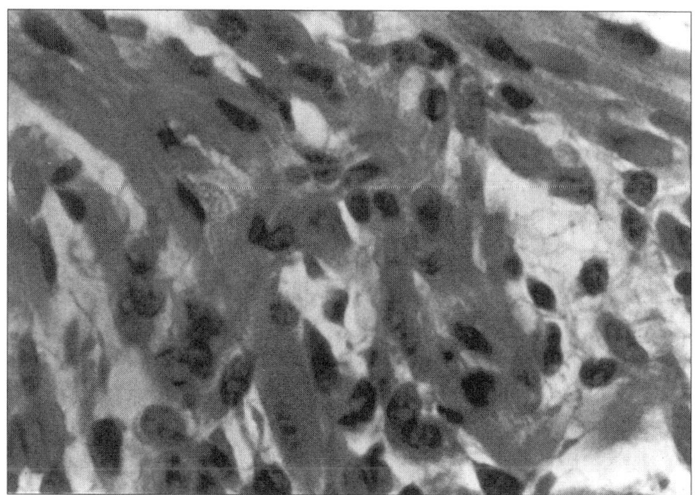

Fig. 18-10. Botryoid sarcoma. Tumor cells showing cross-striation (rhabdomyoblasts).

ADENOCARCINOMA

Adenocarcinoma other than clear-cell carcinoma is rare and includes endometrioid, endocervical-type, intestinal-type, and mesonephric carcinomas. Since the association between in utero diethylstilbestrol (DES) exposure and vaginal clear-cell carcinoma was reported in 1971, the majority of adenocarcinomas recorded have been DES-related and are of clear-cell type. Microscopically, this tumor is composed of clear cells and hobnail cells forming solid, tubulocystic, and papillary patterns. These features are similar to those of clear-cell carcinoma elsewhere. Usually adenosis is found adjacent to the tumor.

BOTRYOID SARCOMA (EMBRYONAL RHABDOMYOSARCOMA)

Botryoid sarcoma is a rare tumor but is the most common sarcoma in the vagina. Grossly, the tumor is composed of grapelike multiple polypoid masses (*botrys* is Greek for *bunch of grapes*). Microscopically, small tumor cells form a bandlike infiltrate ("cambium" layer) beneath the intact squamous epithelium. Rhabdomyoblasts with cross-striation may be found in this layer or a subjacent loose area (Fig. 18-10).

Vaginal polyps (pseudosarcoma botryoides) may resemble botryoid sarcoma. This lesion usually occurs in adults and is composed of loose fibrous tissue without a cambium layer, undifferentiated small tumor cells, or rhabdomyoblasts.

RARE MISCELLANEOUS TUMORS

Yolk sac tumor occurs in infants and clinically may mimic botryoid sarcoma. The histology of this tumor is similar to that of ovarian yolk sac tumor.

Malignant melanoma usually affects white postmenopausal women. Prognosis is generally poor because of deep invasion at the time of diagnosis.

Fallopian Tube Cancer

Fallopian tube cancer is rare and accounts for only 0.2% of female genital malignancies. Most of these are carcinoma.

CARCINOMA

Nearly all carcinomas arising in the fallopian tube are adenocarcinoma. Grossly, the tumor presents as a fusiform swelling of the tube mimicking hydrosalpinx. The lumen is filled with a papillary or solid tumor. It is bilateral in 10–20% of patients. Microscopically, the majority of the tumors are similar to serous papillary carcinoma of the ovary. Presence of main tumor mass within the tubal lumen, absence or minimal involvement of the ovary, and transition between the tubal epithelium and tumor are a key to the diagnosis. Other histologic types such as endometrioid carcinoma, clear-cell carcinoma, squamous cell carcinoma, and transitional cell carcinoma have been reported.

Simultaneous in situ or early invasive adenocarcinoma of the fallopian tube is noted in 5–10% of the patients with ovarian serous carcinoma.

OTHER MALIGNANT TUMORS

Choriocarcinoma occurs rarely in the fallopian tube. Clinically and grossly, it mimics ectopic pregnancy. Malignant müllerian mixed tumor forms a large polypoid mass in the lumen. Germ cell tumor of the tube is mostly mature cystic teratoma, but immature teratoma has been reported.

Selected Readings

Berek JS, Hacker NF, Fu YS et al. Adenocarcinoma of the uterine cervix: Histologic variables associated with lymph node metastasis and survival. *Obstet Gynecol* 65:46, 1985.

Fox H (ed). *Haines and Taylor Obstetrical and Gynaecological Pathology* (3rd ed). Edinburgh: Churchill-Livingstone, 1987.

Hendrickson MR, Ross JC, Kempson RL. Toward the development of morphologic criteria for well-differentiated adenocarcinoma of the endometrium. *Am J Surg Pathol* 7:819, 1983.

Kurman RJ (ed). *Blaustein's Pathology of the Female Genital Tract* (3rd ed). New York: Springer-Verlag, 1987.

Kurman RJ, Norris HJ. Evaluation of criteria for distinguishing atypical endometrial hyperplasia from well-differentiated carcinoma. *Cancer* 49:2547, 1982.

Kurman RJ, Norris HJ, Williamson E. Tumors of the Cervix, Vagina and Vulva. In *Atlas of Tumor Pathology* (3rd series, fascicle 4). Washington, DC: Armed Forces Institute of Pathology, 1992.

Rosai J. *Ackerman's Surgical Pathology* (7th ed). St. Louis: Mosby, 1989.

Scully RE. Tumors of the Ovary and Maldeveloped Gonads. In *Atlas of Tumor Pathology* (2nd series, fascicle 16). Washington, DC: Armed Forces Institute of Pathology, 1979.

Silverberg SG, Kurman RJ. Tumors of the Uterine Corpus and Gestational Trophoblastic Disease. In *Atlas of Tumor Pathology* (3rd series, fascicle 3). Washington, DC: Armed Forces Institute of Pathology, 1992.

Steinberg SS (ed). *Diagnostic Surgical Pathology* (2nd ed). New York: Raven, 1994.

19

Diagnostic Imaging of Gynecologic Malignancies

Paul C. Stomper, Donald L. Klippenstein, and Steven Herman

Modern imaging techniques have an evolving role in the management of patients with gynecologic malignancies. Newer techniques such as contrast-enhanced magnetic resonance imaging (MRI) using an endocervical coil or transvaginal ultrasound with color-flow Doppler analysis provide increased complementary information to physical examination, Papanicolaou (Pap) smear, dilatation and curettage, biopsies, and endoscopic procedures in the evaluation of pelvic malignancies. However, the optimal use, technique, and interpretation of these sophisticated and expensive techniques have not been determined in many gynecologic oncology settings. The most effective use of modern imaging techniques requires a continuous dialogue between the clinical oncologist and diagnostic radiologist. Optimally, the clinician should discuss the purpose of the imaging test with the radiologist in advance and review the images and discuss the findings with the radiologist after it is performed. Not only the selection of an imaging modality but also the technical factors and criteria for interpretation of each imaging test should be discussed in a multidisciplinary format. The diagnostic radiologist's need for adequate clinical information and prior imaging studies is of paramount importance to effectively practice high-quality clinical diagnostic radiology. The diagnostic radiologist's knowledge of physical examination findings, biopsy or surgical findings, and the type and timing of any local or systemic therapeutic interventions is essential. The diagnostic radiologist, through personal consultations and multidisciplinary conferences, must gain an understanding of the treatment strategies, the associated toxicities, and the natural histories of the various malignancies. The diagnostic radiologist should be an active participant in the gynecologic oncology team. Potential roles of imaging in gynecologic malignancy include screening, diagnosis, staging, response assessment, toxicity and complication assessment, and follow-up and surveillance.

Cervical Carcinoma

DIAGNOSIS AND SCREENING

Cervical carcinoma can be demonstrated by ultrasound, computed tomography (CT), and MRI. However, the diagnosis of cervical cancer depends ultimately on cytologic and histologic findings obtained from dilatation and curettage or biopsy, respectively. No cross-sectional imaging modality is currently used in the screening of asymptomatic patients or those at high risk for cervical carcinoma.

On unenhanced CT, detection of cervical carcinoma is limited to those lesions exhibiting cervical enlargement, with or without border irregularity. Obstruction of the endocervical canal may result in a dilated fluid-filled endometrial cavity. Contrast-enhanced CT may demonstrate tumor enhancement or hypodensity, the latter being due to necrosis or ulceration.

On ultrasound, cervical carcinomas appear as cervical enlargement, with or without border irregularity, associated with decreased echogenicity within the neoplasm. Cervical fibroids may be indistinguishable from carcinomas on ultrasound.

MRI is the imaging modality best suited for evaluation of cervical carcinoma location, size, and depth of stromal infiltration. The normal cervix exhibits low signal intensity (dark) on both T1-weighted and T2-weighted pulse sequences, consistent with the increased fibrous tissue content within the cervix. Mucus within the endocervical canal and the contiguous cervical epithelium normally appears as high signal intensity (bright) on T2-weighted images. Cervical carcinomas most commonly appear as regions of T2-hyperintensity relative to the normal low signal intensity of the cervical stroma. While routine contrast-enhanced MRI may not increase the accuracy of tumor detection, contrast tumor enhancement can help distinguish regions of necrosis from viable neoplasm. One study showed that dynamic contrast-enhanced MRI with serial imaging following contrast injection was more accurate in assessing the degree of stromal invasion and tumor size than unenhanced or equilibrium-enhanced MRI.

STAGING

Preoperative chest radiography is routinely performed. Intravenous urography and barium enema studies are usually limited to symptomatic patients with advanced disease. With ongoing improvements in cross-sectional imaging modalities, lymphangiography is performed much less frequently but remains the only imaging modality that allows for assessment of nodal architecture.

For patients with stage IB or IIA neoplasms (International Federation of Obstetricians and Gynecologists [FIGO] staging classification), clinical staging is more accurate than CT staging. By being able to evaluate the entire pelvis and abdomen more easily than MRI, CT is better suited for the initial staging of patients suspected of having clinically advanced disease (stages IIIB–IVB). Parametrial tumor extension is demonstrated on CT as tissue stranding or, in cases of more advanced disease, by distinct masses. Loss of delineation of perirectal and perivesical tissue planes suggests rectal and bladder tumor extension, respectively.

MRI is recommended for the initial staging of stage II tumors. While the overall accuracy of body coil MRI in cervical carcinoma staging has ranged from 76% to 83%, the accuracy of MRI in detecting parametrial tumor extension has been reported as high as 92%, and its accuracy in detecting vaginal extension has been reported as high as 93%.

On T1-weighted MRI images, the pericervical tissues exhibit signal intensity characteristics that are intermediate between the low-intensity cervical stroma and the high-intensity contiguous fat. Slowly flowing blood within the pericervical tissues may result in high signal intensity on T2-weighted images. T2 hyperintense carcinomas that do not extend through the entire thickness of the cervical stroma exhibit preservation of the outer low signal intensity uninvolved stroma. Cervical carcinomas involving the full cervical stroma thickness result in disruption of the outer low signal intensity stroma. Tumor extension into the parametrium is often best visualized on T1-weighted images that maximize the contrast between tumor and parametrial fat. As inflammatory changes associated with cervical cone biopsies may result in signal intensity alterations simulating carcinoma, MRI staging should not be performed during the 6-week interval following the biopsy.

The multiplanar features of MRI allow for coronal and sagittal imaging that results in better visualization of vaginal, bladder, rectal, or lower uterine segment extension. Stage IIA neoplasms, involving the upper two-thirds of the vagina, result in loss of the normal vaginal wall low-intensity signal. Stage IIB neoplasms, involving the parametrium, may exhibit distinct parametrial soft-tissue masses or merely an irregular contour of the lateral cervix. Stage IIIA neoplasms may manifest as a mass lesion in the lower third of the vagina or loss of the normal low-intensity signal from this region. Stage IIIB neoplasms, indicating pelvic side wall involvement, are associated with loss of the normal muscular T2 hypointensity involving the levator ani, pyriformis, or obturator internus muscles. Stage IVA neoplasms, involving the bladder or bowel wall, are associated with loss of tissue planes between these structures as well as loss of the normal low-intensity signal of the organ walls on T2-weighted images.

Gadolinium contrast-enhanced MRI has limited complementary value in the staging of cervical carcinomas, as the studies consistently overestimate tumor size and overestimate vaginal, parametrial, and bladder extension. However, contrast-enhanced studies may be useful in patients in whom the unenhanced images are suboptimal. Accuracy in staging cervical carcinoma may be improved by endorectal surface coils that provide superior resolution and anatomic detail compared to body coil images.

Detection of lymph node metastases by MRI as well as CT is generally limited to recognition of those nodes that are enlarged. Metastases in nonenlarged nodes will result in false-negative staging studies, while nodes that are enlarged due to reactive hyperplasia may result in false-positive studies.

FOLLOW-UP AND SURVEILLANCE

MRI is superior to both CT and ultrasound in the evaluation of patients after surgery, chemotherapy, or radiation therapy. Detection of residual or recurrent tumor is more readily achieved by MRI than the other imaging modalities. With MRI, radiation fibrosis is distinguished from residual or recurrent tumor by its low signal intensity on both T1-weighted and T2-weighted images, versus the high signal intensity of recurrent tumor on T2-weighted images.

Bowel strictures and fistulas between the bowel, bladder, and vagina, resulting from either advanced neoplastic disease or radiation damage, are better evaluated by conventional barium or water-soluble contrast enemas, small-bowel series, plain radiographic studies, or CT than by MRI. In addition to colonic stricture, radiation injury to the colon may manifest as mural thickening or a widened presacral space. The widened presacral space caused by radiation may be due to either thickening of perirectal fibrous tissue or fibrosis between the rectum and sacrum. Ureteral strictures are best evaluated by intravenous or retrograde pyelography or CT.

Endometrial Cancer

SCREENING AND DIAGNOSIS

At present, there is no role for imaging in screening asymptomatic routine or high-risk patients for endometrial cancer.

Transvaginal ultrasound measurement of endometrial thickness has been shown in several studies to be a sensitive method of detecting endometrial pathology in women with postmenopausal bleeding. An endometrial thickness of 4–5 mm or less (including both endometrial layers) indicates a very low risk for endometrial carcinoma or any other major endometrial pathology in women with postmenopausal bleeding. In one study of 120 women with postmenopausal bleeding using an endometrial thickness limit of 5 mm, 82% of the curettage procedures could have been avoided without missing a single case of serious endometrial pathology.

STAGING

Gadolinium-DTPA–enhanced MRI appears to have increased accuracy over iodinated contrast-enhanced CT and ultrasound for the local staging of patients with endometrial carcinoma.

Indications for MRI staging of endometrial cancer include:

1. Suspected advanced disease (grade 3 tumor or papillary serous carcinoma)
2. Patients who are difficult to examine
3. Poor risks for surgical staging

The complementary role of MRI staging to physical examination includes assessment of:

1. Depth of myometrial invasion
2. Cervical invasion
3. Extrauterine extension to bladder or rectum or to extrapelvic structures
4. Lymph nodes by size criteria only

Table 19-1 shows an MRI staging classification for endometrial cancer. The most important factors in the staging of patients with endometrial cancer include the histologic grade of the tumor, the depth of myometrial invasion, the presence or absence of lymph node metastasis, and, in advanced cases, the presence or absence of extrauterine extension. The depth of myometrial invasion and invasion of the cervix correlate with the prevalence of regional lymph node metastases. On the T2-weighted and contrast-enhanced T1-weighted images, the endometrial cancer has a bright or heterogeneous signal relative to the lower signal intensity myometrium or cervical stroma. Contrast enhancement of the endometrial cancer improves differentiation of the tumor from the adjacent endometrium and better distinguishes tumor from areas of necrosis or hemorrhage than noncontrast T1- and T2-weighted MRI images or noncontrast CT images. Imaging in both the axial and sagittal planes relative to the uterus affords the best assessment of tumor volume and penetration. The sagittal plane images allow the best assessment of tumor extension into the endocervical canal.

The accuracy of MRI for the staging of endometrial cancer has been reported from 82% to 92%. The accuracy reported for MRI is better than that reported for CT. Specialized MRI coils such as the

Table 19-1. Magnetic resonance imaging staging classification for endometrial cancer

Stage	*Description*
I	Tumor confined to uterine corpus
IA	Tumor confined to the endometrium
IB	Tumor confined to the inner 50% of the myometrium
IC	Tumor confined to the outer 50% of the myometrium
II	Tumor extension into the cervix
III	Extrauterine tumor spread to the true pelvis
IV	Extension to the bladder and/or rectum

endocervical coil and phased array coil may improve anatomic detail of uterine malignancies.

The most common error in staging of endometrial cancer by cross-sectional imaging tests is the overestimation of the depth of myometrial invasion in cases of large polypoid tumors that distend the uterus so that a thin rim of myometrium is stretched over it rather than being deeply infiltrated by it. Both MRI and CT have similar limitations in lymph node assessment based solely on size due to the presence of microscopic metastases in normal-sized nodes (less than 1 cm in the shortest transaxial diameter) and the presence of enlarged, benign, reactive lymph nodes.

FOLLOW-UP AND SURVEILLANCE

MRI can provide noninvasive assessment of tumor response, detection of recurrent tumor, and, in many cases, differentiation of recurrence from radiation effects.

Ovarian Cancer

DIAGNOSIS

An adnexal mass discovered at pelvic examination or suspected from a patient's symptoms may be identified and characterized by ultrasound, CT, or MRI. Since pelvic ultrasound is less costly and has no ionizing radiation, it is the preferred initial radiologic study for confirmation and evaluation of an ovarian mass. Ovaries were defined as enlarged by ultrasound in one study if their volume was greater than 18 cc in a premenopausal woman and greater than 8 cc in a postmenopausal woman. The volume is estimated using the formula for a prolate ellipse ($0.524 \times D_1 \times D_2 \times D_3$) where the maximum diameters (D_1, D_2, D_3) are measured in orthogonal planes. Transvaginal ultrasound (TVUS) of the pelvis usually shows better detail of the adnexal structures than transabdominal ultrasound and may provide additional information about the uterus and adnexa. Transabdominal ultrasound may be necessary for evaluation of large masses and ovaries displaced by an enlarged uterus or other structures.

Ultrasound features that raise suspicion of malignancy in an adnexal mass include thick septations or papillary processes (≥ 3 ml), irregular walls in a cystic mass, multicystic components within a solid mass, and heterogeneous solid masses. A sensitivity of 62–100% and specificity of 52–100% for malignancy have been achieved applying similar criteria. In several reported series, 0–6% of surgically removed adnexal masses less than 5 cm in diameter were borderline malignant or malignant, but 44–72% of adnexal masses greater than 10 cm were malignant. However, two studies show that malignancy is virtually excluded when masses are classified by TVUS as unilocular simple cysts, including those greater than 10 cm. Morphologic criteria for malignancy have become more important than the size of the mass as the resolution of ultrasound, particularly TVUS, has improved. Benign masses such as dermoids, hemorrhagic cysts, and hydrosalpinges may have virtually pathognomonic ultrasound appearances. Approximately 15% of postmenopausal women are shown to have simple ovarian cysts on TVUS and many of these cysts do not change appreciably on follow-up TVUS. A palpable or enlarged ovary in a postmenopausal woman does not necessarily imply a malignancy.

Ovarian masses have recently been analyzed with color and spectral Doppler. Increased detectable flow by color Doppler and low-resistance flow are expected in malignancies since tumor neovascularity should have increased compliance due to lack of muscular layers. Low resistance in the tumor vessels results in increased diastolic flow on spectral Doppler and a low resistive index (RI) or low pulsatility index (PI). Using cut-off values of 0.40–0.80 for the RI and 0.62–1.25 for the PI, investigators reported sensitivities of 50–100% and specificities of 46–100% for differentiating benign from malignant adnexal masses. One large series using Doppler evaluation to determine whether adnexal masses were malignant showed a sensitivity of 96% and specificity greater than 99% when the lowest resistance vessel within the mass had an RI of 0.40 or less. An adnexal mass is likely to be benign when Doppler evaluation shows no detectable flow, flow only in the periphery of the mass, or a notch in the Doppler waveform in early diastole. Some investigators have recorded significantly higher velocities in the vessels of malignant masses than in the vessels of benign masses, not taking into account the angle of interrogation to determine the true velocities. Premenopausal women should have Doppler evaluation of ovarian masses during days 3–11 in their menstrual cycle as ovarian blood flow in the luteal phase may be low resistance. Although the optimal color Doppler interpretive criteria for differentiation of benign and malignant ovarian masses have not yet been determined, diagnostic accuracy will likely improve when both gray-scale and Doppler findings are considered. Gray-scale and Doppler characteristics may be applied to primary ovarian cancer, fallopian tube primary malignancies, and metastatic disease to the adnexa.

Contrast-enhanced, thin-slice pelvic MRI and CT have demonstrated similar accuracy to TVUS in characterizing ovarian masses as benign or malignant. CT or MRI with fat suppression are helpful in distinguishing teratomas from endometriomas and hemorrhagic cystic lesions. In difficult cases, MRI may be helpful in distinguishing serosal fibroids from ovarian masses. Currently, monoclonal antibody imaging is being investigated for the detection of ovarian cancer. Pilot studies with monoclonal antibody imaging have shown sensitivities up to 95% for primary ovarian malignancies.

SCREENING

Although TVUS may be more sensitive in detecting ovarian malignancy than pelvic examination or serum CA-125, mortality reduction benefit and cost-effectiveness of TVUS ovarian cancer screening has not been proved, even in high-risk women. Many centers are currently performing TVUS at regular intervals in their screening programs for woman at high risk for ovarian cancer.

STAGING

Ovarian cancer staging occurs largely during total abdominal hysterectomy and bilateral salpingo-oophorectomy (TAH/BSO) and cytoreductive surgery. Preoperative staging of the abdomen and pelvis by CT or MRI is usually not indicated. MRI may be helpful in delineating local invasion of pelvic organs. Preoperative CT, ultrasound, bone scan, or gastrointestinal studies may be indicated depending on the patient's symptoms or laboratory abnormalities. A preoperative chest radiograph is routinely performed.

FOLLOW-UP

The frequency and type of radiologic assessment after cytoreductive surgery and chemotherapy is influenced by the clinical examination, the patient's symptoms, serum CA-125 level, or other laboratory abnormalities. CT studies using modern equipment and techniques reveal sensitivities of 78–84% and specificities of 88–100% for detection of peritoneal metastases or tumor recurrence. Studies using intraperitoneal contrast with CT have suggested increased sensitivity for peritoneal spread of tumor. None of these studies have been performed with CT equipment using the latest technical advances. One small series showed a significant improvement in accuracy when CT studies were read by an experienced, specialist radiologist. MRI has shown similar accuracy to CT and may detect smaller peritoneal implants when oral and IV contrast and fat suppression are used. A CT- or ultrasound-guided biopsy of a recurrent mass can save the patient from a second-look laparotomy if the surgery is intended only for restaging purposes. Monoclonal antibody imaging may be more sensitive and specific than CT for persistence or recurrence of ovarian cancer. Signs or symptoms of bowel obstruction, urinary obstruction, or pelvic recurrence warrant further investigation with small-bowel follow through, barium enema, intravenous urogram, renal ultrasound, pelvic ultrasound, or CT.

Selected Readings

Botsis D, Kassanos D, Pyrgiotis E et al. Vaginal sonography of the endometrium in postmenopausal women. *Clin Exp Obstet Gynecol* 19:189, 1992.

Bourne TH, Whitehead MI, Campbell S et al. Ultrasound screening for familial ovarian cancer. *Gynecol Oncol* 43:92, 1991.

Fleischer AC, Rodgers WH, Kepple DM et al. Color Doppler sonography of ovarian masses: A multiparameter analysis. *J Ultrasound Med* 12:41, 1993.

Granberg S, Norstrom A, Wikland M. Tumors in the lower pelvis as imaged by vaginal sonography. *Gynecol Oncol* 37:224, 1990.

Jacquet P, Jelinek JS, Steves MA et al. Evaluation of computed tomography in patients with peritoneal carcinomatosis. *Cancer* 72:1631, 1993.

Kurjak A, Zalud I, Alfirevic Z. Evaluation of adnexal masses with transvaginal color ultrasound. *J Ultrasound Med* 10:295, 1991.

Levine D, Gosink BB, Wolf SI et al. Simple adnexal cysts: The natural history in postmenopausal women. *Radiology* 184:653, 1992.

Lien HH, Blomlie V, Iversen T et al. Clinical stage I carcinoma of the cervix: Value of MR imaging in detecting invasion into the parametrium. *Acta Radiologica* 34:130, 1993.

Lien HH, Blomlie V, Tropé C et al. Cancer of the endometrium: Value of MR imaging in determining depth of invasion into the myometrium. *AJR Am J Roentgenol* 157:1221, 1991.

Stomper PC. *Cancer Imaging Manual*. Philadelphia: Lippincott, 1993.

Surwit EA, Childers JM, Krag DN et al. Clinical assessment of In-CYT-103 immunoscintigraphy in ovarian cancer. *Gynecol Oncol* 48:285, 1993.

Valentin L, Sladkevicius P, Marsal K. Limited contribution of Doppler velocimetry to the differential diagnosis of extrauterine pelvic tumors. *Obstet Gynecol* 83:425, 1994.

VanNagell JR Jr, Higgins RV, Donaldson ES et al. Transvaginal sonography as a screening method for ovarian cancer. *Cancer* 65:573, 1990.

Yamashita Y, Takahashi M, Sawada T et al. Carcinoma of the cervix: Dynamic MR imaging. *Radiology* 182:643, 1992.

VII
Critical Care

20

Critical Care in Gynecologic Oncology

Oscar A. de Leon-Casasola and
Kathleen A. O'Leary

Recent studies have elucidated the pathophysiology of several problems experienced by critically ill patients. The role of cytokines in the clinical presentation of septic shock and systemic inflammatory response syndrome (SIRS) is now more clear. Studies are under way to determine the role of specific therapy targeted against these mediators that ultimately result in organ failure. Thus, until more data are available, treatment of the critically ill patient is limited to providing adequate alveolar ventilation, adequate tissue oxygenation, and nutritional support. If these three goals are achieved, the patient is supported during the healing process.

This chapter discusses current concepts in hemodynamic monitoring and management of patients who develop septic shock and SIRS, and adult respiratory distress syndrome (ARDS). The perioperative management of patients with coagulopathies and the use of blood and blood component therapy is discussed.

Preoperative Evaluation and Optimization

PULMONARY FUNCTION

Preoperative pulmonary screening is used to identify patients at risk for increased morbidity and mortality from pulmonary complications to measure inspiratory and expiratory mechanics and to assess ventilatory reserve.

History and Physical Examination

Several risk factors for pulmonary complications can be identified preoperatively: history of smoking, history of bronchospasm and wheezing, large amount of bronchial secretions, and changes in the color of sputum.

Smoking is a well-recognized preoperative risk factor for the development of postoperative pulmonary complications. Mucus hypersecretion, impairment of tracheobronchial secretion clearance, and small-airway narrowing are three major mechanisms by which smoking may increase perioperative morbidity. Moreover, smokers have a higher closing capacity, increasing the risk of atelectasis. Patients who stop smoking for more than 6 weeks before surgery will experience a decrease in the production of bronchial secretions. Moreover, an increase in the ability to clear secretions will occur due to regeneration of the ciliary epithelium in the tracheobronchial tree. These two factors are associated with a dramatic decrease in the incidence of postoperative pulmonary complications. Conversely, acute smoking abstinence (<2 weeks) will not have an impact on the incidence of postoperative pulmonary complications. However, cessation of smoking for at least 48 hours preoperatively results in a decrease in the levels of carboxyhemoglobin. Carboxyhemoglobin levels in smokers vary between 5% and 8% (nonsmokers = 2.5%). The acute decrease in carboxyhemoglobin results in an increase in tissue oxygen delivery.

Most patients who have bronchospasms (or wheezing) are very aware of the degrees of airway obstruction and chest tightness and the medications that relieve these symptoms. If the amount of bronchospasm reported by the patient in the 48 hours before surgery has increased or the physical examination reveals significant wheezing, optimization of bronchodilator therapy is indicated before surgery.

The amount of bronchial secretions has a direct impact on the incidence of postoperative atelectasis. Thus, if copious amounts are reported by the patient, a few days of pulmonary therapy and secretion removal are indicated.

Finally, if the color of the sputum has changed from clear to yellow or green, sputum culture and sensitivity testing and appropriate antibiotic therapy are indicated.

With these simple measures, the postoperative incidence of atelectasis and pneumonias can be significantly reduced, thus improving patient recovery and final outcome. Moreover, preoperative patients who present with any of the aforementioned variables should undergo further testing in order to stratify their perioperative risk.

Pulmonary Function Tests

Within the context of the proposed surgical procedure, the purpose of pulmonary function testing is to identify those patients at risk of developing postoperative respiratory complications such as atelectasis, pneumonias, increasing dyspnea, cor pulmonale, or acute respiratory failure.

Spirometry

Spirometry will enable the clinician to determine several lung volumes. The discussion of the technique and the different measurements obtained is beyond the scope of this chapter. However, it is important to note the values that increase the risk of postoperative pulmonary complications:

1. Maximum breathing capacity (MBC) less than 50% of predicted value.
2. Forced expiratory volume in one second (FEV_1) of less than 2 liters or 50% of either predicted value or vital capacity (VC).
3. Peak expiratory flow rate of less than 200 liters/min^{-1}.
4. Mid-maximum expiratory flow (MMEF or FEV_{25-75}) of less than 1.2 liters or 40% of the predicted value.

Arterial Blood Gases

Arterial blood gas values associated with a high risk of postoperative morbidity are (1) a $PaCO_2$ greater than 45 mm Hg and (2) a PaO_2 lower than 50 mm Hg.

Doppler Echocardiography

The vast majority of patients with a smoking history will have varying degrees of chronic obstructive pulmonary disease (COPD). Other chronic pulmonary ailments may also result in the chronic alveolar and airway changes of COPD (e.g., asthma). The cardiovascular changes associated with COPD are pulmonary hypertension and increased pulmonary vascular resistance, which may result in varying degrees of right ventricular dilatation, hypertrophy, or even failure (cor pulmonale). Some degree of tricuspid regurgitation is present in the majority of patients with pulmonary artery systolic pressures greater than 35 mm Hg. The noninvasive estimation of pulmonary artery systolic pressure is helpful in the diagnosis and management of all causes of pulmonary hypertension including COPD. The degree of pulmonary hypertension negatively affects perioperative prognosis in patients with COPD. Thus, complete preoperative pulmonary function testing should include tricuspid evaluation via Doppler echocardiography. Moreover, the peak velocity of the tricuspid regurgitant jet may be used to calculate pulmonary artery systolic pressure (PAP) using the formula

$$PAP = 14 + 4(V)^2$$

where PAP is measured in mm Hg and V is the peak tricuspid regurgitant velocity in meters per second.

Once all this information is obtained, the perioperative pulmonary risk associated with general anesthesia and surgery can be estimated. More important, perioperative techniques designed to lower this risk may be used so that surgery can be performed in a safer manner.

CARDIOVASCULAR FUNCTION

Considering the age, obesity, history of smoking, and frequently sedentary life-style of a great percentage of patients affected with gynecologic cancer, it is not surprising that coronary artery disease (CAD) is prevalent in this population. Thus, CAD has important prognostic implications in this population, as it is the most frequent cause of perioperative left ventricular dysfunction. Moreover, the use of chemotherapeutic agents such as doxorubicin may further aggravate perioperative ventricular dysfunction.

It appears that recent (<6 months) myocardial infarction and current congestive heart failure are the only two consistently proven preoperative predictors of perioperative cardiac morbidity. Thus, under ideal circumstances, surgery should be delayed for 6 months after a myocardial infarction and until signs of congestive heart failure have disappeared (e.g., S_3, S_4 gallops, hepatojugular signs, pulmonary edema).

Patients with a history of exposure to doxorubicin or with two or more of the high risk factors for CAD should undergo noninvasive testing (Table 20-1). Two-dimensional echocardiography is a sensitive and specific test for the evaluation of left ventricular ejection fraction (LVEF), valvular function, regional wall motion and thickening (a sign of myocardial ischemia), and intrinsic disease of the heart. Preoperative ventricular dysfunction (ejection fraction <50%) or segmental wall-motion abnormalities predict perioperative ventricular dysfunction. Thus, patients with these abnormalities should have a cardiology consult and undergo further work-up as indicated. Moreover, perioperative hemodynamic monitoring is indicated in these high-risk patients because it is important to determine the degree of cardiac compromise before the surgical procedure and because high-risk patients benefit from supranormal hemodynamics.

Table 20-1. Preoperative cardiac risk factors: Historical

Age: >60 with a poor physiologic status
Previous myocardial infarction (<6 mos)
Previous myocardial infarction (>6 mos)
Angina
Congestive heart failure
Hypertension
Diabetes mellitus
Dysrhythmias
Peripheral vascular disease
Valvular heart disease
High cholesterol
Cigarette smoking
Previous coronary artery bypass graft surgery
Previous percutaneous transluminal coronary angioplasty
Cardiovascular therapy with beta-blocker or calcium channel blocker

Hemodynamic Monitoring

INDICATIONS AND GOALS OF THERAPY

Hemodynamic monitoring of the critically ill patient has been developed to assess intravascular volume (preload), pump function (contractility), and vascular resistance (afterload). New technological advances have introduced oximetry and right ventricular ejection fraction (RVEF) measurements into clinical practice. With this information, a more physiologic evaluation of the critically ill patient is possible.

Instead of delineating clinical conditions as indications for hemodynamic monitoring, a physiologic approach is more rational. Thus, the following are indications for the perioperative insertion of a pulmonary artery (PA) catheter:

1. Assessment of intravascular volume status
2. Measurement of cardiac output
3. Measurement of tissue oxygenation and global use of oxygen (mixed-venous saturation) by the periphery
4. Determination of the impact of therapeutic decisions on derived hemodynamic parameters
5. Achievement of a "supranormal" hemodynamic status

This physiologic approach is based on the suggestion that both the survival and the incidence of multiple organ failure in postsurgical high-risk critically ill patients may be positively affected by achieving "supranormal" therapeutic goals. These goals include: cardiac index (CI) greater than 4.5 $liters.min^{-1}.m^{-2}$, oxygen delivery ($\dot{D}O_2$) greater than 600 $ml.min^{-1}.m^{-2}$, and oxygen consumption ($\dot{V}O_2$) greater than 179 $ml.min^{-1}.m.^{-2}$ Thus, it would appear that postoperative high-risk patients and patients with sepsis or SIRS should have their preload, contractility, and afterload optimized as delineated below to achieve the aforementioned supranormal values.

The concepts of $\dot{D}O_2$ (tissue oxygenation) and $\dot{V}O_2$ (tissue use of oxygen) are examples of how our use of PA catheters has been expanded. It also illustrates that assessing PaO_2 is no longer enough. These two variables can be easily calculated as follows:

$$\dot{D}O_2 = CI \times CaO_2 \text{ (arterial oxygen content)} \times 10$$

$$CaO_2 = \text{hemoglobin} \times \text{arterial oxyhemoglobin saturation } (SpO_2) \times 1.34$$

$$\dot{V}O_2 = CI \times CvO_2 \text{ (mixed venous oxygen content)} \times 10$$

$$CvO_2 = \text{hemoglobin} \times \text{mixed venous oxyhemoglobin saturation } (SpvO_2) \times 1.34$$

Intravascular Volume Status

The first step in the optimization of DO_2 (assuming that SpO_2 >90% and hemoglobin (Hb) >10 g/dl^{-1}) is the optimization of CI. Both in the normal and in the failing heart, preload optimization will result in the improvement of cardiac function, according to the Frank-Starling law. Thus, in patients with hypotension and/or signs of inadequate tissue perfusion, the protocol depicted in Fig. 20-1 is recommended. With the use of the volumetric PA catheter, measurements of RVEF and RV stroke volume index (SVI) will avoid RV overdistention, which results in impairment of LV function and increases myocardial oxygen consumption. With the standard PA catheter, the construction of a curve in which pulmonary artery occlusion pressure (PAOP) is plotted against LVSVI is necessary. When LVSVI increases are not significant despite an increase in PAOP, bolus fluid administration should be stopped because LV distention also results in an increase in LV myocardial oxygen consumption. Moreover, if intracavitary pressures (PAOP) greater than 22–25 mm Hg are achieved, the incidence of myocardial infarction increases. This is presumably because high intracavitary pressures decrease subendocardial blood flow, with myocardial ischemia as the end result.

In summary, it is not physiologically acceptable to set normal or abnormal filling pressure values since each patient will follow a different Starling curve, thus needing a different level of filling pressures. Accordingly, continuous evaluation of the SVI-PAOP relation must be done in every patient to optimize preload.

Cardiac Output

Once preload has been optimized, if DO_2 is still inadequate, myocardial contractility should be evaluated.

In critically ill patients, CI of less than 4.5 liters.min^{-1}.m^{-2} should be aggressively treated. This is particularly important during the first 24 postoperative hours as the incidence of cumulative oxygen deficit that results in multiple organ failure and death will occur during this time interval. Steps to improve myocardial contractility include inotropic support and/or afterload reduction.

Inotropic Agents

SYMPATHOMIMETIC AGENTS. Sympathomimetic agents are potent inotropic agents. Both clinical responses and side effects are the products of stimulation of beta-adrenergic receptors in the myocardium. The most important side effect is the induction of both supraventricular and ventricular dysrhythmias. They usually appear at high dose.

Dopamine is an endogenous catecholamine with dose-dependent effects: 2–3 μg.kg^{-1}.min^{-1} produces mesenteric and renal vasodilata-

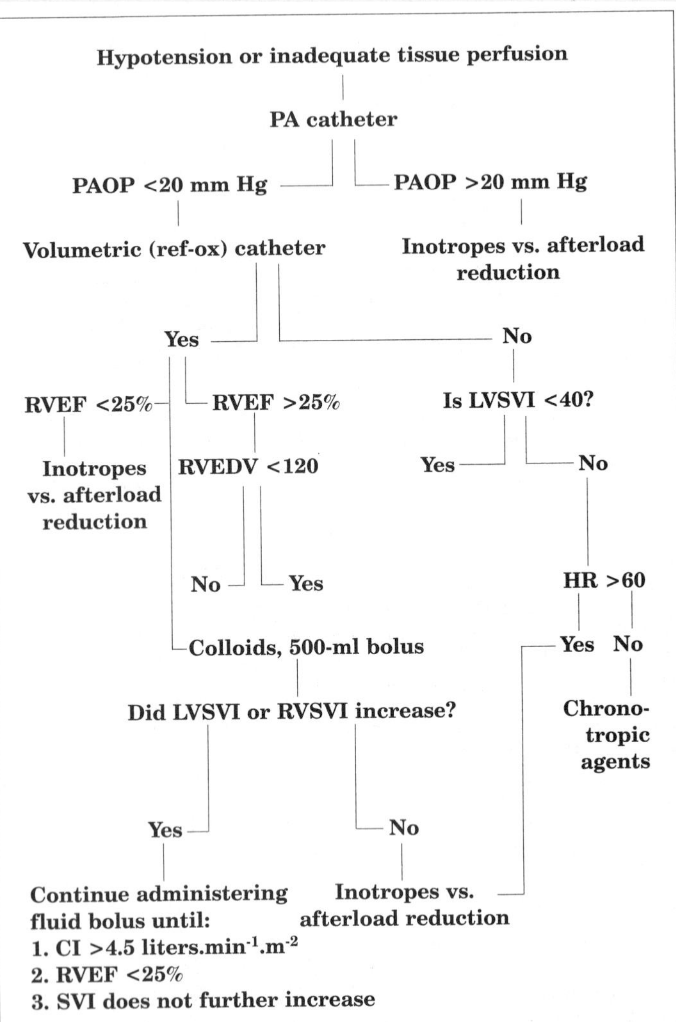

Fig. 20-1. Protocol for inadequate tissue perfusion or hypotension. (PA = pulmonary artery; PAOP = pulmonary artery occlusion pressure; RVEF = right ventricular ejection fraction; LVSVI = left ventricular stroke volume index; RVSVI = right ventricular stroke volume index; RVEDV = right ventricular end diastolic volume; HR = heart rate; CI = cardiac index.)

tion via dopaminergic receptor stimulation. Doses of 5–10 μg.kg^{-1}.min^{-1} produce beta$_1$-adrenergic receptor stimulation. Consequently, cardiac inotropic effects are noted within these doses. Conversely, doses greater than 10 μg.kg^{-1}.min^{-1} are associated with alpha-adrenergic receptor stimulation and peripheral vasoconstriction that may result in a significant decrease of cardiac output.

Dobutamine is a synthetic drug that also stimulates beta$_1$-adrenergic receptors. Thus, dose-dependent direct inotropic stimulation results in reflex peripheral vasodilatations with afterload reduction and increase in cardiac output. Therapeutic effects are seen at doses of 5–10 μg.kg^{-1}.min^{-1}. However, doses of up to 30 μg.kg^{-1}.min^{-1} have been used to achieve a hyperdynamic state. Tachycardia may result from excessive doses, afterload reduction, or a decrease in left ventricular filling pressures, which is associated with improved left ventricular performance. Dobutamine should not be used in patients with low cardiac output due to diastolic dysfunction such as hypertrophic cardiomyopathy or high-output heart failure. Synergistic effects between dopamine and dobutamine have been demonstrated. Thus, they can be used simultaneously when both inotropic support and afterload reduction is desired.

PHOSPHODIESTERASE INHIBITORS. Phosphodiesterase inhibitors produce an increase in myocardial contractility and peripheral vasodilatation by increasing intracellular cyclic adenosine monophosphate (AMP).

Amrinone has hemodynamic effects similar to dobutamine. Following a loading dose of 0.75 mg.kg^{-1} over 2–3 minutes, a continuous infusion of 5–10 μg.kg^{-1}.min^{-1} is used. These doses are also associated with a decrease in calculated pulmonary vascular resistance due to an increase in RV contractility and not to a direct vasodilatory effect on the pulmonary circulation. Synergistic effects may also be obtained when amrinone is combined with dopamine or dobutamine since they differ in the mechanism of action. However, severe peripheral vasodilatation and hypotension may also result. Thus, judicious use of this combination is suggested with continuing evaluations of afterload and blood pressure changes.

Side effects of amrinone include tachycardia and atrial and ventricular dysrhythmias. Hypotension may occur in patients receiving other vasodilators or in patients with inadequate preload optimization. Thrombocytopenia occurs due to a decrease in platelet life span.

Vasodilators

Vasodilators are used to unload the heart and increase cardiac output. Adequate blood flow to vital organs is maintained at perfusion pressures above 60 mm Hg if no local perfusion abnormalities exist.

Nitroglycerin produces an increase in venous capacitance and minimally affects afterload. Onset of action is rapid, and half-life is only 1–3 minutes, allowing for rapid titration. Infusions are commenced at 0.25 μg.kg^{-1}.min^{-1} and titrated up to 4 μg.kg^{-1}.min^{-1}. Higher doses may be associated with severe hypotension without any benefits to coronary flow. Adverse effects include increased intracranial pressure in patients with low intracranial compliance (e.g., edema, tumor) and increased pulmonary shunting (except in patients with severe COPD).

Sodium nitroprusside (SNP) is the most effective afterload-reducing agent. It has a rapid onset, consistent effects, and short half-life. Doses of 0.5–8.0 μg.kg^{-1}.min^{-1} are recommended. Adverse effects include cyanide (CN) and thiocyanate toxicity, rebound hypertension, intracranial hypertension, blood coagulation abnormalities, increased pulmonary shunting with hypoxia (except in patients with severe COPD), and hypothyroidism. Moreover, myocardial, liver, and skeletal muscle oxygen reserves are decreased and the mitochondria may be damaged. Toxic blood CN toxic levels occur when more than 1 $mg.kg^{-1}$ is administered within 2 1/2 hours or when doses greater than 0.5 $mg.kg^{-1}.hr^{-1}$ (8 $\mu g.kg^{-1}.min^{-1}$) are administered within 24 hours. A greater risk of CN toxicity exists in patients with vitamin B_{12} deficiency or with dietary substances containing sulfur. In patients at risk for toxicity or in those receiving high doses of SNP, blood CN and pH measurements are indicated. Treatment of toxicity consists of IV thiosulfate (150–200 $mg.kg^{-1}$) except in patients with abnormal renal function when hydroxicobalamin is recommended.

LIMITATIONS AND PITFALLS

The direct relationship between PAOP and left ventricular end diastolic volume (LVEDV) is the basis for PA catheter monitoring. During diastole, while the mitral valve is open, a static column of blood between the inflated balloon of the PA catheter and the left ventricle is formed. Under these normal circumstances one can assume that PAOP = PVP = left atrial pressure (LAP) = left ventricular end diastolic pressure (LVEDP) = LVEDV. However, several clinical conditions will affect this relationship.

COMPLICATIONS OF PULMONARY ARTERY CATHETERIZATION

Inadvertent arterial puncture, pneumothorax, venous thrombosis or phlebitis (septic or aseptic), local infection, air embolism, cardiac dysrhythmias and bundle branch block, pulmonary infarction, and pulmonary artery rupture are all complications associated with the use of PA catheters. It is noteworthy that patients with a preinsertion left bundle branch block (LBBB) may experience complete heart blocks upon insertion of the PA catheter. Thus, percutaneous pacing should be readily available during insertion of PA catheters in patients with a diagnosis of complete LBBB.

Septic Shock-Systemic Inflammatory Response Syndrome

PATHOPHYSIOLOGY

When bacteria release endotoxins [lipopolysaccharides (LPSs)], an interaction between LPSs and LPS-binding protein (LBP) occurs. This complex then interacts with the surface protein of macrophages, CD-14, which provides the signal for initiation of macrophage function and the synthesis and release of tumor necrosis factor (TNF) and interleukin (IL-1) in bacteremic shock. It appears that the characteristic hemodynamic abnormalities and organ dysfunction in endotoxic shock are produced in response to TNF and IL-1 release stimulated by endotoxins.

DIAGNOSIS

It is important to define the different disorders associated with sepsis for better diagnosis and treatment. *Sepsis* is defined as the suspicion of infection accompanied by the systemic response including tachypnea, tachycardia, and hypothermia or hyperthermia. *Sepsis syndrome* is defined as sepsis with evidence of inadequate organ perfusion. *Septic shock* is defined as sepsis syndrome with hypotension. Septic shock in turn may be hyperdynamic or hypodynamic.

TREATMENT

The results of clinical trials evaluating the effectiveness of human recombinant IL-1 receptor antagonist in the treatment of septic shock have been disappointing. Other agents that could potentially neutralize endotoxins are taurolidine, bactericidal/permeability-increasing protein (BPI), lipid X, and soluble CD14. However, there are no data documenting their effectiveness in humans. Thus, the current treatment of septic shock consists of the prompt initiation of antibiotic therapy and the institution of adequate hemodynamic support. The institution of adequate hemodynamic support is widely accepted. However, what constitutes "adequate" support is controversial since less is known about the mechanisms that regulate systemic hemodynamics and, more important, regional tissue perfusion during sepsis.

The use of supranormal hemodynamic values in septic shock is less than ideal since they do not account for particular oxygen requirements. Current recommendations are aimed at the maximization of DO_2 by preload optimization and the combination of inotropes (see the section on Hemodynamic Monitoring: Indications and Goals of Therapy). However, local metabolic responses, acting via mediators such as adenosine, endothelin, and nitric oxide, may affect neurogenic control of regional flow. Moreover, sepsis may affect cellular metabolism directly, preventing regional tissue oxygen use. Thus, until more sophisticated techniques to evaluate individual organ perfusion and oxygen use are available, the institution of a supranormal state appears to be indicated.

Adult Respiratory Distress Syndrome

DIAGNOSIS

Adult respiratory distress syndrome (ARDS) represents a specific symptom or manifestation of generalized sepsis or SIRS. Pneumonia, aspiration syndrome, and respiratory dysfunction following prolonged surgical procedures may mimic ARDS. However, ARDS specifically occurs as a result of alterations in the capillary membrane, while the others begin within the alveoli.

Patients with ARDS will frequently exhibit alterations in ventilation/perfusion ($\dot{V}/\dot{Q}$) ratios, hypoxemia, decreased lung compliance, and high PA pressures with varying degrees of RV failure.

TREATMENT

Mechanical Ventilation

Mechanical ventilation is the mainstay of therapy to maximize oxygenation. Indications for mechanical ventilation for both ARDS patients as well as for patients in respiratory failure are essentially the same:

1. Inability to maintain adequate oxygenation (SpO_2 >90%) with a partial rebreathing mask despite high levels of FIO_2 (>60%)

2. Rising $PaCO_2$ (>50 mm Hg) with a pH less than 7.3
3. Significant tachypnea (respiratory rate >30/minute) or dyspnea associated with excessive work of breathing

Instituting Mechanical Ventilation

Methods such as conventional controlled mechanical ventilation (CMV), assisted mechanical ventilation (AMV), and inverse I:E ratio ventilation (IRV) provide a fixed level of ventilatory support. Conversely, intermittent mandatory ventilation (IMV), pressure support ventilation (PSV), proportional assist ventilation (PAV), and airway pressure release ventilation (APRV) allow administration of any level of ventilatory support. Choice of a ventilation method depends on the patient's clinical condition. Whenever possible, partial levels of ventilatory support should be used to allow patients to have some spontaneous breathing. This technique will result in lower levels of cardiac impairment, and underdevelopment of respiratory muscles will not occur. Conversely, if the work of breathing is very high, as judged by a rapid respiratory rate, use of accessory muscles of respiratory, and nasal flaring, then fixed ventilatory assistance is indicated. FIO_2 levels should be maintained at the lowest possible level (usually 30–50%) so that oxygen toxicity is avoided. The goal of therapy is to use the lowest level of FIO_2 to produce a PaO_2 greater than 60 mm Hg. The ventilatory rate should be adjusted to maintain a $PaCO_2$ between 35 and 45 mm Hg.

Animal and human investigations over the past two decades have led to the consensus that patients with ARDS should be supported with the lowest levels of positive end-expiratory pressure (PEEP) required to optimize compliance and the FIO_2 to be limited to 0.5 or less. Direct animal data and inferential human data support the notion that overdistention of alveoli leads to further lung injury. Thus, several strategies are in vogue.

CONTROL OF MEAN AIRWAY PRESSURE. The duration of inspiration, peak inspiratory pressures, and levels of PEEP contribute to the control of mean airway pressure (PAW). It is recommended that peak inspiratory pressure and plateau (end-inspiratory occlusion) pressure be kept below 40 and 35 cm H_2O, respectively. Two situations may arise when this strategy is followed:

1. *Permissive hypoxemia.* Traditionally, the goal of therapy has been to maintain the PaO_2 above 60 mm Hg (SpO_2 >90%). However, to avoid high FIO_2 (>50%) or PEEP levels (>15 cm H_2O), PaO_2 levels of 50–60 mm Hg are now accepted, provided cardiovascular function and hemoglobin levels are adequate. Thus, a clinical decision between the risk of lung injury and the effects of cellular oxygenation must be made. However, if patients develop evidence of metabolic acidosis under this therapeutic modality, the management should be modified.
2. *Permissive hypercapnia.* This concept is based on the assumption that with a volume variable ventilation mode, one can use a limiting airway pressure below which alveolar overdistention occurs. While using an appropriate level of PEEP and FIO_2, the tidal volume (5–7 $ml.kg^{-1}$, instead of the traditional 10–15 $ml.kg^{-1}$), the ventilator rate (usually <18 bpm), the I:E ratio, and the working inspiratory pressure are manipulated to optimize minute volume. This avoids auto-PEEP (gas trapping) so that plateau pressures are maintained below 35 cm H_2O. Monitoring auto-PEEP is important because in order for

patients to trigger the ventilator, they need to generate a negative pressure equal to the sum of auto-PEEP plus the level of the ventilator-selected sensitivity. A goal of therapy in patients with permissive hypercapnia without severe cardiac disease is to maintain the arterial blood pH at 7.25 or greater.

To limit plateau and/or peak inspiratory pressures, two techniques are available: limiting the working pressure of the ventilator or using pressure-controlled ventilation. Limiting the working pressure of the ventilator allows the use of any mode of ventilation. Essentially, the tidal volume is limited by a predetermined peak inspiratory pressure. Thus, tidal volume will be determined by the patient's pulmonary compliance and the preset peak airway pressure. Pressure-controlled ventilation differs from limiting the working pressure of the ventilator in that it is *time* initiated and *time* cycled. The final product is the same. Tidal volume is thus affected by the same variables.

LIMITING THE LEVEL OF POSITIVE END-EXPIRATORY PRESSURE. Patients with ARDS benefit from PEEP therapy because of the following:

1. PaO_2 increases due to a reduction in intrapulmonary shunt whereby lung water is redistributed from the alveoli to the interstitial space.
2. The work of breathing and thus $\dot{V}O_2$ are reduced as a result of tidal breathing moving to a more compliant portion of the volume-pressure curve.
3. Further lung injury is possibly decreased as PEEP stabilizes the alveoli, thus avoiding the high shear pressures associated with the repeated closing and opening of alveolar units during high peak ventilatory pressures. However, high levels of PEEP may also potentially result in alveolar overdistention and thus barotrauma, particularly in patients maintained in the supine position. Moreover, decreases in cardiac output and thus $\dot{D}O_2$ may occur due to a decrease in venous return and a decrease in left ventricular compliance. This occurs due to the shift of the interventricular septum into the left ventricle produced by the increase in the RV afterload, and by the increase of juxtacardiac pressure resulting from distended lungs.

In view of these changes, it is suggested that in patients with ARDS, PEEP levels should be maintained lower than 15 cm H_2O. Moreover, patients treated with PEEP levels greater than 7.5–10.0 cm H_2O should receive hemodynamic monitoring with a PA catheter to optimize preload, contractility, and thus $\dot{D}O_2$ and $\dot{V}O_2$.

WEANING FROM MECHANICAL VENTILATION

Weaning from mechanical ventilation is the gradual withdrawal of mechanical ventilatory support. Successful weaning depends on the cardiovascular, respiratory, and nutritional status of the patient, as well as her general condition. Patients who have experienced short periods of mechanical ventilatory support usually wean very easily. Conversely, patients who have received prolonged respiratory support or patients with moderate to severe chronic lung disease, marginal respiratory function, or incompletely resolved respiratory process may experience more difficulty. It is important to recognize that decreasing mechanical ventilatory support too early or too fast during the acute illness that prompted the use of ventilation support may induce respiratory muscle fatigue. Muscle fatigue will invariably result in weaning failure. Concerns that long periods of

Table 20-2. Protocol for endotracheal intubation and initiation of mechanical ventilation

1. Prepare endotracheal tube, laryngoscope, and suction system.
2. Clear the airway of secretions. Place an oral airway.
3. Assist ventilate with an Ambu bag attached to high-flow O_2.
4. Attempt laryngoscopy and tracheal intubation.
5. If unsuccessful within 20 seconds, stop and resume ventilation as in number 3, then repeat attempt.
6. Inflate the cuff and ventilate with the Ambu bag.
7. Auscultate over chest and stomach for proper placement.
8. Get a chest x-ray to confirm position of the tip of the tube.
9. Secure the airway with tape and suction using sterile technique.
10. Order initial ventilation settings:
    FIO_2 80–100%
    Tidal volume 5–10 $ml.kg^{-1}$
    Synchronized intermittent mandatory ventilation or AC mode at 8–12 bpm
11. Ensure proper alarms, humidifier function, and pressure limits.
12. Remain at bedside for initial adjustments based on the patient's level of comfort. Do further adjustments to meet patient's respiratory requirements.
13. Check arterial blood gas 20–30 minutes later. Make additional ventilator adjustments.

respiratory muscle disuse may induce atrophy and cause ventilatory dependence are generally unwarranted. Thus, it is recommended to begin weaning the patient from the ventilator as her overall condition improves. Table 20-2 delineates some guidelines for assessing weaning from ventilatory support, though some patients (particularly COPD patients) may be weaned despite failure to meet these criteria. If the first attempt to wean fails, one or more of the following conditions is usually implicated: incompletely treated pulmonary infection, bronchospasm, excessive tracheobronchial secretions, depressed CI, respiratory muscle weakness (poor nutritional status), small endotracheal tubes, and residual SIRS or sepsis with high mechanical ventilation requirements.

Weaning After Oxygenation Failure

Weaning after oxygenation failure primarily involves the decrease of PEEP (usually in 2.5-cm decrements) and $FIIO_2$ (usually in 5–10% decrements) until the patient can sustain a PaO_2 greater than 60 mm Hg on an FIO_2 lower than 50% and a PEEP lower than 5 cm H_2O. Once this point is reached, extubation can be considered after a trial of 20–30 minutes of unassisted ventilation (T-piece or Briggs).

Weaning After Ventilation Failure

Weaning after ventilation failure involves careful adjustments of tidal volume and rate. Several weaning methods are available that have the advantage of minimizing the hemodynamic adverse effects of positive pressure ventilation by allowing increasing amounts of spontaneous breathing.

Pressure Support Ventilation

PSV may be the preferred method when respiratory muscle weakness appears to be compromising weaning. The patient's spontaneous inspiration triggers the ventilator to provide a variable flow of gas that increases until airway pressure reaches a preselected level. When patient demand for inspiratory flow is reduced (usually 25% of initial value), circuit flow is terminated and airway pressure remains to baseline. Thus, upon the patient's triggering, the assisted breath is pressure-limited and flow-cycled. The ventilator's work of breathing during inspiration depends on the pressure level and the patient's respiratory mechanics. During full assistance (high-pressure support level of usually 20–30 cm), most to all of the work of breathing is performed by the ventilator. Conversely, on low levels (5–8 cm), most of the work of breathing is carried out by the patient. The levels of PSV are individual and change from patient to patient. Thus, bedside titration of the level of support (to a tidal volume of 5–10 $ml.kg^{-1}$) is the best way to determine the initial level of pressure support required. The major theoretical advantage of PSV is adjustable breath to breath ventilatory assistance. This enables controlled weaning from the ventilator's support and facilitates coupling between the patient and the ventilator. Since the patient determines frequency and duration of inspiration, development of respiratory alkalosis is unlikely.

Intermittent Mandatory Ventilation

IMV allows weaning from mechanical ventilation by gradually decreasing the ventilator rate while allowing simultaneous, unrestricted, unassisted spontaneous breathing to occur. Control of ventilation is achieved by increasing the frequency of mandatory breaths, until $PaCO_2$ is lowered below the apneic threshold and the patient's spontaneous respiratory drive ceases. The mandatory breaths during IMV may be delivered in a synchronized or nonsynchronized mode. During synchronized IMV (SIMV), the mechanical breaths are triggered by the patient, if spontaneous respiratory efforts occur as preselected. SIMV was designed to avoid "stacking" of mechanical and spontaneous breaths, which are of no clinical significance.

The major drawback of IMV is that not all spontaneous breaths are assisted. This underscores the importance of the functional characteristics of the circuit. If the ventilatory circuit has high flow resistance, low flow capability, or a poorly functioning demand valve, the resulting spontaneous work of breathing may be so high that it precludes spontaneous breathing. Such ventilators *should not* be used for IMV but only to provide full ventilatory support.

Likewise, in patients with poor pulmonary therapy, the intrinsic respiratory work may be so high to allow for any unassisted breaths. There is a small group of patients in whom, despite optimization of ventilatory mechanics and intrinsic respiratory characteristics, spontaneous work of breathing remains so high that total ventilatory support is required.

Extubation

Once PSV has weaned down to 5–8 cm or IMV down to four breaths per minute and guidelines for assessing the withdrawal of mechanical ventilation have been met, tracheal extubation can be performed.

Extubation and Weaning Failure

Tracheobronchial Secretions

Inadequately treated pulmonary infections and insufficient pulmonary toilet will result in an excessive amount of secretions. They may worsen $\dot{V}/\dot{Q}$ mismatch and increase airway resistance, which results in an increase in the work of breathing and a decrease in gas exchange. Treatment should be directed to the triggering entity, as well as to providing adequate pulmonary toilet.

Inspiratory Muscle Fatigue

Common causes leading to inspiratory muscle fatigue include (1) increased work of breathing due to uncontrolled or persisting underlying disease, (2) poor nutritional status, (3) decreased oxygen delivery (hypoxemia and/or decreased CI), (4) incorrect weaning methods, and (5) metabolic disturbances (severe hypophosphatemia, hypokalemia, or hypomagnesemia).

Upper Airway Obstruction

Glottic and subglottic edema may manifest as inspiratory stridor in the first 24 hours postextubation. A trial dose of 2.5% racemic epinephrine (0.5% ml in 3 ml of normal saline) is indicated if the patient's clinical condition allows it. If successful, treatment may be repeated twice every 20–30 minutes as needed. Conversely, if there is no rapid clinical response, reintubation is indicated. Extubation *should not* be attempted for another 48–72 hours. Steroids are occasionally indicated. However, it is not clear which patients may benefit from this therapy. Patients who experience upper airway obstruction after prolonged intubation periods (>3 weeks) should be evaluated for subglottic stenosis and the need for tracheostomy.

Coagulation Abnormalities

PHYSIOLOGY OF COAGULATION AND PREOPERATIVE CONDITIONS LEADING TO PERIOPERATIVE HEMOSTATIC ABNORMALITIES

The treatment of coagulopathies requires an understanding of normal hemostasis and the factors that can disrupt it. In the critically ill patient, deficiencies of hemostasis are most often due to disseminated intravascular coagulation (DIC), massive blood transfusions, inadequate surgical hemostasis, liver disease, thrombocytopenia, and anticoagulants. Other conditions that should also be considered are vitamin K deficiency and uremia.

The major components of the coagulation system are the vasculature, platelets, protein coagulation cascade, and fibrinolysis.

When vascular endothelium is damaged, platelet exposure to collagen results in the activation and aggregation of platelets. The end result is formation of a platelet plug. The protein coagulation cascade is then activated, with fibrin deposition occurring around the platelet plug in order to build a stable clot. Concurrently, the fibrinolytic process is activated in order to limit clot formation. Thus, perioperative coagulopathies may occur due to platelet quantitative or qualitative defects and/or abnormalities in the coagulation cascade.

Perioperative qualitative platelet dysfunction may result from von Willebrand's disease or the use of nonsteroidal anti-inflammatory drugs (NSAIDs).

Platelets require von Willebrand factor (vWF) for normal adherence to collagen. Patients with von Willebrand's disease appear to lack the stimulus to produce factor vWF rather than the ability to produce it. This congenital disease has an autosomal dominant inheritance pattern with variable penetrance. Typically it is characterized by cyclic variability and severity. Treatment is based on the likelihood or severity of bleeding. In milder cases 1-deamino-8-arginine vasopressin (DDAVP) can produce an increase in vWF activity, at least transiently. For more severe cases, cryoprecipitate is the therapy of choice as it is rich in vWF.

More than half of patients undergoing unexpected surgery are using aspirin and other NSAIDs at the time of surgery. Aspirin irreversibly acetylates and inactivates the enzyme cyclooxygenase, which catalyzes the conversion of arachidonic acid to thromboxane A_2 and other prostaglandin intermediates. Thromboxane A_2 is a potent platelet aggregator. Thus, patients using aspirin will have a defect in platelet aggregation for the lifespan of the platelet (about 10 days), which will be manifested clinically as an increased bleeding time. Other NSAIDs cause similar defects in cyclooxygenase activity, but these are reversible and the effects are present only for the length of time that platelets are exposed to the drugs in the circulation.

Hemophilia A and B, the two most common forms of hemophilia, are sex-linked recessive congenital disorders and will not be found in the gynecologic population. As such, they are not discussed here. Other congenital disorders of coagulation are much more rare. The reader is referred to any textbook of hematology for a discussion of these disorders.

COMMON CAUSES OF COAGULOPATHIES IN THE INTENSIVE CARE UNIT

Disseminated Intravascular Coagulation

DIC is a process in which the coagulation system is activated by an underlying disease. Concurrent fibrin clot formation and fibrinolysis lead to increased consumption of coagulation factors, platelets, and ultimately red blood cells. Clinically, DIC manifests either subclinically with only laboratory abnormalities or as accelerated hemorrhage and/or thrombosis.

The treatment of DIC is to correct the triggering disease process, such as gram-negative septicemia, tumor destruction, hypotension, obstetric complications, fat embolism, and mismatched blood transfusions. Until the underlying process is controlled, administration of platelets, coagulation factors, fibrinogen, and packed red blood cells as needed is necessary. The diagnosis of DIC is made by the presence of increased fibrin degradation products (FDPs); decreased fibrinogen and platelets; and increase in the prothrombin, partial thromboplastin, and bleeding times.

The use of heparin in the treatment of DIC remains controversial. The basis for heparin administration is that it will interfere with clot formation, thus ending the consumption of platelets and coagulation factors. However, the use of heparin in an already bleeding patient is highly risky, particularly in the immediate postoperative period. If the risk-benefit ratio warrants its use, then it should be considered.

Success of therapy is monitored by the patient's clinical status and normalization of fibrinogen levels, FDP levels, platelet count, prothrombin time (PT), and partial thromboplastin time (PTT). DIC cannot be eliminated until the underlying process has been corrected.

Massive Blood Transfusions

Some patients will require significant blood product transfusions in the perioperative period. Up to 80% of the blood volume may be euvolemically lost before coagulopathies develop. Coagulation factors still provide adequate hemostasis, even when present at levels of only 20–30% of normal. Activity of factors V and VIII will decrease in stored whole blood after 21 days to 20–50% of normal, which is still adequate for hemostasis, but if whole blood is used for transfusion, then platelet activity should be considered virtually absent after 72 hours of storage.

Most commonly today, component blood therapy is used and intraoperative whole blood loss is replaced with packed red blood cells. This, in combination with increased platelet consumption due to clot formation, can result in severe thrombocytopenia and resultant coagulopathy in patients requiring massive transfusion. The most common cause of bleeding following massive blood transfusion is thrombocytopenia, not decreased clotting factors. As such, the treatment of bleeding in this situation is platelet transfusion, not fresh-frozen plasma (FFP).

Decreased Factor Formation: Vitamin K Deficiency and Liver Disease

All coagulation factors except factor VIII are synthesized in the liver. In addition, factors II, VII, IX, and X depend on vitamin K for their synthesis. Vitamin K is present in food (e.g., leafy, colored vegetables, fish, and alfalfa) but is also produced endogenously as a by-product of intestinal bacteria metabolism. As vitamin K is fat soluble, it requires bile salts for absorption.

Critically or chronically ill patients frequently experience vitamin K deficiency. Malnutrition, biliary disease, and sterilization of the intestinal tract secondary to antibiotic administration may be present, resulting in vitamin K deficiency and decreased production of the vitamin K–dependent factors. Both PT and PTT levels will be elevated. This coagulopathy will be improved within 4 hours and corrected 12–24 hours after appropriate vitamin K administration. However, if bleeding is present, then immediate transfusion of FFP is warranted to correct the coagulopathy.

If liver disease is present, all coagulation factors may be decreased, but the vitamin K–dependent factors are the most sensitive. In addition, hypersplenism may be present with resultant thrombocytopenia (Banti's syndrome). Moreover, liver disease can directly trigger DIC. As the liver will lack synthetic capabilities, bleeding due to factor deficiencies must be treated with FFP. Cryoprecipitate is indicated in severe cases or when fibrinogen levels are low, as the amount of fibrinogen present in FFP is inadequate to correct the deficit (roughly 200 mg in FFP, compared to 1,500 mg in cryoprecipitate).

Thrombocytopenia

Dilutional thrombocytopenia from massive blood transfusions is the most frequent cause of platelet dysfunction in the perioperative period. Coagulopathy from thrombocytopenia may result if platelet count decreases to less than 50,000/mm^3 in the perioperative period.

Decreased production occurs after the use of cytotoxic drugs and with sepsis. Sepsis can also cause increased destruction or consumption, as can DIC, idiopathic thrombocytopenia purpura, and certain drugs.

Of particular interest in the critically ill patient is heparin-induced thrombocytopenia. It has been reported to occur in 5% of patients treated with heparin, developing 5–10 days after initiation of therapy. This condition may be an asymptomatic laboratory finding or be associated with thrombosis, usually arterial. If thrombosis does occur, it is usually simultaneous with the development of thrombocytopenia.

Bovine heparin appears to produce thrombocytopenia three times more often than porcine heparin. Severe thrombocytopenia, thrombosis, and death have occurred in patients receiving mini-dose heparin, though this is rarely seen in patients treated for less than a week.

The development of severe thrombocytopenia with or without thrombosis necessitates the discontinuation of heparin therapy. This phenomenon can be avoided by concurrently beginning oral anticoagulation therapy to limit the duration of heparin therapy.

Anticoagulant Use

Heparin acts in conjunction with antithrombin III to inhibit factors IXa, Xa, XIa, and IIa. In critically ill patients, heparin is used most frequently in mini-doses of 5,000 units subcutaneously every 8–12 hours. This dosage has been shown to decrease the incidence of deep venous thrombosis in high-risk patients.

Intravenous heparin is used for treatment of deep venous thromboses and pulmonary emboli. Treatment is initiated with a loading dose of 5,000–10,000 units of heparin intravenously, followed by an infusion of 1,000–2,000 units/hour. Adequacy of therapy is monitored by frequent check of PTT levels, adjusting the infusion to maintain PTT at 1.5–2.0 times normal.

Occasionally, patients may appear refractory to heparin therapy. In this situation, antithrombin III deficiency should be suspected. The treatment for this condition is FFP, as it will increase antithrombin III levels and allow for anticoagulation with heparin.

In patients in whom heparin therapy must be quickly reversed due to emergency invasive procedures, bleeding complications, or accidental overdose, protamine administration is the treatment of choice. Protamine, itself an anticoagulant, will bind to heparin and inactivate it. One milligram of protamine neutralizes 80–100 units of heparin activity. However, caution should be exercised in two patient groups: (1) diabetic patients who have received protamine zinc insulin in the past, as they may be sensitized to protamine; and (2) patients with allergies to fish, as protamine is obtained from salmon. Thus, these patients should be observed for evidence of hypersensitivity reactions and anaphylaxis.

In patients receiving oral anticoagulants who develop bleeding complications or in whom invasive procedures are planned, therapy is aimed at restoring normal levels of functional vitamin K–dependent factors. If there is time and liver dysfunction is not suspected, vitamin K therapy should be instituted. Improvement in PT levels will be seen starting 4 hours after the first vitamin K dose. If there must be immediate reversal of drug effects as with ongoing bleeding or urgent invasive procedures, or if severe liver dysfunction is suspected, then FFP can be given to restore adequate levels of vitamin K–dependent factors.

Uremia

Bleeding can be a significant problem in patients with both chronic and acute renal failure. This is due to platelet dysfunction, which improves with dialysis.

Treatment of uremia-induced bleeding has been successful with cryoprecipitate, DDAVP, and conjugated estrogens. DDAVP improvement in platelet function occurs within 1 hour but lasts for only a few hours. Cryoprecipitate effects take 1–12 hours but last for 24 hours. The conjugated estrogens take 5–7 days before maximum effect is noted but last for 2 weeks. Therefore, conjugated estrogens may be the choice for elective procedures in uremic patients, whereas cryoprecipitate and especially DDAVP are more useful in the acute situation.

APPROACH TO THE CRITICALLY ILL PATIENT WITH A COAGULOPATHY

The following systemic approach is a recommended method to evaluate patients with perioperative coagulopathies:

1. Obtain the platelet count, PT, PTT, fibrinogen level, FDP level, and bleeding time.
2. Review the patient's history for the presence of drugs or conditions that may cause platelet dysfunction (e.g., aspirin and other NSAIDs, uremia, von Willebrand's disease).
3. Evaluate predisposing factors contributing to vitamin K deficiency (e.g., malnutrition, biliary tract obstruction, sterile intestinal tract due to broad-spectrum antibiotics).
4. Search for evidence of hepatic disease that may cause impaired synthesis of coagulation factors.
5. Confirm appropriate dosages of anticoagulants, if they are being used.

Once the etiology of the coagulopathy has been discovered or surmised, then therapy is based on the presence or likelihood of bleeding. If bleeding is present or invasive procedures are imminent, then blood component therapy will be necessary. If there is no evidence of bleeding and there is time before the invasive procedure, more conservative management is warranted.

MANAGEMENT OF THE CRITICALLY ILL PATIENT WHO IS BLEEDING

The use of component blood therapy has become much more common than the use of whole blood. Although component therapy is goal-directed, it greatly increases the risk of infection associated with each transfusion, as there is a different donor for each component and frequently multiple donors for certain components. Therefore, it is incumbent upon the treating physician to appropriately transfuse, recognizing the risks and benefits. The current recommendations for use of component therapy are reviewed here as they apply to critically ill patients:

Fresh-Frozen Plasma

FFP is defined as the fluid portion of 1 unit of human blood that has been centrifuged, separated, and frozen solid at −18°C within 6 hours of collection. Each unit of FFP is from a single donor. Its use should be limited to the following conditions:

1. *Replacement of factor deficiencies*. It is efficacious for the treatment of deficiencies of factors II, V, VII, IX, X, and XI when specific component therapy is neither available nor appropriate (e.g., acute liver failure).

2. *Reversal of warfarin effect.* In situations of active bleeding or emergency surgery, FFP should be used to reverse warfarin's effects and achieve immediate hemostasis.

3. *Massive blood transfusion* (>1 blood volume within several hours). Hemorrhage in this situation may also be due to thrombocytopenia. However, if factor deficiency is presumed to be a concurrent event, then FFP should be administered.

4. *Antithrombin III deficiency.* FFP can be used in patients undergoing surgery or in those who require heparin for treatment of thrombosis.

Platelets

Platelets can be harvested from single donors by platelet apheresis or separated from whole blood, with pooling of cells from multiple donors to achieve a therapeutic dose. The number of platelets obtained from a single-donor apheresis is roughly equivalent to the number obtained from five to eight whole blood donations. Transfusion of 1 unit of pooled or single-donor platelets can be expected to raise the platelet count by 7,000–10,000/mm^3.

Indications for platelet transfusion are as follows:

1. *Thrombocytopenia and/or platelet dysfunction in a patient who is actively bleeding.* In actively bleeding patients who have a platelet count of less than 50,000/mm^3, it is recommended to transfuse platelets. However, if the platelet count is greater than 50,000/mm^3, it is unlikely that the bleeding is due to the thrombocytopenia. Bleeding time (BT) can be used to determine platelet dysfunction. A BT of greater than twice normal usually indicates dysfunction of significant magnitude to warrant transfusion. A normal template BT is less than 10 minutes.

2. *Prophylactic platelet transfusion.* This is usually seen with patients receiving myelosuppressive therapy. A common number used as a threshold for transfusion is 20,000/mm^3. However, there are no studies that prove this to be the "correct number." In patients with chronic thrombocytopenia caused by impaired production or accelerated destruction, routine platelet transfusion is not usually needed. In anticipation of invasive procedures, platelet transfusions are frequently given and probably indicated, although there is no conclusive proof that a specific number of platelets are required for appropriate hemostasis.

3. *Massive transfusion.* Following the replacement of one blood volume, 35–40% of platelets usually remain. The majority of patients receiving massive transfusion of one to two blood volumes will not require platelet transfusion, unless there is evidence of increased destruction. In general, after massive transfusion, platelets should only be administered with documented thrombocytopenia and abnormal bleeding.

Packed Red Blood Cells

Packed red blood cells (PRBCs) are indicated *only* to increase oxygen-carrying capacity. The previously held belief that every patient should have a hemoglobin of 10 g.dl^{-1} and hematocrit of 30% has come under close scrutiny. In determining a patient's need for PRBC transfusion, one must evaluate the patient's cardiac and pulmonary status and overall state. In light of adequate cardiac output and oxygenation and the presence of a euvolemic state, the need to transfuse to a hemoglobin of 10 g/dl has not been demonstrated, and in fact, a hemoglobin of 7 g/dl may be adequate. However, in a patient with known myocardial ischemia or other conditions leading to tissue hypoperfusion, anemia is not well tolerated, nor should it be allowed to develop.

Cryoprecipitate

Cryoprecipitate is that fraction of plasma that precipitates when FFP is thawed. It can then be refrozen and stored for future use. It contains high concentrations of factor VIII and contains about 25% of the fibrinogen usually found in one unit of whole blood. Therefore, it is useful in the treatment of hemophilia A, von Willebrand's disease, and hypofibrinogenemic states. The most commonly encountered of these conditions is hypofibrinogenemia due to accelerated DIC.

CONCLUSIONS

Coagulopathies are frequently encountered in the critically ill patient. Careful examination of each of the components in the hemostasis system is necessary to ensure adequate therapy. Evaluation of platelet number and function, drug interactions, the development of DIC, vitamin K deficiency, and liver and renal disease should be performed as these are the most common etiologies of coagulopathies in this population. Knowledge of the risks and benefits of component therapy are also mandatory for safe management of these patients.

Selected Readings

Bone RC. Let's agree on terminology: Definitions of sepsis. *Crit Care Med* 19:973, 1991.

Consensus Conference. Fresh-frozen plasma: Indications and risks. *JAMA* 253:551, 1985.

Consensus Conference. Perioperative red blood cell transfusion. *JAMA* 260:2700, 1988.

Consensus Conference. Platelet transfusion therapy. *JAMA* 257:1777, 1987.

Ellison N. Coagulation. In JW Hoyt, AS Tonnesen, SJ Allen (eds), *Critical Care Practice*. Philadelphia: Saunders, 1991. Pp 295–304.

Guidelines Committee: Society of Critical Care Medicine. Guidelines for the care of patients with hemodynamic instability associated with sepsis. *Crit Care Med* 20:1057, 1992.

Hayes, MA, Timmins AC, Yau EHS et al. Elevation of systemic oxygen delivery in the treatment of critically ill patients. *N Engl J Med* 330:1717, 1994.

Larsen SF, Olesen KH, Jacobsen E et al. Prediction of cardiac risk in noncardiac surgery. *Eur Heart J* 8:179, 1987.

Members of the American College of Chest Physicians-Society of Critical Care Medicine Consensus Conference Committee. Definitions for sepsis and organ failure and guidelines for the use of innovative therapies in sepsis. *Crit Care Med* 20:864, 1992.

Mitchell C, Garrahy P, Peake P. Postoperative respiratory morbidity: Identification and risk factors. *Aust NZ J Surg* 52:203, 1982.

Tobin MT. Mechanical ventilation. *N Engl J Med* 330:1056, 1994.

VIII

Genetics

21

Principles of Tumor Genetics

Richard A. DiCioccio and Thomas B. Shows

The discipline of tumor genetics is a rapidly advancing field with major findings reported almost daily. The purpose of this chapter is to provide a fundamental background to enable clinicians to make sense of the burgeoning research reported in this field. Topics covered include a view of cancer as a genetic disease, genes involved in cancer, the acquisition of genetic changes leading to cancer, the inheritance of cancer, and the mapping and cloning of cancer predisposition genes.

Cancer is a generic name for a large array of diseases featuring abnormal cell growth and development leading to the formation of both solid and liquid cell masses. Benign tumors are restricted to growth in one location, while malignant tumors can spread to nearby and distant places to form secondary tumors—that is, metastases. It is now understood that all forms of cancer have a genetic predisposition as a result of the inappropriate activity of certain genes. These genes may be altered by mutation or may be abnormally affected by viruses. It has been proposed that genetic changes causing cancer occur mostly in two categories of genes: proto-oncogenes and tumor suppressor genes.

Cellular Genes Involved in Cancer

PROTO-ONCOGENES

Changes in genes called proto-oncogenes result in the transformation of a normal cell to a malignant cell by producing an altered or overexpressed gene product. Such changes include simple changes (e.g., nucleotide base changes), chromosome rearrangements (e.g., translocations), and amplifications in gene number. Initially proto-oncogenes referred to normal cellular genes that were used by viruses to transform tissue culture cells. These genes in the viral genome were termed *oncogenes*. However, the term *proto-oncogene* has evolved to mean the normal allele of any cellular gene that, upon genetic mutation or manipulation, generates an allele capable of initiating a cancer phenotype. Genetically altered alleles of proto-oncogenes (i.e., oncogenes) act dominantly because they can transform cells in the presence of gene expression by their normal counterpart (i.e., proto-oncogenes). Over 60 proto-oncogenes have been cataloged—for example, the oncogenes *ras*, *spi*1, *oca*, and *int*2 on chromosome 11 (Fig. 21-1). Protein products of proto-oncogenes include cellular growth factors, growth factor receptors, enzymes (e.g., protein kinases and guanosine triphosphatases [GTPases]) that are signal transducers for growth factor receptors, and DNA-binding proteins that regulate DNA transcription. Clearly, genetic alteration of the expression of these proteins could disrupt normal cell growth.

TUMOR SUPPRESSOR GENES

The normal role of tumor suppressor genes is to prevent cancer. Inactivation or loss of these genes contributes to development of cancer by lack of a functional gene product. This usually requires

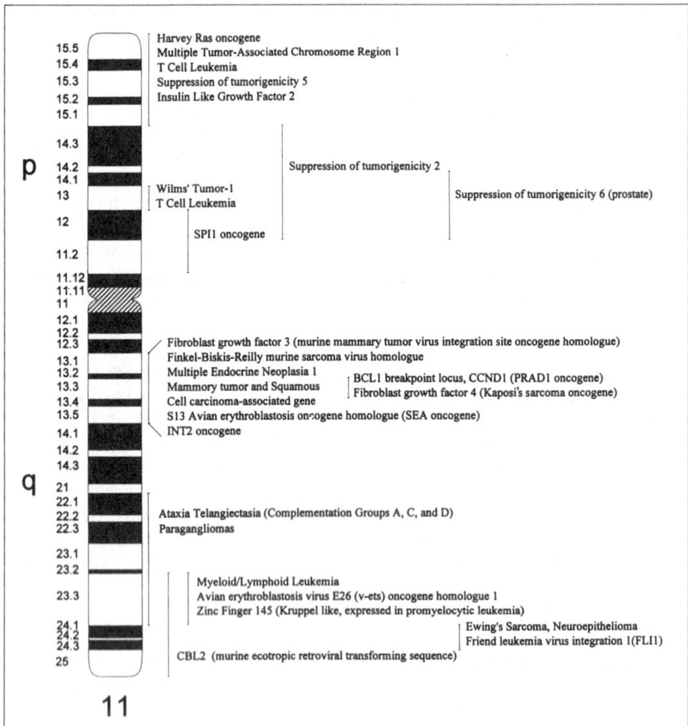

Fig. 21-1. Chromosome 11 cancer-associated loci.

mutations in both alleles or a mutation in one and loss (deletion) of the other allele of a tumor suppressor gene. In these instances, mutant suppressor genes act recessively. At least seven tumor suppressor genes have been described: RB1, WT1, TP53, APC, NF1, NF2, and VHL (Table 21-1). Products of tumor suppressor genes have been proposed to function as regulatory inhibitors of cell proliferation, as DNA transcription factors, and in cell adhesion. Loss of these functions could result in abnormal cell division or gene expression, or increased ability of cells in tissues to detach. These are properties of malignant cells.

Tumorigenesis: A Multistep Process

The progression of a normal cell to a malignant cell can be considered a multistep process that proceeds through a series of genetic alterations involving proto-oncogenes and tumor suppressor genes. For example, a genetic model for colorectal tumorigenesis proposes that normal epithelium sequentially progresses through premalignant conditions such as hyperplasia and early, intermediate, and late adenomas that lead to carcinoma and metastasis. This process likely involves several genes and mutations. Genetic alterations in

Table 21-1. Cloned familial cancer genes

Entity	*Gene symbol*	*Chromosomal location*
Retinoblastoma	RB1	13q14
Wilms' tumor-1	WT1	11p13
Li-Fraumeni syndrome	TP53	17p13
Familial adenomatous polyposis	APC	5q21
Neurofibromatosis type 1	NF1	17q11
Neurofibromatosis type 2	NF2	22q12
von Hippel-Lindau syndrome	VHL	3p25
Multiple endocrine neoplasia type 2	MEN2A or RET	10q11
Hereditary nonpolyposis colon cancer	MSH_2 (COCA1)	2p16
	MLH1 (COCA2)	3p21,3p23
Familial breast and ovarian cancer	BRCA1	17q12

Source: Modified from AG Knudson. All in the (cancer) family. *Nature Genetics* 5:103, 1993.

proto-oncogenes and tumor suppressor genes have been observed in the preneoplastic and neoplastic states. It is proposed that progressive accumulation of such genetic alterations is responsible for the histopathologic progression of tumors. Each alteration apparently confers a selective growth advantage to the mutant cell, resulting in clonal evolution and increased malignant potential. The model for colorectal tumorigenesis serves as a useful prototype for understanding tumor formation in other cancers.

Acquisition of Genetic Changes Involved in Cancer

ENVIRONMENT

Epidemiologic investigations have attributed environmental factors as the cause of at least 80% of human cancer. Many carcinogenic environmental agents (e.g., cigarette smoke tar, ultraviolet light, x-rays, asbestos) directly cause DNA damage and are mutagenic. Other carcinogenic environmental agents (e.g., saccharin) have not, as yet, been shown to directly damage DNA. However, these agents stimulate cell proliferation, which increases the risk of permanent DNA damage (i.e., mutations) caused by endogenously generated cellular mutagens (e.g., free radical oxidants) that are normal by-products of cellular metabolism. In experimental systems, chemical carcinogens have been shown to produce oncogenic mutations in proto-oncogenes, and the mutations reflect the chemical reactivity of the mutagen. In the majority of cases, the mutations occur to DNA of somatic cells as opposed to germ cells, and these so-called somatic mutations are not passed from generation to generation. These analyses suggest that genetic changes that lead to cancer are definitely attributable to environmental agents.

INHERITANCE

Some individuals inherit genetic mutations that predispose them to developing cancer. Thus, the gene mutation occurs or is carried in germ cells and is passed from generation to generation. These individuals may account for up to 5% of cancer cases. Several hundred inherited disorders, most of which are exceptionally rare, have tumors as a feature. It is convenient to consider two broad categories of inherited predispositions to cancer: inherited cancer syndromes and familial clustering of cancer.

Inherited cancer syndromes are mendelian inherited disorders in which cancer is preceded by a recognizable inherited condition or preneoplastic phenotype. For example, xeroderma pigmentosum (XP) is an autosomal recessive disorder featuring extreme sensitivity of skin and eyes to light. Exposure to sunlight results in skin and corneal lesions that frequently progress to cancer. Interestingly, cells from XP individuals have impaired ability to repair ultraviolet light damage to DNA. This contributes to cancer development.

Familial clustering of cancer refers to families with increased incidence of cancer relative to the general population, but for which there is no recognizable inherited phenotype before cancer diagnosis. Familial clustering has been noted for almost all types of cancer including ovarian, endometrial, breast, colon, and brain.

Besides familial clustering of disease, other characteristics indicating genetic inheritance include an early age of onset and multiple, multifocal, or bilateral cancers in one individual. Proof of genetic inheritance requires linkage of disease with an assayable genetic marker.

Inheritance of Cancer Susceptibility

DeMars and Knudson postulated a two-hit hypothesis for inheritance of cancer susceptibility. They proposed that in hereditary cancer, germ-line inheritance of a recessive mutation in a potential cancer-causing gene constituted one hit that predisposes family members to develop cancer. Cancer subsequently develops because of a second hit or somatic mutation in the normal allele of the gene, which renders an individual cell homozygous for the cancer gene. In nonhereditary cancer, both mutations must occur in a single somatic cell, which is a rare event. Later, it was shown that retinoblastoma resulted from functional losses of both alleles of a single gene and that hereditary forms of the disease involved the germ-line loss of one allele and either the physical or functional somatic loss of the other allele of the gene. This information contributed to our understanding of tumor suppressor genes and that inactivation or loss of function of these genes can lead to malignancy.

The above paradigm has provided a conceptual framework to identify, map, and clone familial cancer genes. Thus far, 10 familial cancer genes have been cloned and another nine have been mapped but not yet cloned (Tables 21-1 and 21-2). At least seven of the cloned genes apparently are tumor suppressor genes since inactivation or loss of function of both alleles has been associated with tumors of affected carriers. Additionally, preliminary information suggests that inactivation of both alleles of either MSH_2 or MLH1 may be needed for development of hereditary nonpolyposis colon cancer.

Table 21-2. Uncloned but mapped familial cancer genes

Entity	*Gene symbol*	*Chromosomal location*
Multiple endocrine neoplasia type 1	MEN1	11q13
Familial melanoma	MLM	9p21
Neuroblastoma	NB	1p36
Basal cell nevus syndrome	BCNS	9q31
Beckwith-Wiedemann syndrome	BWS	11p15
Renal cell carcinoma	RCC	3p14
Tuberous sclerosis 1	TSC1	9q34
Tuberous sclerosis 2	TSC2	16p13

Source: Modified from AG Knudson. All in the (cancer) family. *Nature Genetics* 5:103, 1993.

Inheritance of a mutant APC allele predisposes to development of adenomatous polyps that invariably lead to cancer if untreated. Apparently, inactivation or loss of function of only one allele is sufficient for polyp formation. It has been proposed that inactivation of one allele results in a reduced level of APC protein function, which results in a proliferative advantage and polyp development. The accumulation of additional mutations in tumor suppressor genes and oncogenes results in colon cancer.

Hereditary multiple endocrine neoplasia type 2A (MEN2A) is unusual since the germ-line mutation occurs in RET, a proto-oncogene that codes for a receptor tyrosine kinase. It had been thought that the dominant nature of oncogene mutations would not permit germ-line inheritance because expression during embryogenesis would be lethal. Apparently, this is not necessarily the case since evidence suggests that a dominant mutation in one allele of RET may be sufficient to initiate tumors.

BRCA1 has been genetically linked to development of disease in familial occurrences of either breast cancer, breast-ovarian cancer, or ovarian cancer. The BRCA1 gene has not been cloned, but it probably is a tumor suppressor gene since preliminary evidence suggests inactivation or loss of function of both alleles is involved in disease.

Breast cancer presents as a heterogeneous disorder, the severity of which is thought to be a result of an accumulation of mutations at multiple sites controlling growth and proliferation. For example, the oncogenes c-*myc*, c-*erb*^{B}, and HER-2/*neu* and the tumor suppressor genes TP53, RB1, and prohibitin have been implicated in the development and progression of the disease. By comparison to colon cancer, a subset of these alterations may prove to occur in a disease stage–defined manner, with specific alterations occurring early and others occurring as the disease progresses. Also, breast cancer displays differences in patterns of age of onset, disease progression, and histologies of the various categories of breast tumors reflecting the heterogeneity of the disease. Genetic linkage studies have identified a gene at 17q12-21 involved in familial early-onset breast cancer. Loss of heterozygosity (LOH) in this region in both familial and sporadic breast tumors suggest that this locus is a tumor suppressor gene. LOH in breast cancer at several other chromosome loci indicates that other tumor suppressor genes participate in the progression of this disease, perhaps by a mechanism analogous to LOH at chromosomes 5, 17, and 18 in colon cancer. High-frequency LOH for 11p has been observed in adult cancer of the breast, ovary, bladder, testicles, lung, and adrenal cortex, in addition to the childhood tumors rhabdomyosarcoma, Wilms' tumor, hepatoblastoma, and adrenocortical carcinoma. This region has also been shown to contain an interstitial deletion in at least one breast tumor. These studies have defined two regions at p15 that show consistent LOH in breast cancer and other tumor types. The 11p15 region has been defined as being between HBB and TH for breast cancer, and D11S12 to the telomere (pter) for rhabdomyosarcoma and Wilms' tumor. One study has implicated chromosome 11 band p15 to be involved with the metastasis of breast cancer to regional lymph nodes. The 11p15 region is believed to harbor the gene(s) for the Beckwith-Wiedemann syndrome (BWS), which is typified by abnormal growth and susceptibility to a number of childhood cancers. Furthermore, there is an increased risk of breast cancer in mothers of children with rhabdomyosarcoma, which is the hallmark embryonal tumor of BWS. Significantly, constitutional chromosome rearrangements in BWS patients occur in the LOH region, as do somatic rearrangements in breast cancer and other tumors. Chromosome band 11q13 also has been implicated in the tumorigenesis of human breast cancer by the presence of tumor amplicons, which are hypothesized to contain genes providing a selective growth advantage. The presence of amplifications at 11q13 has been correlated with lymph node metastases, an increased risk of relapse, and a shortened disease-free period. Four amplification regions have been identified.

Identification, Mapping, and Cloning Cancer Susceptibility Genes

There are two basic approaches to cloning genes using recombinant DNA technology: functional cloning and positional cloning. Functional cloning relies on knowledge of the protein product (e.g., amino acid sequence or antibody availability) or its specific function for gene isolation and mapping. However, initially, the specific protein product of most putative genes for cancer susceptibility is unknown. Therefore, an alternate strategy, positional cloning, was developed to isolate such genes. Positional cloning relies on the localization or mapping of a gene for disease to a chromosome region, followed by physically searching the region for the gene, isolating it, and then determining its protein product and specific function.

The first step in positional cloning involves the identification of families in which disease apparently segregates as an inherited trait. Genetic inheritance of disease is usually established by linking transmission of disease with a genetic marker whose chromosome location is known. In general terms, a genetic marker is a readily detectable entity that exists in multiple forms—that is, it is polymorphic and segregates in families. A useful analogy for a genetic marker is color (detectable entity), which exists in multiple forms (e.g., blue, green, red). A genetic marker represents a gene and the multiple forms are alleles. Markers used for linkage analysis include proteins and segments of DNA, which can be assayed from blood samples of family members. Linkage analysis in a family is useful only if a marker for a gene exists in two distinguishable forms—that is, alleles. This makes it possible to follow transmission of the putative disease gene and the marker through successive generations. Cotransmission of disease with one form (allele) of the marker through successive generations of a family is evidence of linkage—that is, the disease gene and the marker are located on the same chromosome. If the disease gene and the marker are located on different chromosomes, they will independently assort from each other during meiosis and have only a 50% chance of being cotransmitted. Linkage is more confidently established if disease is cotransmitted with several genetic markers for a specific chromosome region. This also serves to physically locate the disease gene to a chromosome.

Parental chromosomes are not always transmitted intact to offspring. During meiosis, homologous chromosomes sometimes exchange segments of equal length, resulting in the recombination of a parental chromosome pair. The closer two genes (e.g., disease gene and marker gene) lie on the same chromosome, the less likely it is for their alleles to separate and recombine. Thus, if a disease is almost always transmitted with the same form (allele) of a marker, the disease gene and the marker gene must be closely linked to the same region of a chromosome. An occasional independent transmittance of a disease gene and marker allele is indicative of recombination and demonstrates physical distance between the two. Recombination events make it possible to locate or map a disease gene to a region between two genetic markers whose map positions on chromosomes are known.

Mapping generally can localize a gene to a chromosome segment of about one million base pairs, which may contain 30–40 genes. If the chromosome segment with the disease gene also contains previously mapped genes, these genes become "candidate genes" for disease. To determine if a candidate gene may be the disease gene, mutation analysis, often involving DNA sequencing of the candidate genes with DNA samples from linked families and tumors, is required. The consistent presence of a mutation such as a nucleotide substitution in the gene of linked family members and in tumors from affected family members would be evidence for a disease gene. However, if there are no candidate genes or if suspected candidate genes are excluded by mutation analysis as disease genes, then identifying and isolating the anonymous disease gene becomes a more formidable task. This task can be made easier if DNA rearrangements (e.g., chromosome translocations or deletions) have been observed to occur in the chromosome region of the candidate gene, resulting in a disruption of the gene itself. The task, then, is to clone the chromosome breakpoint, which should contain part of the candidate gene. This was the case in cloning disease genes for retinoblastoma and familial adenomatous polyposis. If rearrangements have not been observed in the candidate region, then a brute force physical mapping approach must be taken. This involves isolating the candidate region, cloning all of the genes in the region, and determining which gene is consistently mutated in linked families and tumors. The methods and techniques involved in implementing this strategy are too numerous and sophisticated to be discussed here. However, excellent reviews are available.

Finally, the best proof that an isolated gene causes disease is obtained by functional assays. For example, transfecting a normal allele of a putative tumor suppressor gene into a cell line mutant for these genes should create a cell line that is no longer tumorigenic in laboratory animals. Similarly, transfecting the mutant allele of a putative proto-oncogene into an appropriate nontumorigenic cell line should create a cell line that is tumorigenic.

Cancer-Associated Genes in the Human Genome

Genes, abnormal growth phenotypes, and chromosomal rearrangements associated with cancer have now been mapped to virtually all human chromosomes. Only a few of these genes have actually been cloned or are near cloning (see Table 21-1 and Fig. 21-1). An example of the many cancer-associated loci assigned to just one human chromosome, chromosome 11, is illustrated in Table 21-2. These include several loci with suppression of tumorgenicity phenotypes, chromosomal regions associated with specific cancers, transforming sequences, proto-oncogenes, growth factors and genes abnormally expressed in cancers, abnormal growth disorders, and loci identified by nonrandom breakpoints associated with specific cancers. Any of these loci could result in cancer or be a gene involved in the multistep processes leading to a specific cancer. Many of these loci are, in fact, leading candidate genes for specific tumors. They will be cloned in the near future and examined for changes in DNA from specific tumors for a positive correlation as mentioned above. With these loci on human chromosome 11 as an example, it is very clear that there are large numbers of genes in our genome that are directly or secondarily involved in a cancer phenotype. We can expect from the research activity in this field that the joining of clinical oncology, genetics, and molecular biology will very soon yield information to understand the genetics of cancer.

Significance and Potential Benefits

Rapid technological advances in the field of molecular genetics during the past 5 years have greatly accelerated the development of genome maps and gene discovery. The establishment of an integrated human genome map placing genetic markers within the context of physical DNA clones will provide medical science with the information to not only identify individuals at risk for a disease but also study disease mechanisms and progression. Such clone-based maps provide the framework for structural and biological studies and have been constructed for model organisms including *Caenorhabditis elegans* and *Drosophila melanogaster*. The analysis of the human genome will provide a similar set of detailed maps and the reagents for characterizing and elucidating the function of human genes.

Identification of families and individuals genetically prone to cancer is of great importance both scientifically and clinically, since it affords the possibility of identifying and isolating cancer-predisposing genes. As hereditary and nonhereditary forms of the same cancer are often histologically indistinguishable, gene isolation should lead to understanding genetic mechanisms and biochemical functions that malfunction in both forms of cancer. In turn, this will result in improvements in early screening, detection, and treatment and perhaps in disease prevention.

Selected Readings

Ballabio A. The rise and fall of positional cloning? *Nature Genet* 3:277, 1992.

Bonner LE, Baker SM, Morrison PT. Mutation in the DNA mismatch repair gene homologue hMLH1 is associated with hereditary non-polyposis colon cancer. *Nature* 368:258, 1994.

Bowcock AM. Molecular cloning of BRCA1: A gene for early onset of familial breast and ovarian cancer. *Breast Cancer Res Treatment* 28:121, 1993.

Collins FS. Positional cloning: Let's not call it reverse anymore. *Nature Genet* 1:3, 1992.

DeMars R. Genetic Concepts in Neoplasia. In *Twenty-Third Annual Symposium on Fundamental Cancer Research*. Baltimore: Williams & Wilkins, 1970. Pp 105–106.

Eng C, Ponder BJ. The role of gene mutations in the genesis of familial cancers. *FASEB J* 7:910, 1993.

Hall JM, Lee MK, Newman B et al. Linkage of early onset familial breast cancer to chromosome 17q21. *Science* 250:1684, 1990.

Knudson AG. All in the (cancer) family. *Nature Genetics* 5:103, 1993.

Knudson AG. Mutation and cancer: Statistical study of retinoblastoma. *Proc Natl Acad Sci* (USA) 68:820, 1971.

Miki Y, Swensen J, Shattuck-Eidens P et al. A strong candidate for the breast and ovarian cancer susceptibility gene BRCA1. *Science* 226:66, 1994.

Narod SA, Feunteun J, Lynch HT et al. Familial breast-ovarian cancer locus on chromosome 17q12–23. *Lancet* 338:82, 1991.

Nowak NJ, Shows TB. Genetics of chromosome 11: Loci for pediatric and adult malignancies, developmental disorders, and other diseases. *Clin Invest* (1995, in press).

Smith SA, Easton DF, Evans DGR et al. Allele losses in the region 17q12–21 in familial breast and ovarian cancer involve the wild-type chromosome. *Nature Genet* 2:128, 1992.

Steichen-Gersdorf E, Gallion HH, Ford D et al. Familial site-specific ovarian cancer is linked to BRCA1 on 17q12–21. *Am J Human Genetics* 55:870, 1994.

Takita KI, Sata T, Miyagi M et al. Correlation of loss of alleles on the short arms of chromosomes 11 and 17 with metastasis of primary breast cancer to lymph nodes. *Cancer Research* 52:3914, 1992.

Index

Index